Optical Coherence Tomography of Ocular Diseases

THIRD EDITION

Optical Coherence Tomography of Ocular Diseases

THIRD EDITION

Edited by

Joel S. Schuman, MD
Eye and Ear Foundation Professor and Chairman of Ophthalmology
University of Pittsburgh School of Medicine
Professor of Bioengineering, Swanson School of Engineering, University of Pittsburgh
Director, UPMC Eye Center
Pittsburgh, Pennsylvania

Carmen A. Puliafito, MD, MBA
Dean, Keck School of Medicine
May S. and John Hooval Dean's Chair in Medicine
Professor of Ophthalmology and Health Management
Doheny Eye Institute
University of Southern California
Los Angeles, California

James G. Fujimoto, PhD
Elihu Thomson Professor of Electrical Engineering
Department of Electrical Engineering and Computer Science
Research Laboratory of Electronics
Massachusetts Institute of Technology
Cambridge, Massachusetts

Jay S. Duker, MD
Director, New England Eye Center
Professor and Chairman
Department of Ophthalmology
Tufts Medical Center
Tufts University School of Medicine
Boston, Massachusetts

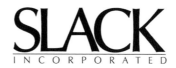

SLACK
INCORPORATED

Published by: SLACK Incorporated
                 6900 Grove Road
                 Thorofare, NJ 08086 USA
                 Telephone: 856-848-1000
                 Fax: 856-848-6091
                 www.Healio.com/books

Contact SLACK Incorporated for more information about other books in this field or about the availability of our books from distributors outside the United States.

Library of Congress Cataloging-in-Publication Data
Optical coherence tomography of ocular diseases / Joel S. Schuman ... [et al.]. -- 3rd ed.
   p. ; cm.
 Includes bibliographical references and index.
 ISBN 978-1-55642-864-7 (alk. paper)
 I. Schuman, Joel S.
 [DNLM: 1. Retinal Diseases--diagnosis. 2. Glaucoma--diagnosis. 3. Tomography, Optical Coherence--methods. WW 270]

 617.7'35075--dc23
                        2012023100

Last digit is print number: 10   9   8   7   6   5   4   3   2

Dedication

To our families, for their dedication and support;
to our teachers and mentors, who gave of themselves so that we could go beyond the state-of-the-art;
to our students and trainees—past and present—
for their commitment to advancing scientific knowledge and clinical care; and
to our patients, who continue to drive us to provide better, safer, and more effective care.

Contents

About the Editors

Joel S. Schuman, MD, is the Eye and Ear Foundation Professor and Chairman of Ophthalmology, the Eye and Ear Institute, University of Pittsburgh School of Medicine, and Director of UPMC Eye Center. He is Professor of Bioengineering at the Swanson School of Engineering, University of Pittsburgh. Dr. Schuman and his colleagues were the first to identify a molecular marker for human glaucoma (*Nature Medicine,* 2001). The NIH has continuously funded him since 1995 as principal investigator of a grant to study novel glaucoma diagnostics. He is an inventor of optical coherence tomography (OCT). He has published more than 250 peer-reviewed scientific journal articles, 8 books, and more than 50 book chapters. In 2012, Dr. Schuman received a Carnegie Science Center Award. He shared the 2012 Champalimaud Award for the invention and development of OCT with James G. Fujimoto, David Huang, Carmen A. Puliafito, and Eric Swanson.

Carmen A. Puliafito, MD, MBA, was appointed Dean of the Keck School of Medicine of the University of Southern California, May S. and John Hooval Dean's Chair in Medicine, and Professor of Ophthalmology and Health Management in November 2007. Since his appointment, he has led the continuing transformation of the Keck School into one of the United States' preeminent research-intensive medical schools. Dr. Puliafito is a renowned ophthalmologist, widely recognized for his innovative advances in treatment, including his co-invention of OCT. In addition to his responsibilities as Dean, he is an active clinician at USC's Doheny Eye Institute and serves as the current editor of *Ophthalmic Surgery, Lasers and Imaging.* A cum laude graduate of Harvard College and a magna cum laude graduate of Harvard Medical School, Dr. Puliafito also earned an MBA from the Wharton School of the University of Pennsylvania. He shared the 2012 Champalimaud Award for the invention and development of OCT with James G. Fujimoto, David Huang, Joel S. Schuman, and Eric Swanson.

James G. Fujimoto, PhD, is the Elihu Thomson Professor of Electrical Engineering and Computer Science at the Massachusetts Institute of Technology. Dr. Fujimoto's group and collaborators are credited with the invention and development of OCT imaging in the early 1990s. He has published nearly 400 peer-reviewed journal articles and is coeditor of more than 10 books and coauthor of more than 20 patents. He is a member of the National Academy of Sciences, the National Academy of Engineering, and the American Academy of Arts and Sciences. Dr. Fujimoto cofounded the startup company Advanced Ophthalmic Devices, which developed OCT for ophthalmic imaging and was acquired by Zeiss. He is also cofounder of LightLab Imaging, which developed intravascular OCT and was recently acquired by St. Jude Medical. He shared the 2012 Champalimaud Award for the invention and development of OCT with David Huang, Carmen A. Puliafito, Joel S. Schuman, and Eric Swanson.

Jay S. Duker, MD, is the Ophthalmologist-in-Chief at Tufts Medical Center, Director of the New England Eye Center, and Chairman of the Department of Ophthalmology at Tufts University School of Medicine. Dr. Duker has been at Tufts Medical Center for 20 years and previously served as Director of the Retina Service. A graduate of Harvard University and Jefferson Medical College, he completed his postgraduate training at Wills Eye Hospital in Philadelphia. His research interests include new treatments of vascular disease, intraocular drug delivery, and imaging of the posterior segment. He has been instrumental in the development of OCT.

Contributing Authors

Bernhard Baumann, PhD (Appendix A)
Research Laboratory of Electronics
Massachusetts Institute of Technology
Cambridge, Massachusetts
New England Eye Center
Tufts Medical Center
Tufts University
Boston, Massachusetts

Vanessa Cruz-Villegas, MD (Chapters 4, 5, 10, 11)
University of Puerto Rico
School of Medicine
San Juan, Puerto Rico

Janet Davis, MD (Chapter 9)
Professor of Ophthalmology
Bascom Palmer Eye Institute
University of Miami Miller School of Medicine
Miami, Florida

Harry W. Flynn Jr, MD (Chapter 5)
Professor of Ophthalmology
J. Donald M. Gass, MD Distinguished Chair
Bascom Palmer Eye Institute
University of Miami Miller School of Medicine
Miami, Florida

Lindsey S. Folio, MS, MBA (Chapters 2, 12; Appendix B)
University of Pittsburgh
Pittsburgh, Pennsylvania

Thomas R. Hedges III, MD (Chapter 13)
Professor of Ophthalmology and Neurology
Tufts University School of Medicine
Director of Neuro-Ophthalmology
New England Eye Center
Boston, Massachusetts

David Huang, MD, PhD (Chapters 1, 14; Appendix A)
Center for Ophthalmic Optics and Lasers
Casey Eye Institute
Department of Ophthalmology
Oregon Health and Science University
Portland, Oregon

Hiroshi Ishikawa, MD (Chapter 2; Appendix B)
Assistant Professor
Departments of Ophthalmology and Bioengineering
University of Pittsburgh
Schools of Medicine and Engineering
Director, Ocular Imaging Center
UPMC Eye Center
Pittsburgh, Pennsylvania

Matthew D. Lazzara, MD (Chapter 13)
Resident in Ophthalmology
New England Eye Center
Tufts University School of Medicine
Boston, Massachusetts

Yan Li, PhD (Chapter 14)
Center for Ophthalmic Optics and Lasers
Casey Eye Institute
Department of Ophthalmology
Oregon Health and Science University
Portland, Oregon

Elias C. Mavrofrides, MD (Chapters 3, 6-9, 11)
Florida Retina Institute
Orlando, Florida

Carlos Mendoza-Santiesteban, MD (Chapter 13)
Adjunct Associate Professor of Ophthalmology
Tufts University School of Medicine
Boston, Massachusetts

Jessica E. Nevins, BS (Chapters 2, 12; Appendix B)
Department of Ophthalmology
UPMC Eye Center
Eye and Ear Institute
Pittsburgh, Pennsylvania

Bing Qin, MD, PhD (Chapter 14)
Center for Ophthalmic Optics and Lasers
Casey Eye Institute
Department of Ophthalmology
Oregon Health and Science University
Portland, Oregon
Department of Ophthalmology
Eye, Ear, Nose, and Throat Hospital of Fudan University
Shanghai, China

Adam H. Rogers, MD (Chapter 3)
Assistant Professor of Ophthalmology
New England Eye Center
Tufts University School of Medicine
Boston, Massachusetts

Philip J. Rosenfeld, MD, PhD (Chapters 7, 10)
Professor of Ophthalmology
Bascom Palmer Eye Institute
University of Miami Miller School of Medicine
Miami, Florida

Heeral R. Shah, MD (Chapters 3-11)
New England Eye Center
Tufts Medical Center
Boston, Massachusetts

Eric Swanson, MS (Chapter 1; Appendix A)
Entrepreneur and MIT Research Affiliate
Gloucester, Massachusetts

Steven N. Truong, MD, FACS (Chapter 3)
Vitreoretinal Surgeon
Pennsylvania Retina Specialists, PC
Camp Hill, Pennsylvania

Natalia Villate, MD (Chapters 7, 9)
Retina Specialist
South Florida Eye Associates
Miami, Florida

Gadi Wollstein, MD (Chapters 2, 12; Appendix B)
UPMC Eye Center
Eye and Ear Institute
Ophthalmology and Visual Science Research Center
Department of Ophthalmology
University of Pittsburgh School of Medicine
Pittsburgh, Pennsylvania

Preface

The history of ophthalmology as a medical specialty began with a collaboration between a physicist and an ophthalmic surgeon when Herrmann von Helmholtz invented the ophthalmoscope in 1851 and Albrecht von Graefe used it to revolutionize ophthalmic diagnosis and therapy. And so it was with optical coherence tomography (OCT), which was born of a collaboration between physical scientists and ophthalmologists (James Fujimoto, David Huang, Charles Lin, Carmen Puliafito, Joel Schuman, and Eric Swanson).

Since the invention of OCT by our groups in the early 1990s and its first scientific description by Huang et al in *Science* (1991;254[5035]:1178-1181), this technology has emerged to become a widely used tool that has already revolutionized the diagnosis and therapy of eye disease. It is now part of the standard armamentarium in eye care. OCT also marks the beginning of a new field that might be called structural imaging of the eye. We believe that these and other technologic developments in ophthalmic structural imaging will produce widespread changes in the way the eye is examined and eye disease is treated.

Several individuals played a special role in the development of OCT. David Huang, MD, PhD, then a student in the Harvard-Massachusetts Institute of Technology (MIT) MD PhD program, conceived the idea of cross-sectional imaging while working on his PhD in Dr. Fujimoto's laboratory at MIT. Joel S. Schuman, MD, who at the time was a fellow in glaucoma at Massachusetts Eye and Ear Infirmary, first conceived of retinal imaging with the precursor to OCT, and together with David Huang did the first retinal scans. Eric Swanson, MS, working at Lincoln Laboratory of MIT, built the first OCT system. Mr. Swanson was also a cofounder, along with Drs. Puliafito and Fujimoto, of the startup company Advanced Ophthalmic Diagnostics, which was acquired by Humphrey Instruments/Carl Zeiss Meditec, Inc, and transferred OCT ophthalmic imaging technology to industry. Michael Hee, MD, PhD, wrote all the original OCT imaging processing algorithms and analysis protocols, which are now in standard clinical use, as well as coauthored the first edition of this book. Charles P. Lin, PhD, and Joseph A. Izatt, PhD, also played important roles in the initial laboratory and clinical investigations. Tony Ko, a student in the Medical Engineering and Medical Physics Program at MIT, made critical contributions to advanced OCT development.

OCT was first implemented as a practical clinical tool at the New England Eye Center of the Tufts University School of Medicine in Boston, Massachusetts, where both Dr. Puliafito and Dr. Schuman were founding faculty members, soon joined by Jay S. Duker, MD. Our valued clinical collaborators at the New England Eye Center have included Cynthia Mattox, MD; Elias Reichel, MD; and Caroline Baumal, MD. Christine Kiernan, Director of Photography at the New England Eye Center from its inception and her photography staff played a vital role.

Dr. Schuman's group established the value of OCT as a valuable tool in eyes with glaucoma. Tamar Pedut-Kloizman, MD; Helena Pakter, MD; Viviane Guedes, MD; and Gadi Wollstein, MD, participated in OCT's development as research fellows. Graduate students Michelle Gabrielle and Larry Kagemann were critical to advancing 3D-OCT imaging in the posterior and anterior segments respectively. Hiroshi Ishikawa, MD, in Dr. Schuman's laboratory, has advanced the analysis algorithms of this device.

The authors are grateful to the retina faculty at the Bascom Palmer Eye Institute for their support in this undertaking. We recognize the invaluable help of Ms. Ditte Hesse, Director of Photography at the Bascom Palmer Eye Institute, and Carl Denis, head OCT technician. We are indebted to Maria Feth, Coordinator and Lead Imager at the Ocular Imaging Center at UPMC Eye Center, for the countless hours she and her staff have spent acquiring excellent images on our patients.

The translation of OCT into a clinical technology would not have been possible without the commitment of industry. The team at Carl Zeiss Meditec played a critical role in engineering the technology and making it available to the general clinical community.

The transition from time-domain (TD) to spectral-domain (SD) OCT in 2006 profoundly affected the widespread clinical utility of the technology, increasing reproducibility and improving longitudinal assessment of eye disease. The introduction of SD-OCT also helped place the technology into more hands globally, accelerated innovation, and expanded the manufacturing of OCT to multiple vendors, spurring a competitive marketplace.

We believe that OCT opens a new window to the eye that promises not only to enable earlier and more sensitive diagnosis of disease, but also to contribute to a better understanding of the mechanisms of disease itself. We hope that this book will prove valuable to both clinicians and researchers who wish to learn more about OCT.

Joel S. Schuman, MD
Carmen A. Puliafito, MD, MBA
James G. Fujimoto, PhD
Jay S. Duker, MD

Section I

Principles of
Operation and Interpretation

Chapter 1

Introduction to Optical Coherence Tomography

James G. Fujimoto, PhD; Joel S. Schuman, MD; David Huang, MD, PhD;
Jay S. Duker, MD; Carmen A. Puliafito, MD, MBA; and Eric Swanson, MS

- Introduction
- Imaging With Light Versus Sound
- Measuring Echoes of Light Using Interferometry
- Axial Scans and Optical Coherence Tomography Image Generation
- Optical Coherence Tomography Instrumentation for Retinal Imaging
- What Optical Coherence Tomography Images Show
- Ultrahigh-Resolution Optical Coherence Tomography and Detailed Retinal Structure
- High-Speed Spectral/Fourier-Domain Optical Coherence Tomography
- Advantages of Spectral/Fourier-Domain Optical Coherence Tomography
- Retinal Structure in Optical Coherence Tomography Images From Commercial Instruments
- Anterior Eye Structure in Optical Coherence Tomography Images
- Conclusion

Introduction

Optical coherence tomography (OCT) is a fundamentally new type of medical diagnostic imaging technology that performs high-resolution, micronscale, cross-sectional imaging of the internal microstructure in biological tissues by measuring the intensity and echo time delay of light.[1-6] OCT is a powerful imaging modality because it enables the real-time, in situ imaging of tissue structure or pathology with resolutions of 1 to 15 µm, 1 to 2 orders of magnitude finer than conventional clinical imaging technologies such as ultrasound, magnetic resonance, or computed tomography. Since its development in 1991, OCT has been explored in a wide range of clinical applications.[7] In ophthalmology, it has emerged as a standard of care, enabling imaging of the retina and anterior eye at resolutions that were previously impossible to achieve with any other noninvasive imaging method.

Figure 1-1 shows the first demonstration of OCT imaging reported by Huang et al showing the human retina ex vivo and corresponding histology.[1] The OCT image in Figure 1-1 has an axial image resolution of ~15 µm, which is almost 10 times finer than ultrasound. Imaging was performed with infrared light at ~800-nm wavelength. The images are displayed using a false-color scale, where different magnitudes of backscattered light are displayed as different colors on a rainbow-color scale. The light signals detected in these OCT images are extremely small, between 4×10^{-10} (0.4 billionths) to 10^{-6} (1 millionth) of the incident light. Figure 1-1 shows an OCT image of the human retina in the region of the optic disc with corresponding histology. This image was acquired ex vivo, and postmortem retinal detachment with subretinal fluid accumulation is evident. The contour of the optic nerve head (ONH)

Schuman JS, Puliafito CA, Fujimoto JG, Duker JS, eds.
Optical Coherence Tomography of Ocular Diseases,
Third Edition (pp 3-26).
© 2013 SLACK Incorporated.

Figure 1-1. The first demonstration of OCT imaging. OCT imaging is analogous to ultrasound B-mode imaging, except light is used instead of sound. A cross-sectional image is generated by scanning a light beam across the tissue and measuring the echo time delay and intensity of backscattered or backreflected light. This figure shows an OCT image of the human retina in vitro and corresponding histology. The axial image resolution is 10 μm, and imaging was performed using infrared light at ~800-nm wavelength. The scale bar is 300 μm. (Reprinted with permission from Huang D, Swanson EA, Lin CP, et al. Optical coherence tomography. *Science.* 1991;254:1178-1181.)

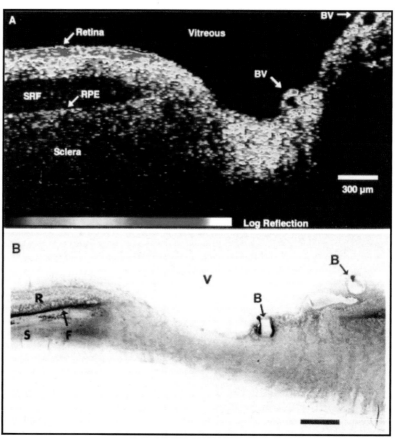

as well as retinal vasculature can be easily seen in the OCT image. The retinal nerve fiber layer (RNFL) can also be visualized and suggested the application of OCT for glaucoma detection.

The eye is the most optically accessible of all organs, and both the anterior and posterior eye can readily be imaged using OCT. Figure 1-2 shows one of the first examples of in vivo OCT imaging of the normal human retina.[3] The axial image resolution was 10 μm in tissue, and imaging was performed with light at ~800-nm wavelength. The OCT image shows the normal contour of the foveal pit and the ONH. The RNFL is seen as a highly backscattering layer that decreases in thickness moving away from the optic disc. The retinal pigment epithelium (RPE) and choroid are evident as a highly backscattering layer posterior to the retina. These early results demonstrated that OCT can image retinal structure with unprecedented resolution.[3-5]

Figure 1-3 shows the first demonstration of OCT imaging of the anterior eye, reported in 1994.[2] The axial image resolution was 10 μm in tissue, and imaging was performed at ~800-nm wavelength. The image spans a transverse dimension of 21 mm, thus allowing cross-sectional imaging of the entire anterior chamber. The OCT image shows the corneal thickness and the depth of the anterior chamber. The curvature of the anterior and posterior surfaces of the cornea can also be measured. However, it is necessary to compensate for image distortion effects from light refraction at the curved surface of the cornea. The sclera and iris are visible as highly optically scattering structures that produce shadowing of posterior features. OCT systems optimized for imaging the anterior eye use light at longer ~1300-nm wavelengths, which reduces optical scattering and improves image penetration depth in the angle.

OCT is especially powerful in ophthalmology because it provides real-time, noncontact, cross-sectional imaging of the retina or the anterior eye with unprecedented resolution. Since OCT generates cross-sectional images of retinal morphology, it can provide vital diagnostic information that is complementary to conventional fundus photography and fluorescein angiography. OCT enables visualization of structural features of the retina, including the fovea and optic disc, as well as the internal architectural morphology of the retina, such as the nerve fiber layer (NFL), ganglion cell layer (GCL), and

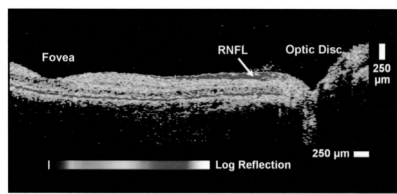

Figure 1-2. Early OCT image of the human retina in vivo. The image shows the normal retinal contour in the fovea and the optic disc region. The RNFL is evident as a highly backscattering layer that emanates from the optic disc and decreases in thickness as it approaches the fovea. The axial image resolution is 10 μm, and imaging was performed using light at ~800-nm wavelength. The image is displayed using a logarithmic false-color scale, which maps the log of the backscattered or backreflected light intensity to a rainbow-color scale. The maximum signal is approximately −50 dB of the incident signal, while the minimum detectable signal is approximately −95 dB. These early results demonstrated the feasibility of using OCT for retinal imaging and suggested its future application in ophthalmology. (Reprinted with permission from Hee MR, Izatt JA, Swanson EA, et al. Optical coherence tomography of the human retina. *Arch Ophthalmol.* 1995;113:325-332.)

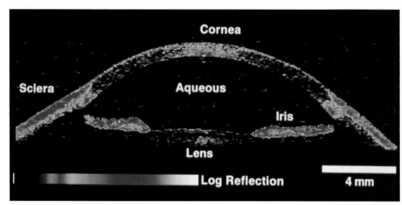

Figure 1-3. OCT image of the anterior chamber in vivo. This image is the first demonstration of anterior eye imaging. The image shows the curvature of the anterior and posterior surfaces of the cornea, as well as the depth of the anterior chamber. The iris is visible, but it scatters light strongly, so deeper structures are shadowed. The axial image resolution is 10 μm, and imaging was performed with light at ~800-nm wavelength. (Reprinted with permission from Izatt JA, Hee MR, Swanson EA, et al. Micrometer-scale resolution imaging of the anterior eye in vivo with optical coherence tomography. *Arch Ophthalmol.* 1994;112:1584-1589.)

photoreceptors.[3] OCT imaging of the anterior eye enables visualization of the cornea, iris, lens, and angle.[2] Early studies established the utility of OCT imaging for the detection and monitoring of a variety of macular diseases, including macular edema, macular holes, central serous chorioretinopathy, age-related macular degeneration, choroidal neovascularization, and epiretinal membranes.[4,8-14]

OCT imaging can also be used to perform quantitative measurements or morphometry of the retina. OCT is especially powerful for the diagnosis and monitoring of diseases such as glaucoma or macular edema because it can provide quantitative information that is a measure of disease progression. Images can be analyzed quantitatively using image processing algorithms to automatically extract features such as retinal thickness or RNFL thickness.[5,15-17] The RNFL thickness, a diagnostic indicator for early glaucoma and disease progression, can be quantified and correlated with measurements of ONH structure or visual function.[17-24] Mapping and display techniques have been developed to represent OCT image data in alternate forms, such as topographic thickness maps, in order to better facilitate interpretation and comparison to fundus images.[14] Finally, since structural image information can be assessed quantitatively, OCT imaging can be used as a diagnostic to predict the probability of disease and to monitor disease progression and the effectiveness of treatment.

Imaging With Light Versus Sound

OCT imaging is analogous to ultrasound B-mode imaging, except that it uses light instead of sound. OCT performs cross-sectional or volumetric imaging by measuring the echo time delay and intensity of backscattered or backreflected light from structures inside tissue. OCT images are 2- or 3-dimensional (2D or 3D) data sets representing variations in optical backscattering or backreflection in a cross-sectional plane or volume of tissue.

Because of the analogy between OCT and ultrasound, it is helpful to compare OCT imaging with ultrasound imaging. Ultrasound is widely used clinically for quantitative measurements of intraocular distances as well as for imaging the anterior eye and globe.[25-29] Since ultrasound imaging depends on the transmission of sound waves into the eye, it requires direct contact of the ultrasound probe to the cornea or immersion of the eye in a liquid. The resolution of ultrasound depends on the frequency or wavelength of the sound waves. For typical ultrasound systems, sound wave frequencies are in the 10-megahertz regime, which yield spatial resolutions of approximately 150 µm. Ultrasound also has the advantage that sound waves are readily transmitted into most biological tissues, and therefore it is possible to image structures deep within the body. High-resolution ultrasound imaging can be performed using higher frequency sound waves to achieve resolutions on the 20-µm scale.[27,28] However, these high-frequency sound waves are strongly attenuated in biological tissues, and imaging can be performed to depths of only 4 to 5 mm. Therefore, high-resolution ultrasound imaging of the retina is not possible.

OCT is an optical imaging technique that uses light rather than sound, and therefore imaging can be performed without requiring contact. The main limitation of using light is that it is highly scattered or absorbed in most biological tissues. Therefore, optical imaging is limited to tissues that are directly optically accessible or that can be imaged using devices such as endoscopes or catheters. OCT is ideally suited for ophthalmology because of the ease of optical access to the eye. In addition, since OCT can be performed without physical contact to the eye, the examination is well tolerated by patients. Imaging using light enables a significantly higher spatial resolution than possible with ultrasound. The first ophthalmic OCT images had axial resolutions of ~10 µm, approximately 10 to 20 times finer than standard ultrasound B-mode imaging.[3] Research OCT systems for ultrahigh-resolution ophthalmic imaging can achieve even finer resolutions of ~2 to 3 µm.[6,30] Current-generation commercial OCT systems using spectral/Fourier (SD/FD) detection have axial image resolutions in the ~5- to 7-µm range. The inherently high resolution of OCT imaging permits visualization of individual retinal layers, thus facilitating the diagnosis of a wide range of retinal pathologies.

When light is directed onto the eye, it is backreflected from tissue boundaries and backscattered with different intensities from tissues with different optical properties. The distances and dimensions of different tissue structures can be determined by measuring the echo time delay of light backreflected or backscattered from structures at varying axial (longitudinal) distances.[31,32] However, it is important to note that the speed of light is almost a million times faster than the speed of sound. Since tissue dimensions are measured using the echo time delay, measuring echoes of light requires ultrafast time resolution.

Figure 1-4 illustrates the distance and time scales for the propagation of light and sound. The speed of sound in water is approximately 1500 m/sec. In contrast, the speed of light is approximately 3×10^8 m/sec (in air). Light travels more slowly in water, and its speed is given by dividing by the index of refraction of water. Distance or axial range information may be measured from the echo time delay according to the formula:

$$\text{Echo time delay} = \frac{(\text{distance the echo travels})}{(\text{velocity of light or sound})}$$

Thus, the measurement of distances or structures with a resolution of ~100 µm, which would be typical for ultrasound, requires a time resolution of ~100 nanoseconds (100×10^{-9} sec). The measurement of structures with a resolution of ~10 µm, which

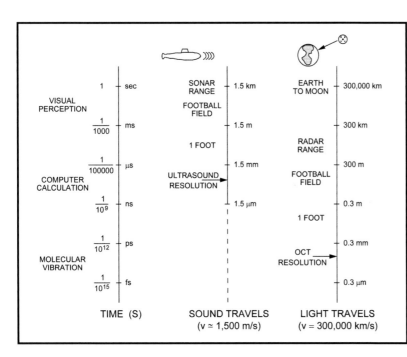

Figure 1-4. Distance and time scales for light and sound. The velocity of sound is approximately 1500 m/sec, while the velocity of light is 3×10^8 (300,000,000) m/sec. Standard ultrasound has a resolution limit of 150 µm, which corresponds to a time measurement of 100 nanoseconds, (100×10^{-9} sec). In contrast, standard OCT imaging has a resolution of 10 µm, corresponding to a time measurement of 30 femtoseconds (30×10^{-15} sec). In order to measure echoes of light from small structures, extremely fine time resolution is required. The scales are logarithmic; each vertical division represents a factor of 1000. Notice that light from the moon takes approximately 1.3 sec to reach Earth.

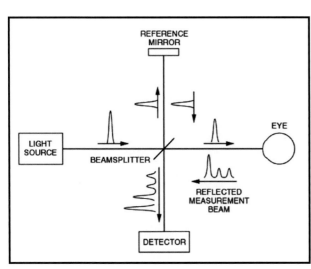

Figure 1-5. Measuring echo time delays of light. The echo delay time of light can be measured with high resolution by comparing or correlating one light beam with another. Light from a source is directed onto a partially reflecting mirror (beamsplitter) and is split into reference and OCT measurement beams. The OCT beam is backreflected or backscattered from the tissue with different echo time delays. The reference beam is reflected from a mirror at a known distance, which produces a known time delay. The light from the tissue, consisting of multiple echoes, and the light from the reference mirror, consisting of a single echo at a known delay, are combined by the interferometer and detected. Previous-generation OCT systems used TD detection, while current-generation systems use SD/FD detection.

is achieved by OCT, requires a time resolution of approximately 30 femtoseconds (30×10^{-15} sec), approximately 1 million times faster. Fortunately, it is possible to perform ultrahigh-resolution time and distance measurements using a simple optical technique known as *interferometry*.

Measuring Echoes of Light Using Interferometry

OCT uses interferometry to perform ultrahigh-resolution time and distance measurements of light. The technique of "low-coherence" or white-light inter-ferometry was first described by Sir Isaac Newton.[33] During the 1980s, low-coherence interferometry was used for performing high-resolution optical measurements in fiber-optic and optoelectronic components.[34-36] In order to perform distance measurements with tens of micron resolution (corresponding to echo delay times of tens of femtoseconds), it is necessary to compare or correlate one optical beam or lightwave with another reference optical beam or lightwave. This type of measurement may be performed using an optical device known as an *interferometer*.

Figure 1-5 shows a schematic of an optical interferometer. This configuration is known as a *Michelson interferometer*. The light source is a laser or

How Time-Domain Optical Coherence Tomography Detection Works

Early OCT systems detected light echoes using what is known as *time-domain* (TD) *detection*. Figure 1-6 shows a schematic of how TD-OCT detection works. When the interferometer reference path is scanned, interference fringes are generated in time at the output of the interferometer.[37-40] This process can also be understood by noting that the scanning reference mirror produces a Doppler shift of the light. If a traditional laser light source that emits a narrow band of optical frequencies is used, the interference will occur over a wide range of path length differences. However, in order to detect light echoes, a low-coherence or broad-bandwidth light source is required. Low-coherence light can be characterized as having statistical phase discontinuities over a distance known as the *coherence length*, which is inversely proportional to the frequency bandwidth of the light. When low-coherence light is used, interference is only observed when the reference path is matched to the light signal from the eye to within the coherence length of the light. The interferometer measures the correlation of the electric field of the light. The magnitude and time delay of light echoes can be measured by scanning the reference arm and detecting the interference signal. Echoes from different depths are detected sequentially as the reference arm is scanned. The coherence length of the light source determines the axial image resolution. Since it is possible to have light sources with a few-microns coherence length, this enables the measurement of echoes of light with femtosecond timescale resolution.

Figure 1-6. How TD-OCT detection works. The echo time delay of the backreflected or backscattered light signal can be measured using low-coherence interferometry with a scanning reference arm. When a narrowband light source is used, the output of the interferometer consists of interference fringes. However, when a broadband or low-coherence light source is used, interference occurs only when the path lengths of the reference and signal are equal. Detecting the interference signal as the reference path is scanned sequentially measures echoes from different depths. This generates an axial scan, which is analogous to ultrasound A-mode measurements.

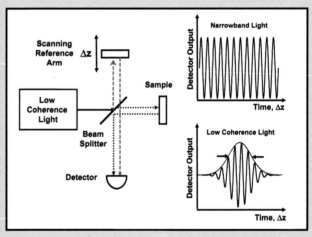

other device that emits short coherence-length light. The optical beam from the light source is incident onto a partially reflecting mirror (beamsplitter), which splits the light into 2 paths. One light beam is sent to the patient's eye and is backreflected or backscattered from intraocular structures at different distances. The light returning from the eye consists of multiple echoes that give information about the distance and thickness of these intraocular structures. The second beam is reflected from a reference mirror at a known distance and acts as a time reference. This reflected reference light beam travels back to the partial mirror (beamsplitter), where it combines or interferes with the light from the eye. The detector measures the interference or correlation of the light echoes from the eye with an echo that has traveled a known reference path delay. Different methods can be used to detect echo time delays of light using interferometry. Previous-generation OCT systems used TD, or time-domain, detection, while current-generation OCT is based on SD/FD detection.

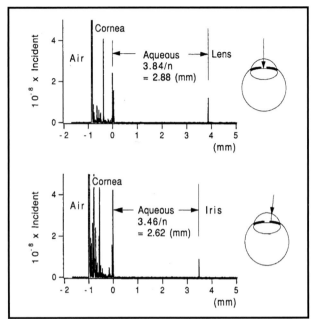

Figure 1-7. Axial scan measurement of anterior chamber depth using low-coherence interferometry. The plots display the magnitude of the backreflected or backscattered optical intensity as a function of echo delay or distance. A large reflection is observed from the anterior surface of the cornea, while smaller reflections originate from the posterior corneal surface (cornea-aqueous boundary) and the lens or iris. Note the presence of scattered light that originates from within the cornea. The graphs show the structural features that occur along the axis of the optical beam. If the transverse position of the optical beam is changed, then different features are measured (the depth of the anterior chamber versus the depth to the iris). (Reprinted with permission from Huang D, Wang J, Lin CP, Puliafito CA, Fujimoto JG. Micron-resolution ranging of cornea and anterior chamber by optical reflectometry. *Lasers Surg Med.* 1991;11:419-425.)

Axial Scans and Optical Coherence Tomography Image Generation

The simplest measurement that can be performed by OCT is analogous to an ultrasound A-mode (axial) scan, which gives information on tissue thickness. Figure 1-7 shows an early example of axial distance measurements or axial scans of the anterior chamber.[38] The plot shows the intensity of the backreflected or backscattered light from different structures within the anterior eye as a function of echo time delay or axial (longitudinal) distance.

Echoes are generated from the anterior and posterior surfaces of the cornea, as well as from the anterior capsule of the lens. The intensity of the reflected light depends on the difference in refractive index between different tissues. The reflection from the anterior surface of the cornea is relatively large; however, reflections from internal surfaces (such as between the cornea and aqueous or different layers of the retina) are small. In addition, different tissues (such as the cornea, lens, and sclera of the anterior eye or the different layers of the retina) will produce varying amounts of optical backscattering depending on the structure of the tissue. This backscattering is detected in the OCT axial scan measurement.

The axial (longitudinal) distance measurement shown in Figure 1-7 permits a direct measurement of the corneal thickness as well as anterior chamber depth. The thickness of the tissue is calculated by measuring the optical echo delay and multiplying it by the speed of light in the tissue. The speed of light in the tissue is given by the speed in vacuum, divided by the index of refraction of the tissue. Therefore, measuring the physical thickness in OCT relies upon knowing or assuming the tissue index of refraction. The measured thickness would be scaled by dividing by the index of refraction of the tissue. The intensity of the backreflected or backscattered light is extremely small, approximately 10^{-5} to 10^{-9} (-50 to -90 dB) of the incident intensity. Thus, very high detection sensitivity to extremely weak reflected light echoes is required in order to measure structures within the eye.

Once an axial scan or A-mode scan is obtained, the relative positions of different structures may be measured by scanning the optical beam in the transverse direction. Figure 1-7 shows a second axial measurement with the optical beam aimed at the iris rather than at the anterior capsule of the lens. Because the light beam can be focused to a small spot size, the transverse position of the beam can be known with high precision. Thus, information on both the axial (longitudinal) and the transverse microstructure of tissue can be measured. The transverse resolution is determined by the focused spot size of the light and has a resolution similar to the transverse resolution in conventional microscopy.

OCT cross-sectional (B-mode) imaging is performed by acquiring successive axial (longitudinal) measurements or A-scans of the tissue at different transverse positions, as shown in Figure 1-8.[1-3,41] Successive, rapid axial measurements or A-scans are performed while scanning the optical beam in the transverse direction. The result is a set of axial scans,

Figure 1-8. How OCT images are generated. OCT is analogous to ultrasound B-mode imaging. OCT images are generated by performing rapid, successive axial (longitudinal) measurements at different transverse positions. Each axial measurement represents the echo delay of backreflected and backscattered light from microstructures inside tissue and gives a measurement of tissue dimensions along the optical beam. By scanning the beam transversely while performing successive axial measurements, a 2D data set can be acquired. These data are a cross-sectional map of the backreflection and backscatter within the tissue and can be displayed as a cross-sectional image.

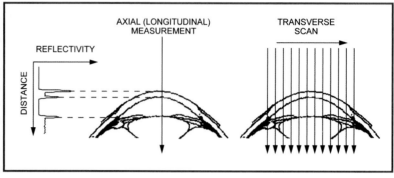

where each scan represents the optical backreflection or backscattering as a function of depth in the tissue at a different transverse position. This 2D data set is displayed as a grayscale or false-color OCT image and is often referred to as a *B-scan* or *line scan*. The image in Figure 1-3 is an example of an OCT of the anterior eye that would be achieved using the scan pattern in Figure 1-8. Multiple B-scans with different directions can be acquired to cover a volume of the eye. 3D volumetric images can be acquired by scanning a raster pattern consisting of multiple B-scans displaced in the perpendicular direction.

Optical Coherence Tomography Instrumentation for Retinal Imaging

Retinal imaging requires that the OCT beam be focused and scanned on the retina. The instrument design for retinal imaging is similar to a fundus camera and is shown schematically in Figure 1-9. It is helpful to briefly discuss this instrument in order to understand how to achieve optimum image quality in OCT images and avoid imaging artifacts. A high-power objective lens, similar to a hand-held 78-diopter lens, is used to relay an image of the retina onto an image plane inside the instrument. The instrument then relays the retinal image onto a video camera that enables real-time operator viewing of the fundus. Some instruments have an integrated scanning laser ophthalmoscope (SLO),

which provides a real-time fundus view. The OCT imaging beam is coupled into the optical path of the instrument using a partially reflective mirror (beamsplitter) and is focused onto the retinal image plane using another lens. The focused OCT beam is then relay imaged onto the retina by the objective lens and the patient's eye. The size of the incident OCT beam on the pupil is typically ~1.5 mm, and the transverse spot size on the retina is typically ~15 to 20 μm. The instrument must be aligned horizontally and vertically so that the OCT beam passes through the pupil of the eye. Prior to OCT image acquisition, the objective lens position is adjusted to focus the OCT beam on the retina. This also focuses the video fundus image. The instrument also illuminates the fundus to enable viewing.

The transverse position of the OCT beam is scanned by 2 perpendicular x-y scanning mirrors that are inside the instrument. The optical system is designed so that the OCT beam pivots about the pupil of the eye when it is scanned, as shown in Figure 1-9. This prevents the OCT beam from being vignetted by the pupil and enables access to a wide field of view on the retina. In order to ensure that the OCT pivots about the pupil of the eye, the patient's eye must be located at a given distance from the ocular objective lens. If the instrument is too close or too far from this position, the OCT beam will change transverse position instead of pivoting about the pupil and vignetting will occur. Vignetting causes reduction in the signal of OCT images near the edges of the scan and can lead to interpretation artifacts.

OCT imaging can be performed at different locations on the fundus by controlling the scanning

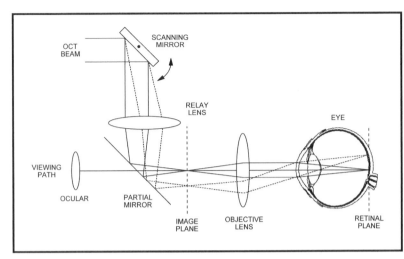

Figure 1-9. Schematic of OCT instrument for retinal imaging. The OCT instrument is analogous to a fundus camera. An objective lens relays an image of the retina to a plane inside the instrument. Operator viewing of the fundus is performed by a video camera. A computer-controlled, 2-axis scanning mirror scans the OCT beam. A relay lens focuses the OCT beam onto the image plane, and the objective lens directs the OCT beam through the pupil onto the retina. The OCT beam is focused on the retina by adjusting the objective lens. When the OCT beam is scanned, it pivots about the pupil of the eye in order to minimize vignetting.

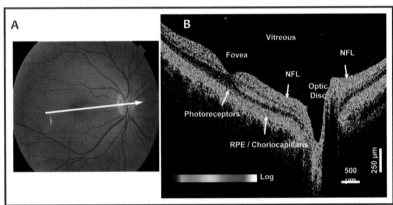

Figure 1-10. (A) OCT image of a normal fovea and optic disc taken along the papillomacular axis. This image is performed using the previous generation of OCT technology based on TD detection and has an axial resolution of 8 to 10 μm. (B) The OCT scan is 10-mm long and its location is shown on a corresponding fundus photograph. The fovea and optic disc are identifiable by their characteristic morphology, and the layered structure of the retina is apparent. The RNFL is highly reflective and increases in thickness toward the disc.

of the OCT beam. The location of the OCT image also can be controlled by changing the patient's point of fixation. The instrument has an internal fixation target, visible to the patient's eye that is being imaged, which can be adjusted under computer control. Many instruments enable the operator to view the fundus image in real time, which is displayed in a window on the computer monitor. Instruments also have special modes of operation for alignment where the instrument scans a special pattern of OCT images, usually a combination of horizontal (temporal-nasal) and vertical (superior-inferior) images, and displays the images in real time to enable precise aiming of the OCT imaging beam. The OCT beam is also visible to the patient as a thin red line, whose position in the patient's visual field corresponds to the points on the retina that are being scanned. Different scan patterns have

been designed that are optimized for the diagnosis and monitoring of different retinal diseases. The use of different scan patterns to image retinal features is described in more detail in later chapters. Figure 1-10 shows an example of an OCT image along the papillomacular axis. The figure shows an example of an image acquired with the previous generation of OCT using TD detection. The axial image resolution is 8 to 10 μm.

Retinal imaging is performed using infrared light at 800-nm wavelengths. The allowable retinal exposure limits for safe exposure have been thoroughly investigated and are governed by international standards such as those of the American National Standards Institute (ANSI standard). The maximum safe, permissible exposure depends upon the wavelength, the spot size, the duration of exposure, as well as repeated exposures. Because OCT instruments have extremely high detection sensitivities, low power levels of ~750 uW can be used and are well within safe exposure limits.

What Optical Coherence Tomography Images Show

Image contrast in OCT depends upon differences in optical backreflection or backscattering between different tissue structures. Since light that reaches deeper tissue layers must pass through more superficial layers, shadowing effects, similar to those in ultrasound, can occur. Light incident onto tissue can be transmitted, absorbed, reflected, or scattered.[42-45] Transmitted light remains unaffected and continues traveling into deeper tissue layers. Absorbed light is essentially removed from the incident beam. Absorption occurs because tissue chromophores, such as hemoglobin or melanin, absorb specific wavelengths in the incident light. Reflections occur where there are sharp boundaries between different tissues that have different indices of refraction. Reflections are highest when the OCT beam is perpendicular to the structure and occur at the foveal pit and the junction between the inner (IS) and outer segments (OS) of the photoreceptors. Optical scattering is a property of a heterogeneous medium and occurs because of microscopic spatial variations in the refractive index within tissue. These refractive index variations can be caused by subcellular structures, such as nuclei, cytoplasm, or cell membranes, or bundles of smaller structures, such as nerve fibers or axons. Structures such as the NFL, plexiform layers, and pigment epithelium appear brighter in OCT images because they scatter more light than other layers. Optical scattering causes incident light to be redirected in multiple directions. Light that completely reverses direction when scattered is called *backscattered light*.

In tissues that are strongly absorbing or scattering, the intensity of the incident beam decreases exponentially with depth. In tissues other than the eye, attenuation of the optical beam from scattering limits the OCT image penetration depth, although the high sensitivity of OCT enables the detection of light from depths up to ~2 mm in most scattering tissues.[46,47] In ophthalmic imaging, the retina backscatters weakly, generating very small optical signal levels. In this case, the high sensitivity of OCT allows these weak optical signals to be detected so that retinal tissues can be imaged even though they are virtually transparent.

OCT images are mostly composed of "single backscattered" light, light that has propagated into tissue, been backscattered once from the structure being imaged, and then propagated out of the tissue. The strength of the OCT signal from a tissue structure at a given depth is defined by a combination of the amount of incident light that is transmitted without absorption or scattering to that depth, the fraction of this light that is directly backscattered, and the fraction of the directly backscattered light that propagates out of the tissue and returns to the detector. Direct backreflections can also occur at the boundary of 2 materials that have different indices of refraction, such as between the cornea and the aqueous in the anterior eye (see Figure 1-3), the foveal pit, or the boundary between the IS and OS of the photoreceptors. When there is strong absorption or scattering, such as from blood vessels, hemorrhage, or the RPE, light is strongly attenuated and shadowing of deeper structures can occur.

It is important to note that although OCT images display the true dimensions of the structures being imaged (after correcting for index of refraction and refraction effects), contrast in OCT images comes from different mechanisms than in histology. In histology, selective stains are used to identify specific cellular or subcellular features. In OCT, image contrast occurs from intrinsic differences in tissue optical properties. Thus, care must be taken when interpreting OCT images since they are not analogous to conventional histology. In addition, it is important to note that the false-color scale used to display OCT images indicates differences in light signal levels. While different tissues can have different OCT signal levels because they have differences in backscattering or backreflection, the color in OCT images may not necessarily correspond to different types of tissue.

Ultrahigh-Resolution Optical Coherence Tomography and Detailed Retinal Structure

Since the introduction of commercial OCT instrumentation for retinal imaging in 1996, OCT technology has undergone multiple generations of product development. Ultrahigh-resolution OCT retinal imaging was demonstrated in 2001 and provided insight into the interpretation of retinal images.[30] Using specially designed broadband light sources and OCT instruments, it was possible to achieve axial image resolutions of ~3 μm,

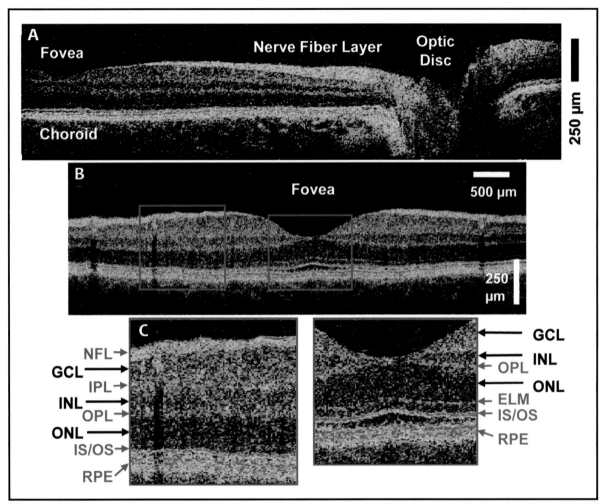

Figure 1-11. Ultrahigh-resolution OCT images of the macular region. Imaging is performed with 3-μm axial resolution. (A) OCT image with 6-mm transverse width and 512 transverse pixels. (B) High-magnification OCT image with 3-mm transverse width and 512 transverse pixels. (C) Enlargements of the fovea and parafoveal regions. The images are displayed expanded in the vertical direction for better visibility of the retinal layers. The retina can be divided into 10 distinct layers, including 4 cell layers and 2 layers of neuronal interconnections. Proceeding from the inner retina to the outer retina these layers are as follows: the inner limiting membrane (not shown), the nerve fiber layer (NFL), ganglion cell layer (GCL), inner plexiform layer (IPL), inner nuclear layer (INL), outer plexiform layer (OPL), outer nuclear layer (ONL), the external limiting membrane (ELM), the inner (IS) and outer segments (OS) of the photoreceptor layer, and the retinal pigment epithelium (RPE). The choriocapillaris and choriod are immediately posterior to the RPE. Ultrahigh-resolution imaging enables an excellent visualization of retinal microstructure and provides additional confirmation for the interpretation of standard-resolution images. (Adapted from Drexler W, Morgner U, Ghanta RK, Kärtner FX, Schuman JS, Fujimoto JG. Ultrahigh-resolution ophthalmic optical coherence tomography. *Nat Med.* 2001;7:502-507.)

significantly finer than the 10-μm axial resolution that was available in commercial instruments at that time.[30,48-50] Figure 1-11 shows an example of an ultrahigh 3-μm axial resolution image.[30]

Ultrahigh-resolution OCT enables visualization of individual retinal layers and correlates with the well-known morphology of the retina.[51-54]

Histologically, the retina can be viewed as divided into 10 distinct layers, including 4 cell layers and 2 layers of neuronal interconnections. The interpretation of OCT imaging is supported by studies that compare OCT to histology as well as ultrahigh-resolution OCT imaging studies.[55-60] The interpretation of features in OCT images is also confirmed by imaging pathologies that produce known alterations of retinal architecture.[48-50]

The NFL and plexiform layers consist of axonal structures that are highly optically backscattering and appear as red in the false-color OCT images. In contrast, nuclear layers are weakly backscattering and appear as blue-black. The first highly backscattering layer, visible adjacent to the fovea, is the NFL. This layer is thin in the macular region. The 3 weakly reflective layers are the GCL, inner nuclear layer (INL), and outer nuclear layer (ONL). The GCL increases in thickness in the parafoveal region. The moderately backscattering inner plexiform layer (IPL) is adjacent to the GCL and INL. The obliquely running photoreceptor axons, sometimes considered as a separate layer in the outer plexiform layer (OPL) known as *Henle's fiber layer*, are highly backscattering. The external limiting membrane (ELM) can be visualized as a thin backscattering layer posterior to the ONL and anterior to the boundary between the photoreceptor IS and OS. The ELM is not a physical membrane but is an alignment of structures between the photoreceptors and the Müller cells.

The boundary between the photoreceptor IS and OS is visible as a thin, highly backscattering band immediately anterior to the RPE and choroid. The reflection arising from this structure may be the result of a refractive index difference between the photoreceptor IS and the highly organized structure of the OS, which contains stacks of membranous discs, rich in the visual pigment rhodopsin.[54,61] The thickness of the photoreceptor IS and OS increases in the foveal region, corresponding to the well-known increase in the length of the OS of the cones in this region. The RPE, which contains melanin, is a very strongly backscattering layer. The RPE can have a banded structure that is related to the rod and cone distribution and interdigitation of the RPE cells between the photoreceptors.

Recent studies performed with ultrahigh-resolution SD/FD-OCT revealed that the banded appearance of the RPE on OCT images is the result of reflections from the photoreceptor OS tips and follows the expected rod and cone distribution across the macula.[60] The ability to image the photoreceptor morphology and its impairment is especially interesting as a marker of disease progression.[48,50,62]

Bruch's membrane, which is only 1- to 4-μm thick, is difficult to visualize in the normal retina because it is adjacent to the highly scattering RPE. In cases where there is an RPE detachment or drusen, Bruch's membrane is sometimes visible.

Finally, the choriocapillaris is vascular and strongly backscattering. The vascular structures of the choriocapillaris and choroid are highly optically scattering and produce shadowing effects that limit the OCT imaging depth for deeper structures. In some cases, retinal blood vessels can be identified by their increased backscatter and by their shadowing of deeper structures.

High-Speed Spectral/Fourier-Domain Optical Coherence Tomography

In addition to improvements in image resolution, new detection techniques now enable dramatic improvements in imaging speed.[63-69] Previous-generation OCT instruments used an interferometer with a scanning reference delay arm, a technique known as TD detection. However, it is also possible to detect echoes of light in the FD or frequency domain by measuring the interference spectrum. This concept was first proposed almost 2 decades ago in 1995.[63] The first demonstration of retinal imaging was performed in 2002.[64] This result showed that SD/FD detection could achieve sufficient sensitivity to image the retina and motivated a renewed interest in this technology. In 2003, 3 different research groups, working independently, demonstrated that FD detection has a powerful sensitivity advantage over TD detection, since FD detection essentially measures all of the echoes of light simultaneously.[70-72] The sensitivity enhancement is approximately given by the ratio of the axial resolution to the axial imaging depth. For most OCT systems, this yields a sensitivity increase of 50 to 100 times, enabling a corresponding increase in imaging speeds. Studies in 2004 demonstrated video rate retinal imaging using SD/FD-OCT to achieve 29,000 axial scans per second with 6-μm axial image resolution as well as ultrahigh-resolution retinal imaging with ~2-μm axial resolution at 19,000 axial scans per second.[67,68] These and other advances stimulated rapid growth in OCT research and commercial development.

Advantages of Spectral/Fourier-Domain Optical Coherence Tomography

SD/FD detection essentially measures all of the echoes of light simultaneously, while TD detection

How Spectral/Fourier-Domain
Optical Coherence Tomography Detection Works

Figure 1-12 shows a schematic of how SD/FD-OCT detection works. This detection technique uses a broadband light source with an interferometer and measures the interference spectrum using a spectrometer and a high-speed line scan camera. In SD/FD detection, different echo time delays of light are encoded as different oscillation frequencies in the spectrum of an interference signal. The echo time delays of light can be measured by Fourier transforming the interference spectrum to extract the oscillation frequencies. SD/FD can be understood by noting that an interferometer acts like a periodic frequency filter, where the periodicity of the frequency filter depends on the difference Δz between the sample and reference paths. The output from a broadband light source is split into 2 beams. One beam is directed onto the tissue to be imaged and is backreflected or backscattered from structures at different depths. The second beam is reflected from a fixed (not scanned) reference mirror. The signal beam and the reference beam have a relative time delay determined by the path length difference Δz, which is related to the depth of the structure in the tissue. The interference of the 2 beams will have a spectral modulation or oscillation that can be measured using a spectrometer. The periodicity of this oscillation will be inversely related to the echo time delay Δz. Larger echo delays will produce higher frequency spectral oscillations. The echo delays can be measured by Fourier transforming the interference signal. This produces an axial scan measurement (A-scan) of the magnitude and echo delay of the light signal from the tissue.

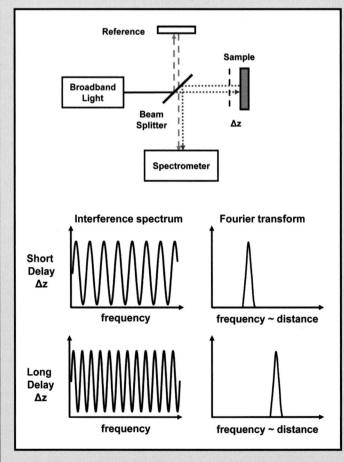

Figure 1-12. SD/FD-OCT detection. SD/FD-OCT uses an interferometer with a broadband light source and measures the spectrum of the interference output with a spectrometer and a high-speed line scan camera. Echo time delays of light are measured by noting that the interferometer acts like a spectral filter, which has a periodic output spectrum depending on the path length mismatch Δz (away from the zero delay position shown as dashed line). Larger path length differences generate higher frequency interference oscillations, where the frequency is proportional to the delay (bottom). Fourier transforming the spectral interference extracts the frequency and measures the delay (axial scan information). SD/FD detection essentially measures all of the echoes of light simultaneously and therefore has a significant sensitivity advantage compared with TD detection.

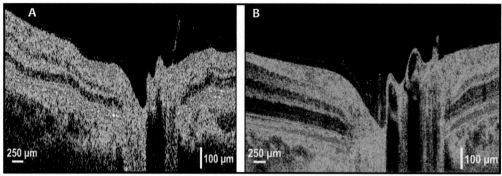

Figure 1-13. Comparison of OCT with TD detection with high-speed, ultrahigh-resolution OCT using SD/FD detection. (A) Previous-generation OCT image of the optic disc with ~10-μm axial image resolution and 512 axial scans, acquired in ~1.3 sec. (B) High-speed, ultrahigh-resolution SD/FD-OCT image with ~2-μm axial resolution and 2048 axial scans, acquired in 0.13 sec. The rapid acquisition speed preserves the retinal contour and enables a high-definition imaging with a large number of axial scans (transverse pixels). Images shown here are from a research prototype system. Typical commercial instruments have 5- to 7-μm axial image resolution.

measures the echoes sequentially as a function of delay. This property gives SD/FD-OCT a dramatic advantage in detection sensitivity, which enables OCT imaging ~50 to 100 times faster than previous OCT systems. High-speed SD/FD-OCT has a number of advantages, including improved image quality, preservation of true retinal topography, improved retinal coverage, and accurate registration of the OCT image set to fundus features. In general, for a given acquisition time, high-speed imaging can increase the number of axial scans or transverse pixels per image to yield high-definition images, as well as to increase the number of cross-sectional images acquired in a sequence to improve retinal coverage. Figure 1-13 shows a comparison of standard OCT using TD detection and high-speed, ultrahigh-resolution OCT using SD/FD detection from reference.[69] Figure 1-13A shows a standard OCT image with TD detection, having 10-μm axial image resolution with 512 axial scans, acquired in ~1.3 sec. Figure 1-13B shows an example of a high-speed, ultrahigh-resolution image using a research SD/FD instrument having ~2-μm axial resolution and 2048 axial scans, acquired in 0.13 sec. The ultrahigh axial resolution and greater number of transverse pixels in the OCT image improves the visualization of internal retinal structure. Increased imaging speed minimizes eye motion artifacts and enables the true topography of the ONH to be better preserved.

The ability of SD/FD-OCT to achieve both ultrahigh resolution and high pixel density has improved the understanding and interpretation of retinal structure in OCT images. Figure 1-14 shows ultrahigh-resolution images acquired from the parafovea and periphery from reference.[60] Details of the photoreceptor OS and RPE can be visualized as a multilayered structure. Reflections from the ELM and the boundary between the photoreceptor IS and OS can be seen. In addition, it is possible to resolve the cone outer segments (COS) and rod outer segments (ROS) as well as the RPE and Bruch's membrane. Studies were performed that mapped the thickness of these layers in a normative population and were consistent with expected rod and cone distribution in the normal retina.[60] Commercially available instruments have axial resolutions in the 5- to 7-μm range and therefore cannot always visualize these fine structures. However, studies with ultrahigh-resolution research prototype instruments can provide guidelines for image interpretation.

In addition to improvements in resolution, high-speed OCT imaging enables the acquisition of 3D-OCT data sets in a time comparable to that of previous OCT protocols that acquired several individual images. Figure 1-15 shows 3D-OCT raster scan imaging of the optic disc from reference.[69] The 3D-OCT volumetric data set contains comprehensive structural information. An en face view or OCT fundus image, identical to a standard retinal fundus view, can be generated by summing the data in the axial direction.[69,73] Individual cross-sectional OCT images (B-scans) can be precisely and reproducibly registered to en face features of the retina.

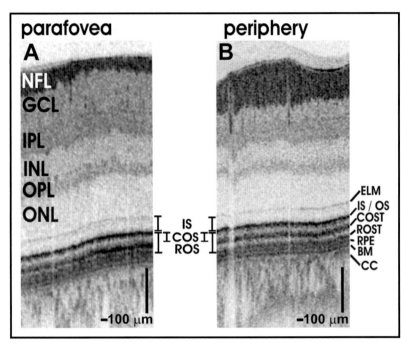

Figure 1-14. Ultrahigh-resolution SD/FD-OCT retinal images from the parafovea ~1.5 mm from foveal center (A) and the periphery ~5.2 mm from foveal center and superior to the nerve head (B) of a normal retina. The external limiting membrane (ELM) and reflection from the photoreceptor inner segment (IS) and outer segment (OS) boundary is clearly visible. Detailed structure including the rod outer segments (ROS) and cone outer segments (COS) as well as their tips can be visualized. The retinal pigment epithelium (RPE) and Bruch's membrane (BM) are also visible. The thickness of the photoreceptor OS follows the expected rod and cone distribution. These findings provide support for the interpretation of features in OCT images. (Reprinted with permission from Srinivasan VJ, Monson BK, Wojtkowski M, et al. Characterization of outer retinal morphology with high-speed, ultrahigh-resolution optical coherence tomography. *Invest Ophthalmol Vis Sci.* 2008;49:1571-1579.)

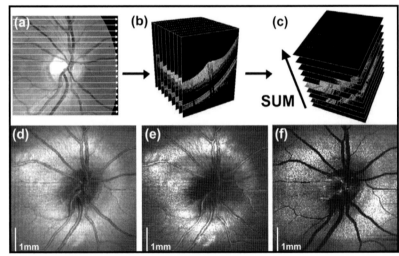

Figure 1-15. 3D-OCT fundus image generated with raster scan. (A, B) High-speed OCT enables acquisition of 3D-OCT data that contain comprehensive volumetric information. (C, D) An OCT en face retinal fundus image can be generated from 3D-OCT data by summing the signal along the axial direction. (E, F) OCT en face images can be generated by displaying individual retinal layers such as (E) the NFL or (F) RPE. Individual OCT cross-sectional images can be precisely and reproducibly registered to features on the fundus image. (Reprinted with permission from Wojtkowski M, Srinivasan V, Fujimoto JG, et al. Three-dimensional retinal imaging with high-speed ultrahigh-resolution optical coherence tomography. *Ophthalmology.* 2005;112:1734-1746.)

The 3D-OCT data enable the generation of an NFL thickness map similar to that obtained by scanning laser polarimetry, except that OCT measures the NFL thickness using cross-sectional image information, while scanning laser polarimetry measures the NFL thickness using birefringence. This map can provide information on the radial as well as circumpapillary variations in the NFL thickness. Figure 1-16 shows a plot of the NFL thickness variation measured along a 3.4-mm circle centered about the optic disc.

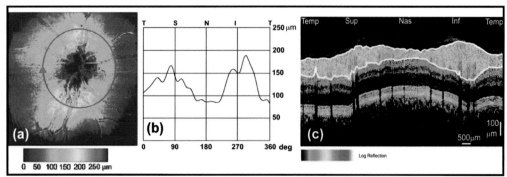

Figure 1-16. Circumpapillary measurement of the NFL from 3D-OCT volumetric data. (A) False-color map of NFL thickness generated from 3D-OCT data. (B) Measurement of NFL thickness along a circumpapillary scan. (C) Virtual OCT circumpapillary image that is extracted from the 3D-OCT volumetric data set. The position of the circumpapillary image can be adjusted in post processing to reduce errors from registration. (Reprinted with permission from Wojtkowski M, Srinivasan V, Fujimoto JG, et al. Three-dimensional retinal imaging with high-speed ultrahigh-resolution optical coherence tomography. *Ophthalmology.* 2005;112:1734-1746.)

Circumpapillary OCT images of any diameter as well as radial OCT images can be generated. Figure 1-16 also shows an example of a 3.4-mm diameter circumpapillary OCT image generated from the 3D-OCT data. OCT images and NFL maps can be precisely and repeatably registered to the fundus by using the OCT fundus image generated from the same 3D-OCT data.[69,73] This addresses a limitation in previous generations of OCT systems where variations in the scan position can produce variations in measured NFL thickness values.

Artifacts in Spectral/Fourier-Domain Optical Coherence Tomography Imaging

Although OCT using SD/FD detection has powerful advantages in terms of imaging speed, it also has important limitations that are not present in previous-generation OCT systems using TD detection. SD/FD-OCT is subject to "mirror" artifacts in the images, when the eye is positioned incorrectly or when retinal features span a large depth range. This can be understood by referring back to Figure 1-12. SD/FD detection measures the echo time delays of light by comparing backreflected or backscattered light from the eye to light from a reference path delay, which determines a "zero delay." SD/FD detection cannot distinguish between positive versus negative time delays compared to this zero delay. Therefore, if the axial position of the eye is exactly at the reference zero delay position or if retinal features cross this zero delay, the OCT image appears folded about this zero delay with a mirror artifact.

Figure 1-17 shows a series of OCT retinal images that illustrate the mirror artifact. The different images, from the top to the bottom, are acquired by moving the OCT instrument toward the eye so that the distance to the eye is decreasing. The echoes of light from the retina are measured with respect to a specific delay, the zero delay position from the instrument, which is determined by the setting of the reference path of the interferometer. The retina appears in a normal position when it is farther than the zero delay. When the instrument is moved toward the eye so that the retina is exactly at the zero delay reference position, the portions of the retina that cross the zero delay appear folded over or mirror imaged. Finally, when the instrument is moved still closer to the eye, the retina is closer than the zero delay reference position and the retina appears inverted. The mirror image artifact also frequently occurs when imaging structures that span a large range of depths, such as eyes with high myopia where there is a high curvature of the retina, or pathology such as retinal detachment, posterior vitreous detachment, pronounced edema, or elevated tumors.

(continued)

Artifacts in Spectral/Fourier-Domain Optical Coherence Tomography Imaging
(continued)

Instrument operators should be careful to recognize the mirror artifact in OCT image data and to repeat the image acquisition with the OCT instrument or reference delay position adjusted correctly so that the structure to be imaged does not overlap the zero delay position. Special care must also be exercised when interpreting OCT images, especially in cases where the retina is tilted at an angle to the imaging frame or where there are structures that span a large depth range. These features can often cross the zero delay position and appear as mirror images.

In addition to mirror image artifacts, SD/FD detection also has an artifact that the detection sensitivity varies within the instrument measurement range. The instrument is most sensitive to echoes that are close to the zero reference delay position and sensitivity decreases farther from zero delay. This phenomenon occurs because the spectrometer in SD/FD detection has a limited spectral resolution. Echoes that are farther from the zero delay position produce progressively high-frequency spectral oscillations that begin to exceed the spectrometer resolution. The resulting sensitivity variation can be seen in the images of Figure 1-17, where the retina appears brighter when it is near zero delay. Conversely, features that are farther from zero delay appear dimmer. Depending upon the application, it may be desirable to have increased sensitivity to signals from deeper in the retina in order to assess features below the RPE such as choroidal thickness or choroidal neovascularization. For other applications, it may be desirable to have higher sensitivity to structures anterior to the retina, such as epiretinal membranes or posterior vitreous detachment.

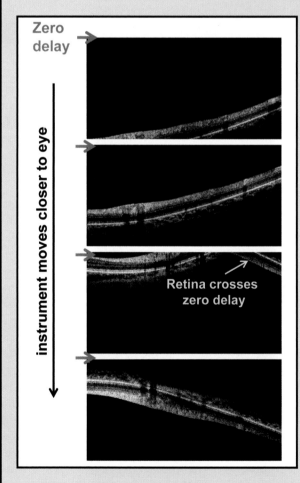

Figure 1-17. Artifacts in SD/FD-OCT detection. SD/FD detection cannot distinguish between echoes from positive or negative time delays, producing a mirror image artifact. Series of OCT images (top to bottom) as the instrument is moved closer to the eye. When the retina crosses the zero delay position of the interferometer, from positive to negative delays with respect to the zero reference position, it appears as if it is in front of the zero delay. This produces a folded or mirror image appearance in the OCT image. When the instrument is moved even closer to the eye, such that the retina is in back of the zero delay, the image appears inverted. Care must be taken to avoid misinterpreting mirror image artifacts in OCT images.

Figure 1-18. Example of OCT images of the normal retina using a commercial instrument. (A) Single OCT image from a raster scan with 512 axial scans (transverse pixels). (B) High-definition image consisting of 4096 axial scans (transverse pixels). Imaging with a higher density of axial scans improves continuity of retinal layers. (C) Averaged image consisting of 16 individual OCT images. Image averaging reduces speckle noise, giving the retinal layers a more homogenous appearance. Signal to noise is also improved, yielding increased image penetration into the choroid.

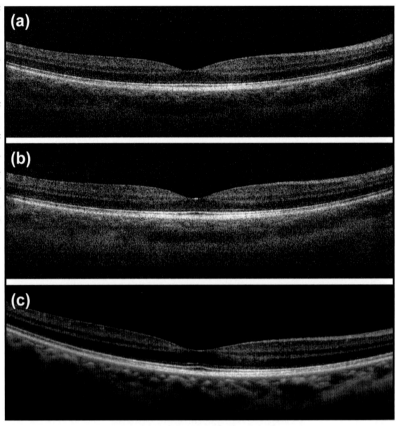

Retinal Structure in Optical Coherence Tomography Images From Commercial Instruments

Figure 1-18 shows OCT example images of the normal retina acquired with a typical commercial SD/FD-OCT instrument. The images have a 5- to 7-μm axial image resolution and are acquired using different imaging protocols. The images are shown in grayscale in order to avoid artifacts from false-color scale and to better visualize differences in the images. Figure 1-18A has 512 axial scans (transverse pixels) and is from a raster scan protocol. Figure 1-18B is a high-definition image with 4096 axial scans. The large number of axial scans improves the image quality by increasing the number of images pixels in the transverse direction. Figure 1-18C is an average of 16 individual OCT images, each consisting of 1024 axial scans. Image averaging reduces speckle noise and gives a smoother appearance to the retinal layers.[74] Image averaging also increases signal to noise, yielding a brighter image with improved image penetration

below the RPE and into the choroid. However, care must be used because image averaging can produce blurring of fine image features if there is eye motion. Some instruments use eye tracking in combination with image averaging to track changes in the fixation, so that multiple images are from the same position on the fundus.

Figure 1-19 shows 2x enlargements of the high-definition OCT image (4096 axial scans) and the averaged OCT image (16 images of 1024 axial scans). The images of the macula show the normal foveal contour with reduced total retinal thickness and increased ONL thickness. Increased thickness of the photoreceptor OS is also evident and can be seen from the reflection from the photoreceptor IS/OS junction. All major retinal layers can be visualized including the NFL, GCL, IPL, INL, OPL, ONL, ELM, junction between the photoreceptor IS and OS, RPE, and choroid. The averaged image, Figure 1-19B, shows a multilayer appearance of the RPE, which arises from variations in the cone and rod photoreceptor tips and the normal cone and rod distribution in the retina.[60] These structures are near the resolution limit of commercial OCT instruments and may not be visible in all patients.

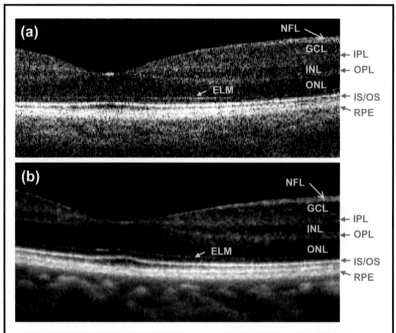

Figure 1-19. OCT images of the normal retina. (A) High-definition image and (B) averaged image. Retinal layers are visible including the nerve fiber layer (NFL), ganglion cell layer (GCL), inner plexiform layer (IPL), inner nuclear layer (INL), outer plexiform layer (OPL), outer nuclear layer (ONL), the external limiting membrane (ELM), the inner (IS) and outer segments (OS) of the photoreceptor layer, and the retinal pigment epithelium (RPE).

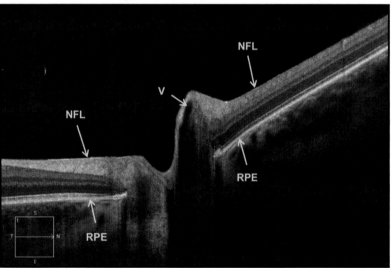

Figure 1-20. OCT image of the normal optic disc. The NFL is visible and increases in thickness approaching the disc rim. The termination of the RPE/choriocapillaris and photoreceptors near the lamina cribrosa can be clearly visualized. Disc parameters such as cup and disc diameter, neuroretinal rim area, and cup-to-disc ratio may be measured using this feature as a landmark. The lamina cribrosa and blood vessels (v) near the disc are also visible.

Generally speaking, these results show that OCT images can provide detailed information about retinal pathology with resolutions that approach that of histopathology on the level of architectural morphology. With the development of OCT atlases that establish a correspondence of OCT images to retinal disease, it should ultimately be possible to read OCT images in a manner that approaches the way that pathologists interpret histological micrographs.

Figure 1-20 shows an OCT image of the normal optic disc. The OCT image shown is a high-definition image consisting of 4096 axial scans.

The contour of the optic disc is demarcated by the boundary between the low backscattering vitreous and the highly backscattering NFL. The normal cupping of the disc is evident. The OCT image shows an increase in NFL thickness approaching the neuroretinal rim where the NFL is nearly the entire thickness of the retina. The retinal nerve fibers have a directional dependent reflectance. The reflected light intensity from the nerve fibers decreases at the disc rim, where the nerve fibers are no longer perpendicular to the incident OCT optical beam but bend into the ONH.

Figure 1-21. 3D-OCT imaging of the normal retina. Multiple windows are used to present the 3D-OCT volumetric data. An en face OCT fundus image is shown in the upper left. Cross-sectional images (B-scans) in the horizontal (temporal-nasal) or vertical (superior-inferior) direction can be displayed (top right, bottom left), which are registered to features in the fundus. A 3D-animation window (bottom right) shows a rendered view of the 3D-OCT data set.

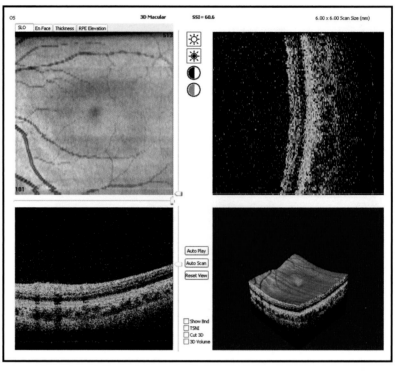

The RPE and choriocapillaris are visible as a highly backscattering layer that terminates at the lamina cribrosa. The boundary between the photoreceptor IS and OS is also visible as a thin, highly backscattering feature immediately anterior to the RPE and choroid. The photoreceptor layer and RPE terminate in the region approaching the disc and can be used as a landmark to define the disc margin. The IPL and OPL are moderately reflective while the INL and ONL are weakly reflective.

OCT imaging of the ONH and neuroretinal rim is valuable in assessing glaucoma or neuro-ophthalmic diseases. In evaluating the contour of the disc, it is important to note that OCT images are usually displayed with an expanded scale in the axial direction in order to allow better visualization of the thin retinal layers while still encompassing a several-millimeters transverse scan. Quantitative morphometry of the images using the correct axial and transverse scales are therefore important.

Figure 1-21 shows an example of 3D-OCT data of the normal macula. The data are acquired using a raster scan covering a 6-mm x 6-mm retinal area, consisting of 101 images (B-scans), each with 513 axial scans. The total volume data set consists of 101 x 513 or about 51,000 axial scans and is acquired in ~2.2 sec. Volumetric OCT data contain comprehensive information about retinal structure. An en face fundus image can be generated by summing the OCT signal in the axial direction. This image provides a view of the fundus similar to an SLO. Cross-sectional images (B-scans) can be extracted from the 3D-OCT volumetric data set. The figure shows images along the temporal-nasal and superior-inferior directions. These individual images are registered to features on the fundus. The figure also shows a rendering of the 3D-OCT volumetric data. The rendering can be manipulated to display the retina from a virtual perspective, and cut-away views can be generated.

3D-OCT volumetric data also enable quantitative mapping of retinal features. Almost all commercial instruments have software that enables automated "segmentation" or identification of retinal thickness, NFL thickness, the RPE, and a subset of internal retinal layers. After segmentation, retinal layer thicknesses can be quantitatively measured or the elevations of the layer scan be displayed using false-color or contour maps. Figure 1-22 shows an example of an analysis of 3D-OCT from the macula. The data are acquired using a raster scan covering a 6-mm x 6-mm retinal area, consisting of 128 images (B-scans), each with 512 axial scans. The total volume data set consists of 128 x 512 or about 65,000 axial scans and is acquired in ~2.5 sec. The analysis shows the total retinal thickness (from the RPE to the inner

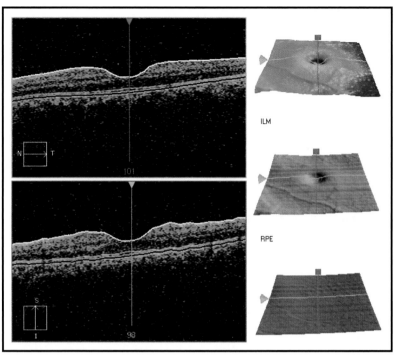

Figure 1-22. Analysis of 3D-OCT data sets. 3D-OCT data sets enabling mapping regions of the fundus. Retinal layers can be automatically "segmented" or identified. This example shows segmentation of the ILM and RPE. The retinal thickness can be measured and displayed as a false-color topographic map, superimposed on the fundus image. The elevation of the ILM and RPE can be measured with respect to its normal position. RPE elevation provides a way to quantitatively assess pathology such as drusen or choroidal neovascularization.

limiting membrane [ILM]) as a false-color topographic map, superimposed on the fundus image. The average thickness within ETDRS regions is also displayed. 3D surface maps show the elevation of the RPE and ILM. The RPE elevation can be helpful in assessing pathology such as drusen or choroidal neovascularization. In addition to segmentation and quantitative mapping, most commercial instruments also have software that enables quantitative longitudinal measurement of changes in retinal structures across multiple examinations. These features can provide quantitative indicators of disease progression and response to therapy.

Anterior Eye Structure in Optical Coherence Tomography Images

Many OCT instruments can perform imaging of the anterior eye using adapter modules that attach to the objective lens of the instrument. Other instruments are designed explicitly for anterior eye imaging. Under normal operation, scanning the retina involves pivoting a collimated beam about the pupil plane of the eye, as shown previously in Figure 1-9. Corneal adaptor modules focus the OCT beam onto the cornea and also produce a parallel (telecentric) displacement of the OCT beam as it is

scanned, similar to the scan shown previously in Figure 1-8. Since the OCT beam is refracted when it is incident on the curved surface of the cornea, special software is required to "dewarp" the OCT image in order to display the true curvature of structures behind the cornea.

Figure 1-23 shows an example image of the cornea. Imaging is performed at 800 nm with 5- to 7-µm axial image resolution. The image has been dewarped to correct for refraction at the anterior corneal surface and shows the curvature of anterior and posterior surfaces of the cornea. A strong reflection is evident at the center of the cornea where the air-cornea interface is exactly perpendicular to the incident OCT beam. This strong reflection produces echo artifacts in the OCT image that are visible in the A-scan lines at the center of the image. An enlargement of the OCT image shows a reflection from the anterior surface as well as the epithelial layer, which is demarcated by low scattering. The corneal stroma has scattering in a striated pattern resulting from collagen organization.

Figure 1-24 shows an example of an image of the normal anterior angle. Image averaging was performed to reduce speckle noise and improve sensitivity, increasing the image penetration. The corneal epithelium joins with the sclera in the region of the corneoscleral limbus. Schwalbe's ring is on the posterior surface of the cornea at the termination of Descemet's membrane and is a useful landmark

Figure 1-23. Imaging the cornea. RTVue image of the cornea. 2x enlargement shows details of the corneal epithelium (ep), stroma, and endothelium (en). The strong reflection from the central portion of the cornea, where the OCT beam is backreflected into the instrument, has an elevated background along the entire length of the axial scan and shows multiple echoes from the strong reflection.

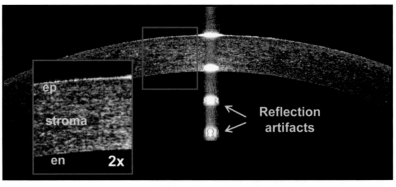

Figure 1-24. OCT image of the normal anterior angle. Image is averaged 16 times to reduce speckle noise and enhance signal. The epithelium (ep), corneal limbus (cl), iris (ir), and Schwalbe's ring (sr) at the termination of Descemet's membrane and Schlemm's canal (sc) can be visualized. The trabecular meshwork is shadowed by the sclera.

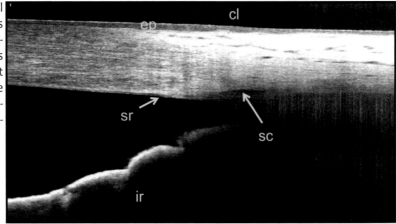

for measuring the anterior angle. Schlemm's canal is visible. The iris is highly pigmented and shadows deeper structures.

Examples of scan protocols for imaging the anterior chamber and clinical applications are discussed in later chapters.

Conclusion

This chapter has presented a brief summary of the history of OCT in ophthalmology as well as an overview of how OCT technology works, including both TD detection and SD/FD detection. A discussion of what OCT images show and their general interpretation was also presented. The recent advances in OCT technology enable a dramatic improvement in OCT image quality, allowing visualization of individual retinal layers. As additional clinical studies become available, OCT images may eventually be used to assess detailed retinal pathology on the level of architectural morphology, such as that used by pathologists. The high imaging speeds that are now possible enable the acquisition of 3D-OCT volumetric data sets that have com-

prehensive information on retinal structure. OCT en face fundus images can be generated that are analogous to SLO images. Cross-sectional (B-scan) images can be extracted from 3D-OCT data sets and are precisely registered to features on the fundus. This capability will allow more accurate tracking of changes in retinal pathology from visit to visit. The high acquisition speeds also enable more accurate assessment of true retinal topography. Quantitative measurement of retinal features including retinal thickness, RNFL thickness, and other intraretinal layers is also possible with improved accuracy and reproducibility. These capabilities promise to improve the sensitivity for disease diagnosis as well as the ability to monitor disease progression and response to treatment.

References

1. Huang D, Swanson EA, Lin CP, et al. Optical coherence tomography. *Science.* 1991;254:1178-1181.
2. Izatt JA, Hee MR, Swanson EA, et al. Micrometer-scale resolution imaging of the anterior eye in vivo with optical coherence tomography. *Arch Ophthalmol.* 1994;112:1584-1589.

3. Hee MR, Izatt JA, Swanson EA, et al. Optical coherence tomography of the human retina. *Arch Ophthalmol.* 1995;113:325-332.

4. Puliafito CA, Hee MR, Lin CP, et al. Imaging of macular diseases with optical coherence tomography. *Ophthalmology.* 1995;102:217-229.

5. Schuman JS, Hee MR, Arya AV, et al. Optical coherence tomography: a new tool for glaucoma diagnosis. *Curr Opin Ophthalmol.* 1995;6:89-95.

6. Drexler W, Fujimoto JG. State-of-the-art retinal optical coherence tomography. *Prog Retin Eye Res.* 2008;27:45-88.

7. Drexler W, Fujimoto JG. *Optical Coherence Tomography Technology and Applications.* New York, NY: Springer; 2008.

8. Puliafito CA, Hee MR, Schuman JS, Fujimoto JG. *Optical Coherence Tomography of Ocular Diseases.* Thorofare, NJ: SLACK Incorporated; 1996.

9. Hee MR, Puliafito CA, Wong C, et al. Quantitative assessment of macular edema with optical coherence tomography. *Arch Ophthalmol.* 1995;113:1019-1029.

10. Hee MR, Puliafito CA, Wong C, et al. Optical coherence tomography of macular holes. *Ophthalmology.* 1995;102:748-756.

11. Hee MR, Puliafito CA, Wong C, et al. Optical coherence tomography of central serous chorioretinopathy. *Am J Ophthalmol.* 1995;120:65-74.

12. Hee MR, Baumal CR, Puliafito CA, et al. Optical coherence tomography of age-related macular degeneration and choroidal neovascularization. *Ophthalmology.* 1996;103:1260-1270.

13. Wilkins JR, Puliafito CA, Hee MR, et al. Characterization of epiretinal membranes using optical coherence tomography. *Ophthalmology.* 1996;103:2142-2151.

14. Hee MR, Puliafito CA, Duker JS, et al. Topography of diabetic macular edema with optical coherence tomography. *Ophthalmology.* 1998;105:360-370.

15. Schuman JS, Hee MR, Puliafito CA, et al. Quantification of nerve fiber layer thickness in normal and glaucomatous eyes using optical coherence tomography. *Arch Ophthalmol.* 1995;113:586-596.

16. Schuman JS, Pedut-Kloizman T, Hertzmark E, et al. Reproducibility of nerve fiber layer thickness measurements using optical coherence tomography. *Ophthalmology.* 1996;103:1889-1898.

17. Schuman JS, Pedut-Kloizman T, Pakter H, et al. Optical coherence tomography and histologic measurements of nerve fiber layer thickness in normal and glaucomatous monkey eyes. *Invest Ophthalmol Vis Sci.* 2007;48(8):3645-3654.

18. Bowd C, Weinreb RN, Williams JM, Zangwill LM. The retinal nerve fiber layer thickness in ocular hypertensive, normal, and glaucomatous eyes with optical coherence tomography. *Arch Ophthalmol.* 2000;118:22-26.

19. Zangwill LM, Williams J, Berry CC, Knauer S, Weinreb RN. A comparison of optical coherence tomography and retinal nerve fiber layer photography for detection of nerve fiber layer damage in glaucoma. *Ophthalmology.* 2000;107:1309-1315.

20. Bowd C, Zangwill LM, Berry CC, et al. Detecting early glaucoma by assessment of retinal nerve fiber layer thickness and visual function. *Invest Ophthalmol Vis Sci.* 2001;42:1993-2003.

21. Schuman JS, Wollstein G, Farra T, et al. Comparison of optic nerve head measurements obtained by optical coherence tomography and confocal scanning laser ophthalmoscopy. *Am J Ophthalmol.* 2003;135:504-512.

22. Guedes V, Schuman JS, Hertzmark E, et al. Optical coherence tomography measurement of macular and nerve fiber layer thickness in normal and glaucomatous human eyes. *Ophthalmology.* 2003;110:177-189.

23. Wollstein G, Schuman JS, Price LL, et al. Optical coherence tomography (OCT) macular and peripapillary retinal nerve fiber layer measurements and automated visual fields. *Am J Ophthalmol.* 2004;138:218-225.

24. Wollensak G, Aurich H, Wirbelauer C, Pham DT. Potential use of riboflavin/UVA cross-linking in bullous keratopathy. *Ophthalmic Res.* 2009;41:114-117.

25. Olsen T. Calculating axial length in the aphakic and the pseudophakic eye. *J Cataract Refract Surg.* 1988;14:413-416.

26. Olsen T. The accuracy of ultrasonic determination of axial length in pseudophakic eyes. *Acta Ophthalmologica.* 1989;67:141-144.

27. Pavlin CJ, Sherar MD, Foster FS. Subsurface ultrasound microscopic imaging of the intact eye. *Ophthalmology.* 1990;97:244-250.

28. Pavlin CJ, Harasiewicz K, Sherar MD, Foster FS. Clinical use of ultrasound biomicroscopy. *Ophthalmology.* 1991;98:287-295.

29. Pavlin CJ, Foster FS. Ultrasound biomicroscopy. High-frequency ultrasound imaging of the eye at microscopic resolution. *Radiol Clin North Am.* 1998;36:1047-1058.

30. Drexler W, Morgner U, Ghanta RK, Kärtner FX, Schuman JS, Fujimoto JG. Ultrahigh-resolution ophthalmic optical coherence tomography. *Nat Med.* 2001;7:502-507.

31. Fujimoto JG, De Silvestri S, Ippen EP, Puliafito CA, Margolis R, Oseroff A. Femtosecond optical ranging in biological systems. *Opt Lett.* 1986;11:150-153.

32. Stern D, Lin WZ, Puliafito CA, Fujimoto JG. Femtosecond optical ranging of corneal incision depth. *Invest Ophthalmol Vis Sci.* 1989;30:99-104.

33. Born M, Wolf E, Bhatia AB. *Principles of Optics: Electromagnetic Theory of Propagation, Interference and Diffraction of Light.* 7th expanded ed. Cambridge, England: Cambridge University Press; 1999.

34. Youngquist R, Carr S, Davies D. Optical coherence-domain reflectometry: a new optical evaluation technique. *Opt Lett.* 1987;12:158-160.

35. Takada K, Yokohama I, Chida K, Noda J. New measurement system for fault location in optical waveguide devices based on an interferometric technique. *Appl Opt.* 1987;26:1603-1608.

36. Gilgen HH, Novak RP, Salathe RP, Hodel W, Beaud P. Submillimeter optical reflectometry. *IEEE J Lightwave Technol.* 1989;7:1225-1233.

37. Fercher AF, Mengedoht K, Werner W. Eye-length measurement by interferometry with partially coherent light. *Opt Lett.* 1988;13:1867-1869.

38. Huang D, Wang J, Lin CP, Puliafito CA, Fujimoto JG. Micron-resolution ranging of cornea and anterior chamber by optical reflectometry. *Lasers Surg Med.* 1991;11:419-425.

39. Hitzenberger CK. Measurement of corneal thickness by low-coherence interferometry. *Appl Opt.* 1992;31:6637-6642.

40. Swanson EA, Huang D, Hee MR, Fujimoto JG, Lin CP, Puliafito CA. High-speed optical coherence domain reflectometry. *Opt Lett.* 1992;17:151-153.

41. Swanson EA, Izatt JA, Hee MR, et al. In vivo retinal imaging by optical coherence tomography. *Opt Lett.* 1993;18:1864-1866.

42. Patterson MS, Chance B, Wilson BC. Time resolved reflectance and transmittance for the non-invasive measurement of tissue optical properties. *Appl Opt.* 1989;28:2331-2336.

43. Flock ST, Patterson MS, Wilson BC, Wyman DR. Monte Carlo modeling of light propagation in highly scattering tissues. I. Model predictions and comparison with diffusion theory. *IEEE Trans Biomed Eng.* 1989;36:1162-1168.

44. Flock ST, Wilson BC, Patterson MS. Monte Carlo modeling of light propagation in highly scattering tissues. II. Comparison with measurements in phantoms. *IEEE Trans Biomed Eng.* 1989;36:1169-1173.

45. Cheong WF, Prahl SA, Welch AJ. A review of the optical properties of biological tissues. *IEEE J Quantum Electron.* 1990;26:2166-2185.

46. Fujimoto JG, Brezinski ME, Tearney GJ, et al. Optical biopsy and imaging using optical coherence tomography. *Nat Med.* 1995;1:970-972.

47. Schmitt JM, Knuttel A, Yadlowsky M, Eckhaus MA. Optical-coherence tomography of a dense tissue: statistics of attenuation and backscattering. *Phys Med Biol.* 1994;39:1705-1720.

48. Drexler W, Sattmann H, Hermann B, et al. Enhanced visualization of macular pathology with the use of ultrahigh-resolution optical coherence tomography. *Arch Ophthalmol.* 2003;121:695-706.

49. Ko TH, Fujimoto JG, Duker JS, et al. Comparison of ultrahigh- and standard-resolution optical coherence tomography for imaging macular hole pathology and repair. *Ophthalmology.* 2004;111:2033-2043.

50. Ko TH, Fujimoto JG, Schuman JS, et al. Comparison of ultrahigh- and standard-resolution optical coherence tomography for imaging macular pathology. *Ophthalmology.* 2005;112(11):1922.e1-15.

51. Hogan H, Alvarado JA, Weddell JE. *Histology of the Human Eye: An Atlas and Textbook.* Philadelphia, PA: WB Saunders; 1971.

52. Gass JDM. *Stereoscopic Atlas of Macular Diseases: Diagnosis and Treatment.* 3rd ed. Vol 1. St. Louis, MO: CV Mosby; 1987:46-65.

53. Krebs W, Krebs I. *Primate Retina and Choroid: Atlas of Fine Structure in Man and Monkey.* New York, NY: Springer Verlag; 1991.

54. Spalton DJ, Hitchings RA, Hunter PA. Anatomy of the retina. In: Spalton DJ, eds. *Atlas of Clinical Ophthalmology.* 2nd ed. St. Louis, MO: Mosby; 1994.

55. Toth CA, Narayan DG, Boppart SA, et al. A comparison of retinal morphology viewed by optical coherence tomography and by light microscopy. *Arch Ophthalmol.* 1997;115:1425-1428.

56. Huang Y, Cideciyan AV, Papastergiou GI, et al. Relation of optical coherence tomography to microanatomy in normal and rd chickens. *Invest Ophthalmol Vis Sci.* 1998;39:2405-2416.

57. Li Q, Timmers AM, Hunter K, et al. Noninvasive imaging by optical coherence tomography to monitor retinal degeneration in the mouse. *Invest Ophthalmol Vis Sci.* 2001;42:2981-2989.

58. Gloesmann M, Hermann B, Schubert C, Sattmann H, Ahnelt PK, Drexler W. Histologic correlation of pig retina radial stratification with ultrahigh-resolution optical coherence tomography. *Invest Ophthalmol Vis Sci.* 2003;44:1696-1703.

59. Anger EM, Unterhuber A, Hermann B, et al. Ultrahigh resolution optical coherence tomography of the monkey fovea. Identification of retinal sublayers by correlation with semithin histology sections. *Exp Eye Res.* 2004;78:1117-1125.

60. Srinivasan VJ, Monson BK, Wojtkowski M, et al. Characterization of outer retinal morphology with high-speed, ultrahigh-resolution optical coherence tomography. *Invest Ophthalmol Vis Sci.* 2008;49:1571-1579.

61. Sidman R. The structure and concentration of solids in photoreceptor cells studied by refractometry and interference microscopy. *J Biophys Biochem Cytol.* 1957;3:1530.

62. Drexler W. Ultrahigh-resolution optical coherence tomography. *J Biomed Opt.* 2004;9:47-74.

63. Fercher AF, Hitzenberger CK, Kamp G, Elzaiat SY. Measurement of intraocular distances by backscattering spectral interferometry. *Opt Commun.* 1995;117:43-48.

64. Wojtkowski M, Leitgeb R, Kowalczyk A, Bajraszewski T, Fercher AF. In vivo human retinal imaging by Fourier domain optical coherence tomography. *J Biomed Opt.* 2002;7:457-463.

65. Wojtkowski M, Bajraszewski T, Gorczynska I, et al. Ophthalmic imaging by spectral optical coherence tomography. *Am J Ophthalmol.* 2004;138:412-419.

66. Cense B, Nassif N, Chen TC, et al. Ultrahigh-resolution high-speed retinal imaging using spectral-domain optical coherence tomography. *Opt Express.* 2004;12:2435-2447.

67. Nassif NA, Cense B, Park BH, et al. In vivo high-resolution video-rate spectral-domain optical coherence tomography of the human retina and optic nerve. *Opt Express.* 2004;12:367-376.

68. Wojtkowski M, Srinivasan VJ, Ko TH, Fujimoto JG, Kowalczyk A, Duker JS. Ultrahigh-resolution, high-speed, Fourier domain optical coherence tomography and methods for dispersion compensation. *Opt Express.* 2004;12:2404-2422.

69. Wojtkowski M, Srinivasan V, Fujimoto JG, et al. Three-dimensional retinal imaging with high-speed ultrahigh-resolution optical coherence tomography. *Ophthalmology.* 2005;112:1734-1746.

70. Leitgeb R, Hitzenberger CK, Fercher AF. Performance of Fourier domain vs. time domain optical coherence tomography. *Opt Express.* 2003;11:889-894.

71. De Boer JF, Cense B, Park BH, Pierce MC, Tearney GJ, Bouma BE. Improved signal-to-noise ratio in spectral-domain compared with time-domain optical coherence tomography. *Opt Lett.* 2003;28:2067-2069.

72. Choma MA, Sarunic MV, Yang CH, Izatt JA. Sensitivity advantage of swept source and Fourier domain optical coherence tomography. *Opt Express.* 2003;11:2183-2189.

73. Jiao S, Knighton R, Huang X, Gregori G, Puliafito CA. Simultaneous acquisition of sectional and fundus ophthalmic images with spectral-domain optical coherence tomography. *Opt Express.* 2005;13:444-452.

74. Sander B, Larsen M, Thrane L, Hougaard JL, Jorgensen TM. Enhanced optical coherence tomography imaging by multiple scan averaging. *Br J Ophthalmol.* 2005;89:207-212.

Chapter 2

Interpretation of the Optical Coherence Tomography Image

Gadi Wollstein, MD; Lindsey S. Folio, MS, MBA;
Jessica E. Nevins, BS; Hiroshi Ishikawa, MD;
Carmen A. Puliafito, MD, MBA; James G. Fujimoto, PhD; and Joel S. Schuman, MD

Introduction

Optical coherence tomography (OCT) provides noncontact, real-time, and high-resolution imaging of the eye. The device generates cross-sectional images of in vivo tissue structures by measuring the echo time delay and intensity of backscattered or backreflected light.[1-5] Time-domain (TD) OCT uses low-coherence light that is split into 2 beams at a partially reflecting mirror. One beam is directed at the tissue of interest, while the other beam is directed at a mirror attached to a moving reference arm. The beams then recombine at a photodetector, and the interference is assessed to evaluate the intensity of the backreflected light, which relates directly to the structural measurements of the tissue. Spectral-domain (SD) OCT, also known as *Fourier-domain* (FD) OCT, assesses the signal without moving the reference arm, greatly reducing acquisition time. SD-OCT encodes the time delay at each depth simultaneously by taking the Fourier transform of the interference spectrum of the light signals. In addition, the device uses a broader wavelength that allows further improvements to image resolution. Taken together, this allows SD-OCT to acquire greater amounts of data at higher speed and better resolution than TD-OCT, making it a remarkable tool for intraocular disease evaluation.[6-8]

OCT images provide diagnostically important information on a wide range of ocular pathologies, including macular edema, retinal detachment, alterations in the vitreoretinal interface, macular hole, age-related macular degeneration, diabetic retinopathy, glaucoma, and others. A wide range of OCT scanning protocols may be used to obtain optimum diagnostic information on specific structures such as the macula or optic disc. In addition to providing direct visualization of both the volumetric structure and the cross-sectional layers of retina, computer image processing can be applied to identify and measure layers of the retina automatically. Quantitative measurements obtained with SD-OCT may be displayed with topographic maps, such as retinal thickness or retinal nerve fiber layer (RNFL) thickness maps, which facilitate direct comparison and registration with fundus images or fluorescein

Schuman JS, Puliafito CA, Fujimoto JG, Duker JS, eds.
Optical Coherence Tomography of Ocular Diseases,
Third Edition (pp 27-66).
© 2013 SLACK Incorporated.

Figure 2-1A. Papillomacular image (obtained with Spectralis HRA+OCT, Heidelberg Engineering, GmbH, Heidelberg, Germany).

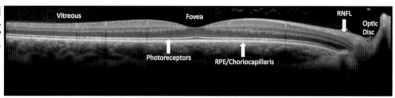

angiography. Some SD-OCT devices incorporate scanning laser ophthalmoscopy (SLO) or fundus photography into their systems, thus offering simultaneous OCT scanning and fundus imaging to enhance the evaluation of retinal pathologies and disease.[9] The ability of OCT to provide direct visualization as well as quantitative information makes it useful to longitudinally track small alterations in tissue structure associated with the progression or resolution of disease.

This chapter provides a brief explanation of how light propagates through tissue, guidelines on how to interpret OCT images of the retina and normal anterior eye, and an overview of OCT image processing for quantitative structural measurement.

Interpreting Optical Coherence Tomography Images of the Normal Retina

Papillomacular Bundle

OCT can visualize the cross-sectional structure of the retina and posterior eye.[2,10-15] Figure 2-1A shows a large field-of-view OCT tomogram of the normal retina, including both the macular and peripapillary region. The image was performed with 7-µm axial resolution at an 870-nm wavelength and spans 8.7 mm. The image is composed of 18 repetitive cross sections (B-scans), marked by the green line on the infrared confocal scanning laser ophthalmoscopy (CSLO) image of Figure 2-1B. SD-OCT has the ability to average repetitive B-scans to greatly reduce image noise and produce a sharper appearing cross-sectional image. Retinal tracking, a method of correcting for eye motion during scanning, is available in some SD-OCT devices, which can further reduce the motion-related artifacts in images.

Structurally, the retina is a very thin layer, but the OCT image is intentionally expanded in the axial direction in order to better visualize the microstructure of the retina. Large-scale anatomic features of the retina, such as the fovea, optic disc, retinal profile, and curvature, are evident, and they can be

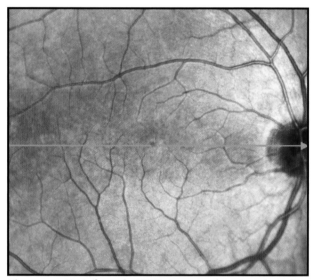

Figure 2-1B. Infrared CSLO image showing location of papillomacular image (obtained with Spectralis HRA+OCT).

identified by their characteristic morphology. The vitreoretinal interface is identified by the increase in backscattering between the transparent vitreous and the surface of the inner retina. The fovea appears as a characteristic thinning of the retina with the absence of inner retinal layers and an increase in thickness of the photoreceptor layer reflecting the high density of cones in the macula. The optic disc appears with the characteristic contour of the optic nerve. A highly scattering layer delineates the posterior boundary of the retina in the tomogram and corresponds to the retinal pigment epithelium (RPE) and choriocapillaris. A second, closely spaced, highly scattering layer, which is immediately anterior, arises from a reflection between the inner (IS) and outer segments (OS) of the photoreceptors. These posterior layers terminate at the margin of the optic disc and are consistent with the termination of choroidal circulation at the lamina cribrosa. Posterior to the choriocapillaris, relatively weak signals are visible from the deep choroid and sclera due to attenuation of the optical beam after passing through the retina, RPE, and choriocapillaris. A variable thickness, highly scattering layer at the

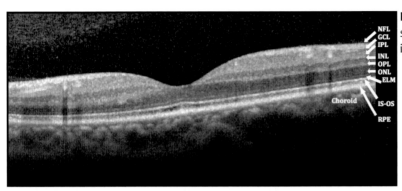

Figure 2-2A. Macular vertical cross-line scan in grayscale showing layers of the retina (obtained with Spectralis HRA+OCT).

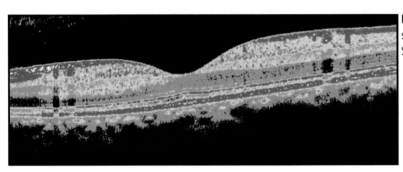

Figure 2-2B. Macular horizontal cross-line scan false-color image (obtained with Spectralis HRA+OCT).

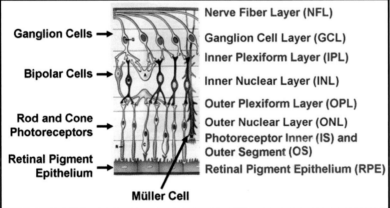

Figure 2-2C. Drawing of layers of the retina.

inner margin of the retina corresponds to the RNFL. The RNFL is thicker in the region of the optic disc and becomes thinner toward the macula, in agreement with well-established retinal morphology.

Retinal Microstructure

Due to the higher axial resolution and greater scan density, SD-OCT images can visualize the microscopic anatomy of the retina in greater detail than TD-OCT images. Figure 2-2A shows an SD-OCT image of the normal macula in grayscale. The image is 8.7 mm in transverse width, consists of 1536 trans-

verse pixels, and is oriented in the superior-inferior direction. Figure 2-2B shows the same image, but represented with the false-color analysis, where warmer colors indicate higher reflectivity of retinal structures. The microstructure of the various retinal layers can be differentiated in the OCT image and correlates with the well-known morphology of the retina in the foveal and parafoveal region.[16-19] For comparison, Figure 2-2C shows a schematic of the different retinal layers. Histologically, the retina can be divided into 10 distinct layers, including 4 cell layers and 2 layers of neuronal interconnections. These layers can be resolved in ophthalmic OCT images. The interpretation of OCT imaging is supported by studies that compare OCT to histology.[20-24] The interpretation of features in OCT images is also confirmed by imaging pathologies that produce known alterations of retinal architecture.

The RNFL and plexiform layers consist of axonal structures that are highly optically backscattering and appear as red in the false-color OCT image (see Figure 2-2B). In contrast, nuclear layers are weakly backscattering and appear as blue-green. The first highly backscattering layer, visible outside the fovea, is the RNFL. The 3 weakly backscattering layers are the ganglion cell layer (GCL), inner nuclear layer (INL), and outer nuclear layer (ONL). The GCL increases in thickness in the parafoveal region reflecting the high density of photoreceptors in the fovea connected to this layer. The moderately backscattering inner plexiform layer (IPL) is adjacent to the GCL and INL. The obliquely running photoreceptor axons, sometimes considered as a separate layer in the outer plexiform layer (OPL) known as *Henle's fiber layer*, are highly backscattering.

The boundary between the photoreceptor IS and OS is visible as a thin, highly backscattering band immediately anterior to the RPE and choroid. The reflection arising from this structure may be the result of a refractive index difference between the photoreceptor IS and the highly organized structure of the OS, which contains stacks of membranous discs, rich in the visual pigment rhodopsin.[18,19,25] The thickness of the photoreceptor IS and OS increases in the foveal region, which corresponds to the well-known increase in the length of the OS of the cones in this region.

The external limiting membrane (ELM) can also be visualized as a thin backscattering layer posterior to the ONL and anterior to the boundary between the photoreceptor IS and OS. The ELM is not a physical membrane but is an alignment of structures between the photoreceptors and the Müller cells.

The RPE, which contains melanin, is a very strongly backscattering layer. Bruch's membrane, which is only 1- to 4-μm thick, cannot be visualized as an independent structure. Finally, the choriocapillaris is vascular and strongly backscattering. Since the RPE is in close contact with the choriocapillaris, it is often not distinguishable as a separate layer in the OCT images. The vascular structures of the choriocapillaris and choroid are highly optically scattering, and they produce shadowing effects that limit the OCT imaging depth for deeper structures.

Retinal blood vessel locations can be identified by their increased backscatter and by their shadowing of the deeper structures.

Optic Nerve Head

OCT images can directly visualize the contour of the optic disc in both 2 and 3 dimensions (2D and 3D). Figure 2-3A shows an OCT image of the normal optic disc, and Figure 2-3B shows the same optic disc obtained with a volumetric scan. The 3D image can be manipulated to view any slice of the cube of data acquired in the scan. 3D imaging of the disc and macula will be discussed in more detail in a following section. In Figure 2-3A, the contour of the optic disc region is demarcated by the boundary between the low backscattering vitreous and the highly backscattering RNFL and optic nerve head (ONH) surface. The normal cupping of the disc is evident. The OCT image shows an increase in RNFL thickness approaching the optic disc margin where the RNFL is nearly the entire thickness of the retina. The retinal nerve fibers exhibit a directional reflectance. The reflected signal intensity from the nerve fibers decreases at the disc rim, where the nerve fibers are no longer perpendicular to the incident OCT optical beam but bend into the ONH.

The RPE and choriocapillaris are visible as a highly backscattering layer that terminates at the disc margin. The boundary between the photoreceptor IS and OS is also visible as a thin, highly backscattering feature immediately anterior to the RPE and choroid. The photoreceptor layer and RPE terminate in the region approaching the disc and can be used as a landmark to define the disc margin. The IPL and OPL are moderately reflective, while the INL and ONL are weakly reflective.

OCT imaging of the optic nerve and neuroretinal rim is valuable in assessing glaucoma and neuro-ophthalmic diseases. In evaluating the contour of the disc, it is important to note that OCT images are often displayed with an expanded scale in the axial direction in order to allow better visualization of the thin retinal layers while still encompassing a several-millimeter transverse scan. In this manner, the depth of the disc cup is exaggerated and quantitative morphometry of the images using the correct axial and transverse scales is, therefore, important. The use of algorithms to assess the morphology of the optic disc will be discussed in a later section.

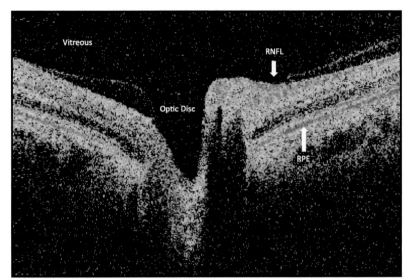

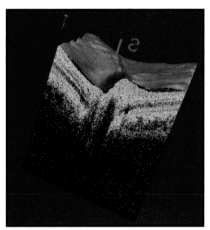

Figure 2-3B. 3D image of ONH with SLO shown as overlay (obtained with RTVue-100).

Figure 2-3A. ONH B-scan (obtained with RTVue-100, Optovue, Inc, Fremont, CA).

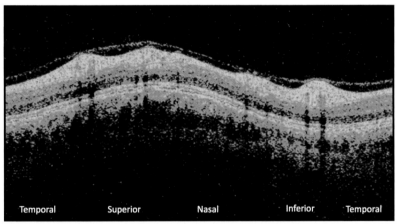

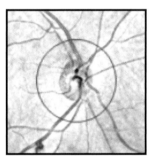

Figure 2-4B. Fundus image indicating location of circumpapillary scan (obtained with Cirrus HD-OCT).

Figure 2-4A. Image on 3.4-mm circle around optic disc (obtained with Cirrus HD-OCT, Carl Zeiss Meditec, Inc, Dublin, CA).

Peripapillary Region

Documentation of RNFL thickness in the peripapillary region is important in the diagnosis and clinical management of glaucoma. SD-OCT devices use a protocol similar to that of TD-OCT, which was introduced in 1995, to assess the RNFL.[26-28] Circumpapillary SD-OCT scans can be performed, creating cylindrical sections of the retina centered around the optic disc so that all nerves emanating from the nerve head cross the OCT image plane. SD-OCT circumpapillary scans can also be sampled from a cube scan acquired in the circumpapillary region (see Figure 2-3B). The 3.4-mm circle can be placed anywhere within this region to ensure cen-

tration of the ONH and accurate measurement of RNFL thickness. Figure 2-4A shows a circumpapillary OCT scan with a diameter of 3.4 mm centered on the ONH. The circle sampled from the cube scan is marked in red in Figure 2-4B, the corresponding OCT fundus image. Figure 2-4A is displayed "unwrapped," and the superior, inferior, temporal, and nasal quadrants around the ONH are labeled. The SD-OCT scan of the circumpapillary region has been shown to be a good tool to detect abnormalities of the retina caused by glaucoma.[29] The circle scan sampled from the cube scan offers advantages over the circle scan in that the scan location can be corrected to match previous TD- or SD-OCT scan locations for longitudinal analysis.[30]

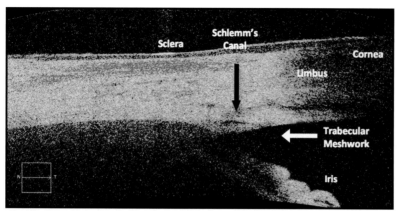

Figure 2-5A. Anterior chamber angle (obtained with Cirrus HD-OCT).

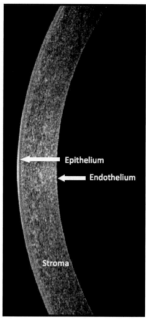

Figure 2-5B. Vertical line scan of the cornea (obtained with RTVue-100).

In Figure 2-4A, the RNFL is visible as a well-demarcated, highly backscattering layer in the OCT image. The thickness of the RNFL varies with position around the ONH, with the thickest RNFL corresponding to the superior and inferior nerve fiber bundles. The RPE and choriocapillaris, as well as the junction between the IS and OS of the photoreceptors, are evident as thin, highly backscattering layers at the posterior surface of the retina. Retinal vessels originating from the optic disc can be visualized in cross section and are evident by their increased backscatter and by their shadowing of deeper structures. The RNFL can be detected automatically using segmentation algorithms with boundary detection, and its thickness can be quantitatively measured. These image-processing and analysis techniques will be discussed in a later section.

Interpreting Optical Coherence Tomography Images of the Normal Anterior Eye

In addition to retinal imaging, OCT can also be used to image the anterior eye.[3,31,32] Figure 2-5A shows SD-OCT imaging of the anterior chamber angle of a normal human eye. The image has 5-μm axial resolution, using a wavelength of 840 nm, and spans 3 mm. In this case the image was acquired with a retinal imaging SD-OCT device with anterior segment imaging capabilities and therefore an 840-nm light source is used to obtain this image, instead of a higher wavelength light source used in dedicated anterior chamber OCT. Other strictly anterior segment imaging devices use longer wavelengths to reduce the attenuation from optical scattering and enable increased image penetration depth and better visualization of the angle.[14,15,33] Since the safe ocular exposure limit is higher for longer wavelength light, higher incident powers can be used to image the anterior eye.

Figure 2-5A shows clearly identifiable structures, including the cornea, sclera, iris, trabecular meshwork, Schlemm's canal, and the corneoscleral limbus. Structures in the angle region, such as the trabecular meshwork and Schlemm's canal, are not visualized as well, since light is attenuated after penetrating the overlying scleral tissue. The strongest signals arise from the epithelial surface of the cornea and the highly scattering sclera and iris. The limbus appears as the angled interface between the cornea and the sclera. Structures in the angle are also visible. Because light is refracted or bent when it is incident at an angle between 2 media with different indices of refraction, such as the air and the cornea, the OCT image of the anterior chamber must be corrected for this refraction in order to correctly show the geometry of the anterior chamber. This correction can be performed with computer image-processing techniques.[31] Figure 2-5B shows an SD-OCT image of the cornea of a healthy patient obtained by scanning 6 mm in the vertical direction.

Table 2-1

Commercially Available Spectral-Domain Optical Coherence Tomography Systems in North America

Device	Company
3D OCT-1000	Topcon Medical Systems, Inc (Oakland, NJ)
Bioptigen SD-OCT	Bioptigen, Inc (Research Triangle Park, NC)
Cirrus HD-OCT	Carl Zeiss Meditec, Inc (Dublin, CA)
Copernicus SOCT	Canon (Middlesex, United Kingdom)
RTVue-100	Optovue, Inc (Fremont, CA)
Spectral OCT SLO	OPKO, Inc (Miami, FL)
Spectralis OCT	Heidelberg Engineering, GmbH (Heidelberg, Germany)

Here the epithelium, endothelium, and stroma are clearly identifiable. Clinically relevant parameters may be quantitatively extracted from these images, including corneal thickness and curvature, anterior chamber depth, and anterior chamber angle.

Optical Coherence Tomography Scanning and Imaging Protocols

Image Pixel Density and Acquisition Speed

SD-OCT images are generated by performing a sequence of rapid axial measurements of backreflected or backscattered light at successive transverse positions. Since SD-OCT stores the depth of the signal intensity in the frequency domain, it is capable of acquiring all points along each A-scan at the same time. This provides much faster acquisition speeds for SD-OCT as compared to TD-OCT and allows line scans as well as high-density raster scans to be performed. Fast image acquisition time implies a lower pixel density, while higher pixel density requires a longer image acquisition time. However, the transverse pixel density of the image is limited by the maximum transverse resolution.

Current SD-OCT instruments scan at a rate that ranges between 18,000 to 50,000 axial scans per second, approximately 40 times faster than the scanning rate of TD-OCT.[6] Table 2-1 lists the current Food and Drug Administration-approved SD-OCT devices. While the axial resolutions of these devices remain on the range of 4 to 7 μm, axial resolutions of 2 μm have been reported.[7] Figures 2-6A and B demonstrate the resulting

images acquired with transverse pixel densities of 512 A-scans per 6 mm (Figure 2-6A) and 200 A-scans per 6 mm (Figure 2-6B). The image in Figure 2-6A shows a higher level of detail of the macular structures than Figure 2-6B, which has a lower transverse pixel density. Higher transverse pixel density (512 and higher transverse pixels) images are typically used to image macular pathology because they display more retinal detail, but they take longer to acquire and are increasingly subject to eye motion artifacts. Lower transverse pixel density images can be acquired very rapidly and are less sensitive to eye motion. These images are typically used when mapping the ONH contour or retinal thickness in order to minimize eye motion artifacts. The transverse resolution of the OCT instrument is determined by the spot size of the OCT light beam on the retina. Typical ophthalmic OCT instruments employ a spot size of approximately 15 to 20 μm. A typical OCT scan across the macula is 6 mm in length, so an image containing 200 transverse pixels has a transverse pixel size of 6 mm/200 = 30 μm. In contrast, a 512-pixel image has a transverse pixel size of 6 mm/512 = 11.7 μm. However, as stated previously, the pixel density is limited by the transverse resolution of the OCT. Therefore, the appearance of a higher pixel density is actually generated by overlapping adjacent points where the improvement in image quality derives from averaging multiple overlapping points.

In the axial direction, a typical retinal OCT image is 2-mm deep in tissue and consists of 1024 pixels, leading to a longitudinal pixel size of 2 mm/1024 = 1.9 μm. In contrast, the fundamental axial or longitudinal resolution of the instrument is approximately 5 μm and is determined by the coherence length of the light source. Therefore, the pixel size in the axial

Figure 2-6A. Macular B-scan (obtained with Cirrus HD-OCT macular cube 512 x 128 scan).

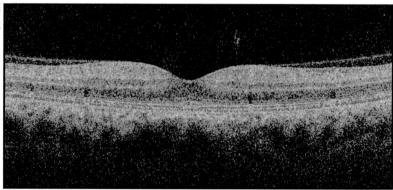

Figure 2-6B. Macular B-scan (obtained with Cirrus HD-OCT macular cube 200 x 200 scan).

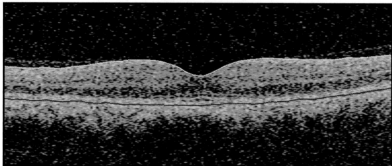

direction is much finer than the axial resolution of the instrument, thus providing good visualization of fine features. A more detailed discussion of the imaging parameters governing resolution and pixel density is presented in Appendix A.

Scans of the Macula

Three-Dimensional Cube Scans

In analogy to other imaging modalities, such as X-ray, computed tomography, or magnetic resonance imaging, information on 3D structure can be obtained by using SD-OCT to acquire volumetric cubes of data. Figure 2-7 shows a 4- x 4-mm² macular cube scan of a healthy patient obtained with RTVue-100, consisting of 101 horizontal B-scans, each composed of 512 A-scans. Scans of this type are often helpful in visualizing the 3D extent and volume of structural alterations of the macula caused by pathologies such as macular holes or edema. These types of scans, however, are more prone to artifact caused by eye movement, due to the extended acquisition time, but when combined with computer image correction techniques, artifacts can be minimized. The cube scans allow registration and alignment techniques to be implemented for longitudinal analysis. This ensures that the images acquired and

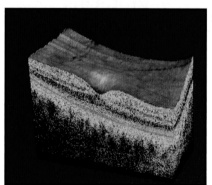

Figure 2-7. 3D macular scan (obtained with RTVue-100).

measurements recorded are from a consistent location from visit to visit. Additional 3D cube scans of healthy macula are shown in Figure 2-8 obtained with Cirrus HD-OCT, consisting of 200 horizontal B-scans each composed of 200 A-scans spanning a 6- x 6-mm² cube. Figure 2-9 was obtained with Spectralis HRA+OCT, consisting of 49 horizontal B-scans each composed of 1024 A-scans, spanning a 6- x 6-mm² area, and Figure 2-10 was obtained with 3D OCT-1000, consisting of 256 B-scans each composed of 256 A-scans, spanning a 6- x 6-mm² area.

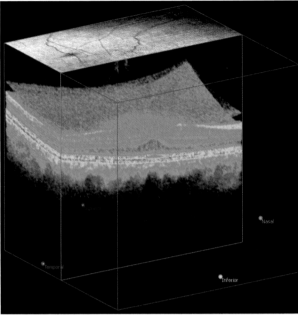

Figure 2-8. Macular cube 200 x 200 scan with LSO fundus image shown above (obtained with Cirrus HD-OCT).

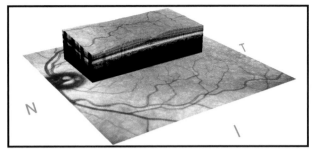

Figure 2-9. 3D macular cube scan shown with infrared CSLO image (obtained with Spectralis HRA+OCT).

Line and Cross-Line Scans

OCT imaging can be performed with an arbitrary orientation of the cross-sectional imaging plane. SD-OCT line scans consist of one B-scan that is generally composed of a higher number of A-scans per B-scans than in a 3D cube scan. This is due to the shorter length of time required to complete one line scan compared to a cube scan, where images have to be taken in multiple consecutive planes. Line scans are clinically useful for acquiring images in high detail of the retinal tissue because of the high sampling density. Figure 2-2A, shown previously, shows a vertical line scan of the macula, consisting of one B-scan and 1536 A-scans, obtained with Spectralis HRA+OCT. Figure 2-11 shows the images acquired from a cross-line scan of the macula obtained with RTVue-100. Figure 2-11A is the vertical line scan directly across the fovea, and Figure 2-11B is the horizontal line scan obtained from the same scan protocol.

Raster Scans

Raster scans of the macula, similar to the serial raster scans acquired with TD-OCT, can be acquired with SD-OCT and are capable of high transverse image resolution. Each of the Cirrus HD-OCT 5 B-scans that make up the raster scan shown in Figure 2-12A are 6-mm long, spaced 0.25-mm apart, and are made of 4096 A-scans. Figure 2-12B shows the center serial section, and the 4 images in Figure 2-12C show the 4 remaining B-scans. Characteristic features of the retina appear consistently in all 5 serial sections. The anterior and posterior surfaces of the neural retina are demarcated by backscattering at the RNFL and the highly backscattering red layer that represents the RPE and choriocapillaris. The sequence of images shows cross sections of the foveal depression, which reaches its maximal depth at the fovea centralis, shown in Figure 2-12B. As expected, the ONL is thickest and most pronounced in the

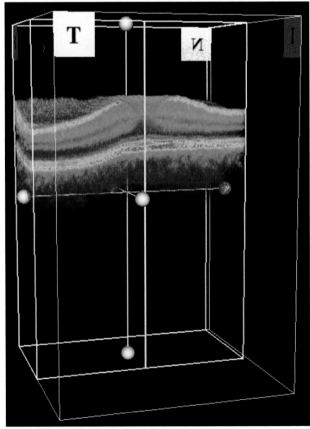

Figure 2-10. 3D macular cube scan (obtained with 3D OCT-1000, Topcon Medical Systems, Inc, Oakland, NJ).

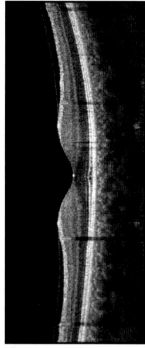

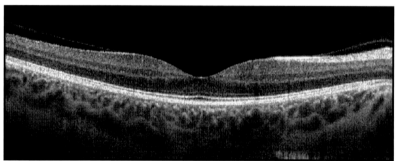

Figure 2-11B. Horizontal cross-line scan of macula (obtained with RTVue-100).

Figure 2-11A. Vertical cross-line scan of macula (obtained with RTVue-100).

image through the fovea centralis. Figure 2-12B also shows the RNFL is thickest nasally, where the scan is sampling through the papillomacular bundle close to the ONH. Figure 2-13 shows the center B-scan image acquired with a 5-line raster scan using Spectralis HRA+OCT. Again, the multilayer architecture of the macula is evident with the thickest RNFL in the nasal region. The high image resolution of 5-line raster scans provides an excellent image for viewing macular pathologies in the retinal layers.

Mesh Scans

Macular mesh scanning patterns have also been developed to improve clinically relevant information that can be retrieved from an OCT scan. They combine the use of vertical and horizontal B-scans over the retinal area of interest. Figure 2-14 shows the RTVue-100 MM5, a mesh scanning pattern of the macula centered on the fovea and its corresponding thickness analysis. The MM5 consists of an inner and outer grid, shown as white grid lines. The outer grid consists of 11 horizontal and 11 vertical B-scans, each composed of 668 A-scans, spanning 5 mm and spaced 0.5-mm apart. The

inner grid consists of 6 horizontal and 6 vertical B-scans, each composed of 400 A-scans, spanning 3 mm and spaced 0.5-mm apart. In Figure 2-14, the accompanying vertical and horizontal 5 mm in length B-scans are from the center grid lines, shown in red.

Radial Scans

A similar radial scanning protocol to that used by TD-OCT can be used to assess the macula. Six to 12 OCT images can be taken through radial planes with different angular orientations, each passing through the fovea. This set of images provides a means of imaging the entire macula, including extrafoveal pathologies, while still allowing each individual image to intercept the fovea. In combination with segmentation or boundary detection algorithms, this scanning protocol enables macular thickness to be topographically mapped.[7,34] Figure 2-15 shows the RTVue-100 MM6, a radial scanning pattern of the macula centered on the fovea and its corresponding thickness analysis. The MM6 is composed of 12 radial scans, shown as white lines, each with 1024 A-scans over a 6-mm region. Similar to the MM5, both OCT B-scans shown correspond to the vertical and horizontal radials in red. Figure 2-16 shows the radial macular scan obtained with Spectralis HRA+OCT. Like the MM6, the scan is centered on the fovea; however, it is composed of 6 radial scans, instead of 12, and uses pixel averaging, as shown in Figure 2-16A. Each B-scan consists of 1024 A-scans and spans 6.4 mm, shown in the vertical B-scan (Figure 2-16B). Figure 2-17 shows all 6 images obtained using a radial scanning pattern on the 3D OCT-1000. Here the layers of the retina are clearly identifiable. Also of note is that the fovea appears directly in the center of all 6 images, indicating the scan has been correctly centered.

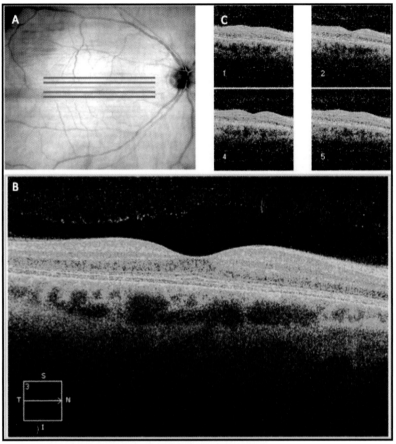

Figure 2-12. Five-line raster scan (obtained with Cirrus HD-OCT). (A) LSO fundus image showing location of raster scan across macula. (B) Center B-scan. (C) Top and bottom B-scans.

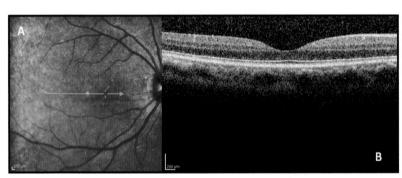

Figure 2-13. Five-line raster scan (obtained with Spectralis HRA+OCT). (A) CLSO fundus image showing location of raster scan across macula. (B) Center B-scan.

All of the macular scanning patterns can be used to measure the macular retinal thickness at different regions of the macula, such as the foveal thickness and temporal, superior, nasal, and inferior inner and outer thicknesses. However, it should be noted that in order to fill in the missing information between adjacent radial scans the software is using extrapolation. Therefore, the reliability of findings closer to the fovea where all scans are closely spaced is higher than in the periphery where the scans are widely apart. More detail on the quantitative measurement analysis will be discussed in a later section.

Scans of the Optic Disc

Three-Dimensional Cube Scans

Similar to the macular cube scans, 3D cube scans can also be acquired of the ONH region. Figure 2-3B, shown previously, was obtained with RTVue-100 3D disc scan. The cube spans a 4- x 4-mm² region and consists of 101 B-scans each composed of 512 A-scans. The image shown in Figure 2-3B is a B-scan in temporal-to-nasal orientation. 3D-OCT images can be manipulated on their respective devices to section the cube of data at different B-scans.

Figure 2-14. Macular mesh scanning pattern (obtained with RTVue-100 MM5).

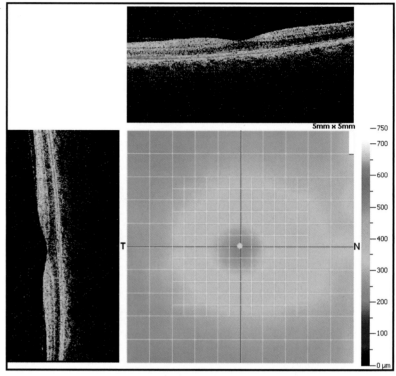

Figure 2-15. Macular radial scanning pattern (obtained with RTVue-100 MM6).

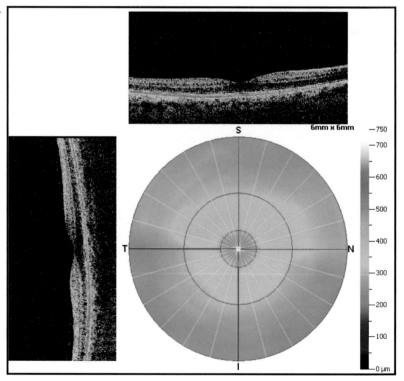

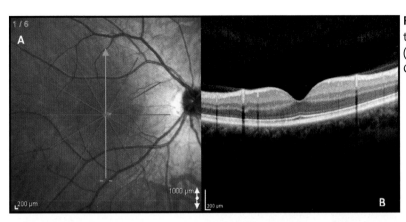

Figure 2-16. Macular radial scanning pattern (obtained with Spectralis HRA+OCT). (A) Radial scanning pattern on infrared CSLO. (B) Vertical B-scan across macula.

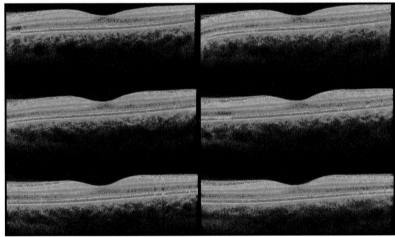

Figure 2-17. Six-line radial scan of macula (obtained with 3D OCT-1000).

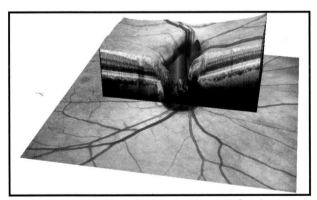

Figure 2-18. 3D ONH cube scan with CSLO fundus image (obtained with Spectralis HRA+OCT).

Figure 2-18 shows the 3D ONH cube image obtained with Spectralis HRA+OCT, consisting of 193 B-scans each composed of 512 A-scans, spanning a 6- x 6-mm² area, and its corresponding CSLO image. Figure 2-19 shows the Optic Disc Cube scan obtained with Cirrus HD-OCT, consisting of 200 B-scans each composed of 200 A-scans, spanning a 6- x 6-mm²

area, and its laser scanning ophthalmoscopy (LSO) fundus image. Figure 2-20 shows the 3D ONH image obtained with 3D OCT-1000, consisting of 256 B-scans each composed of 256 A-scans, spanning a 6- x 6-mm² area. All of the 3D cubes can be viewed in either grayscale or false color and can be "cut" at different positions to view a cross section of the cube of data. Advanced algorithms can be applied to measure features of the optic disc such as the disc, cup, and rim areas; cup-to-disc ratios; and volumetric measurements of the ONH.

Radial Scans

Radial scans of the ONH can be acquired to create images that intersect the ONH. These contain a various number of B-scans, most generally 4, 6, or 12, that have equispaced angular orientations all centered on the ONH. Figure 2-21 displays OCT images taken through radial planes with 45-degree angular orientations, each passing through the center of the ONH. The orientation of each image is shown against the corresponding CSLO fundus

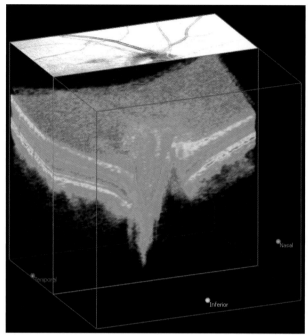

Figure 2-19. Optic Disc Cube scan with LSO fundus image (obtained with Cirrus HD-OCT).

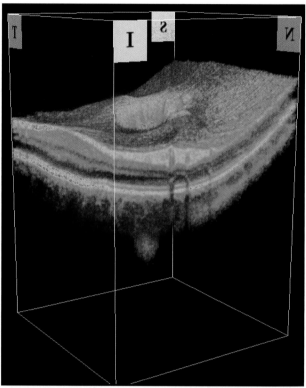

Figure 2-20. 3D ONH scan (obtained with 3D OCT-1000).

image. Figure 2-21 was obtained with Spectralis HRA+OCT and consists of 4 B-scans each composed of 768 A-scans, spanning 4.7 mm. In the vertical B-scan (Figure 2-21B), high backscattering is visible from the RNFL and from a band defining the posterior boundary of the sensory retina, which corresponds to the RPE and choriocapillaris. The OCT image shows the RNFL increasing in thickness toward the optic disc to occupy nearly the entire retinal thickness, which is commensurate with the presence of the inferior and superior arcuate nerve fiber bundles. In comparison, the horizontal B-scan (Figure 2-21C) exhibits a thinner RNFL, which is consistent with smaller nerve fibers in the temporal aspect of the disc and fewer nerve fibers in the nasal region. In all regions, RNFL thickens as it approaches the disc margin. The surface contour and normal cupping of the disc are visualized in both tomograms with prominent vasculature appearing as circular spaces with shadowing underneath. The termination of the RPE and choroid, as well as the photoreceptors at the disc margin, is also visible. Similar to the radial scans of the macula, ONH radial scans are generally acquired with a higher pixel density than 3D cube scans, creating a higher image resolution for evaluating tissue detail.

Circumpapillary Scans

A circumpapillary scanning pattern, which is typically 3.4 mm in diameter, can be used to acquire an image that samples the retinal tissues surrounding the ONH. This type of scan is effective in assessing glaucomatous damage because it intercepts all of the nerve fibers that emanate from the optic disc and avoids inaccurate measurements resulting from sampling through peripapillary atrophy.[26-29] Figure 2-4A, shown previously, shows the circumpapillary image obtained with Cirrus HD-OCT Optic Disc Cube 200 x 200 scan. Where TD-OCTs' circumpapillary scans consisted of a single circle scan, SD-OCTs' high scan speed allows the circle to be sampled from data within the boundaries of a cube scan. The placement of the image obtained in Figure 2-4A is shown as a red circle on Figure 2-4B. Some SD-OCTs, however, do use the circle scanning pattern or a combination of circular and radial scans, instead of sampling from a cube of data. Figure 2-22 shows the image obtained with Spectralis HRA+OCT 3.4-mm diameter circumpapillary scan consisting of 1536 A-scans, using eye movement tracking and scan averaging to reduce image noise. Figure 2-23 shows the image acquired with 3D OCT-1000 circumpapillary scan on a 3.4-mm diameter circle, consisting of

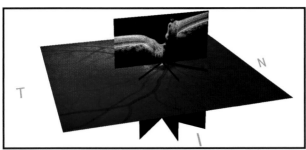

Figure 2-21A. ONH radial scan shown with CSLO fundus image (obtained with Spectralis HRA+OCT).

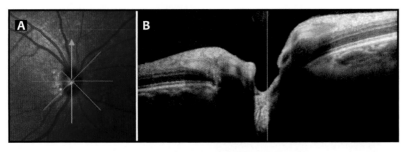

Figure 2-21B. ONH vertical radial scan. (A) CSLO fundus image. (B) ONH B-scan (obtained with Spectralis HRA+OCT).

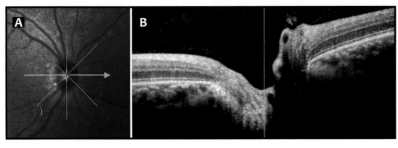

Figure 2-21C. ONH horizontal radial scan. (A) CSLO fundus image. (B) ONH B-scan (obtained with Spectralis HRA+OCT).

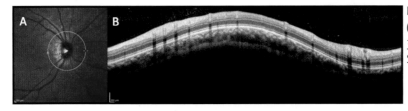

Figure 2-22. ONH circumpapillary scan. (A) CSLO fundus image. (B) B-scan on 3.4-mm diameter circle (obtained with Spectralis HRA+OCT).

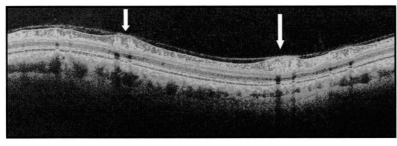

Figure 2-23. ONH circumpapillary scan on 3.4-mm diameter circle (obtained with 3D OCT-1000).

1024 A-scans. The highly reflective RNFL is shown as the anterior-most layer in red, and the RPE and choriocapillaris are shown as the highly reflective posterior layer. Of note is the increase in thickness of the RNFL in the superior and inferior regions, shown as the humps marked by the white arrows, compatible with the known thickening adjacent to the optic disc poles.

Figure 2-24. ONH scan. (A) SLO image showing scan centered on ONH. (B) Vertical radial B-scan across ONH. (C) Circumpapillary scan with 3.4-mm diameter. (D) Volumetric and thickness analysis of normal ONH. (E) 3.4-mm diameter circumpapillary scan centered on ONH. (F) Quantitative measurements of RNFL and ONH. (G) Summary of OCT RNFL thickness by quadrant (above) and clock hour (below). (H) RNFL thickness profile. Green represents age-adjusted 5th to 95th percentile, yellow 1st to 5th percentile, and red below the 1st percentile. (A-D obtained with RTVue-100; E-H obtained with Cirrus.)

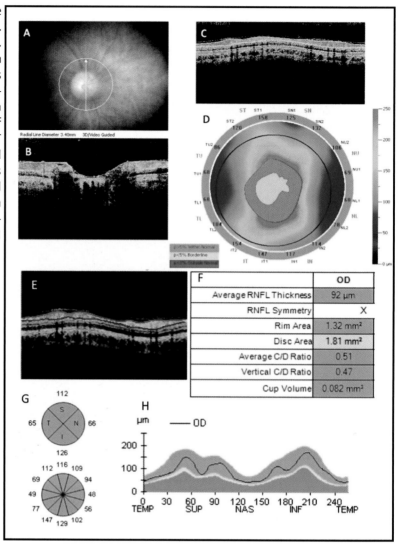

The circumpapillary and radial combination scanning pattern is shown in Figure 2-24. This scan, called the ONH scan, is composed of 12 radial scans each 3.4 mm in length consisting of 452 A-scans and 6 concentric circle scans with diameters of 2.5, 2.8, 3.1, 3.4, 3.7, and 4.0 mm, each composed of 587 to 775 A-scans, all centered on the ONH, as shown in Figure 2-24A. The vertical radial scan is shown in Figure 2-24B, and the circumpapillary scan at 3.4 mm is shown in Figure 2-24C. The combination of radial and circle scans allows volumetric analysis to be conducted of the ONH, as shown in Figure 2-24D.

Similar to the macular scanning patterns, the circumpapillary and optic disc scanning patterns can be used to quantitatively measure the structure of the optic disc such as the disc area, cup area, rim area, cup volume, rim volume, and cup-to-disc ratios. The quantitative measurements of the retinal tissue sur-

rounding the ONH can also be measured as will be described in the next section.

Quantitative Measurements of Retinal Morphology

Detection of Retinal Layers by Segmentation

OCT is especially powerful for diagnosing and monitoring conditions such as RNFL atrophy in glaucoma or macular edema associated with diabetic retinopathy because it can provide quantitative information most accurately from layered structures. SD-OCT images can be analyzed quantitatively and processed using advanced algorithms to extract features such as retinal or RNFL thickness.[7,26-29,34,35] Images acquired with SD-OCT have a more superior axial resolution than TD-OCT images, therefore, visualization and segmentation of the layers and quantitative measurement reproducibility is improved.[30] SD-OCT also employs a faster scanning rate than TD-OCT, therefore, more data can be acquired in a shorter period of time, with less motion artifact, allowing more comprehensive analysis of the macula and ONH. Mapping and display techniques have been developed to represent the image data in alternative forms to better facilitate clinical interpretation. Normative distributions of retinal thickness measurements have also been produced to offer a standard to compare the measurements made by each scan.

Retinal Thickness Measurement

Computer image-processing algorithms have been developed to automatically identify the superficial and deep neurosensory retinal boundaries to measure retinal thickness. The measurement of retinal thickness is important in quantifying macular edema or abnormal fluid accumulation within the neurosensory retina, which often leads to retinal thickening. Macular edema is a potential consequence of many ocular conditions, such as diabetic retinopathy, epiretinal membrane (ERM) formation, ocular inflammation, retinal vascular occlusion, and following cataract extraction. It is important to measure macular thickness in order to track the progression and treatment of macular edema. Macular thickness measurement might also be a potentially useful screening method for the development of macular edema, especially in patients with diabetes.

The challenge is to identify the retinal boundaries, despite varying intraretinal morphology and varied signal level in the images. Retinal morphology may be disrupted in many diseases. Diabetic retinopathy, in particular, often leads to the presence of hard exudate and cyst formation, which manifest as abnormally high or low intraretinal backscattering, respectively. Signal level can vary with instrument alignment, cataracts, and other media opacity. In scans with high signal or in the presence of ocular inflammation, intravitreal reflections might be confused with retinal reflections. A common example is prominent posterior vitreous detachment, which sometimes is interpreted by the software as the vitreoretinal interface. In conditions with low signal, retinal reflections are minimally visible, particularly in the fovea. The signal level can vary within a given OCT image (eg, if the pupil

obstructs part of the scanning beam). Although automated image-processing algorithms are reasonably robust, if the OCT image quality is sufficiently degraded, it is possible to have incorrect measurements or artifacts. Therefore, it is important to assess the quality of OCT images and the results of automated image processing. The impact of image quality on the performance of image-processing algorithms will be discussed in more detail in a later section.

The first step in quantitatively measuring retinal thickness is boundary detection, which is also known as *segmentation*. Boundary detection algorithms have been developed that consist of the following steps: smoothing, edge detection, and error correction. Special consideration is required to achieve good performance in low signal level. Figure 2-6B shows an example of a processed image of the macula that has been segmented to detect retinal thickness. The segmentation lines in the image are produced automatically by the image-processing algorithm. The anterior boundary of the retina is assumed to lie at the vitreoretinal interface, marked by the white line, and is detected from the increase in backscattering signal that occurs at this interface. The RPE boundary is identified by detecting the thin, high backscattering boundary at the posterior retina, marked by the black line in Figure 2-6B.

After the anterior and posterior boundaries of the retina have been detected on the OCT image, the retinal thickness at any transverse position in the cube scan can be measured. The image resolution of TD-OCT created difficulties in differentiating between high backscattering signals of the junction between the photoreceptor IS and OS and the RPE/choriocapillaris. SD-OCT, however, with its higher pixel density can better delineate the 2 boundaries.[36]

C-Mode Post-Processing

The fast acquisition speed of SD-OCT allows 3D volumes of data to be acquired. The volumetric images can be viewed both in the axial plane (similar to TD-OCT) and in a plane perpendicular to the scanning axis, otherwise known as *C-mode*. Post-processing software can be used to segment the volumetric images in C-mode, so only certain layers of retina are shown to offer better visual assessment of retinal pathologies.[37] This post-processing technique is shown in Figures 2-25A through D, where the C-mode plane is determined from the tissue curvature. The C-mode in Figure 2-25A is highlighting

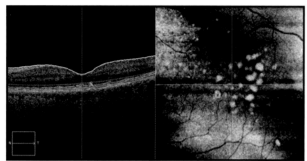

Figure 2-25A. C-mode plane, pink dotted lines, fit to RPE layer highlighting drusen as white deposits (obtained with Cirrus HD-OCT).

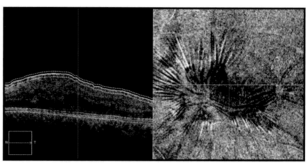

Figure 2-25B. C-mode plane, white dotted line, fit to ILM curve to show vitreomacular traction syndrome with retinal folds (obtained with Cirrus HD-OCT).

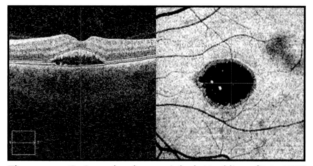

Figure 2-25C. C-mode plane, pink dotted line, fit to RPE layer to show neuroretinal detachment (obtained with Cirrus HD-OCT).

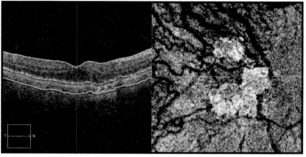

Figure 2-25D. C-mode plane, yellow line, fit to RPE to show choroidal neovascularization membrane (obtained with Cirrus HD-OCT).

the drusen as white deposits. The curvature of the inner limiting membrane (ILM) is used to determine the C-mode plane in Figure 2-25B. The traction on the retina is clearly shown as striations, over the macular region, in the C-mode image. Figure 2-25C shows the RPE detachment in the C-mode image. The curvature of the C-mode boundaries in Figure 2-25D is determined from the RPE plane and is shown as a yellow line, which has been added to the image for better visualization, in the choroid region. Here the C-mode image clearly shows the choroidal neovascularization in the macular region.

Retinal Topographic Mapping and Analysis

The utility of OCT in clinical practice depends on the ability of the physician to accurately and quickly interpret the OCT results in the context of conventional clinical examination. In standard ophthalmoscopic examination, retinal features are assessed on the appearance of the fundus. Therefore, if the topographic methods of displaying retinal and RNFL thickness obtained from OCT are combined

with the fundus, they can be directly and intuitively compared for clinical evaluation. In these methods, the segmented 3D data sets are used to extract the retinal or RNFL thickness measurements. Then the thicknesses are used to form a 2D topographic data set that can be displayed in false color as an overlay on the OCT fundus or LSO, as shown in Figure 2-26A. Retinal thickness values between 0 and 500 μm are displayed by colors ranging from blue to red, as shown in the bar index.

Measurement of retinal thickness in the macula is particularly important in patients with diabetic macular edema, where it is necessary to determine whether macular thickening involves the fovea. Thus, scanning patterns such as the 3D cube, mesh, and radial, as described previously, can be used to obtain measurements of the central fovea, where accurate information is most important. A protocol for displaying macular thickness with TD-OCT was developed by Hee et al.[34] This macular thickness display is also used for SD-OCT scans, as shown in Figure 2-26B. For quantitative interpretation, the macula is divided into 9 regions, including a central circle of 500-μm radius (the foveal region), and an inner and outer ring, each

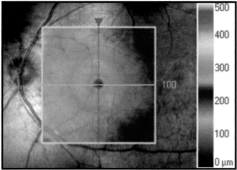

Figure 2-26A. Macular thickness analysis from macular cube 200 x 200 scan overlaid on LSO image (obtained with Cirrus HD-OCT).

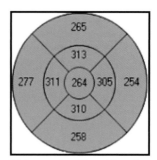

Figure 2-26B. Macular thickness analysis from macular cube 200 x 200 scan indicating a normal thickness in all sectors measured (obtained with Cirrus HD-OCT).

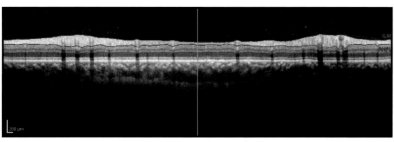

Figure 2-27. RNFL segmented circumpapillary image from 3.4-mm diameter circle (obtained with Spectralis HRA+OCT).

divided into 4 quadrants. An average retinal thickness is reported for each of the 9 regions.

The ability to reduce image information to numerical information is important for documentation, comparison between successive images, and it allows a normative database to be developed and statistics to be calculated. The topographic thickness mapping protocol demonstrates how SD-OCT images can be processed to yield different levels of diagnostic information and detail. On the coarsest level, the foveal thickness—a single number—can provide a diagnostic indicator of central macular edema in a patient. This type of information might be useful in a screening context in which a high-risk patient population (eg, patients with insulin-dependent diabetes) is screened for macular edema in a nonspecialist setting. On the next, more detailed level, regional retinal thickness values can be used to more specifically localize the presence of macular edema and to improve the statistical accuracy of the assessment. The topographic false-color map provides more graphic information that can be compared directly to the fundus or SLO image of the retina. Finally, the original OCT images contain the most specific information on retinal pathology and

can be interpreted to diagnose the presence of other retinal pathologies, in addition to macular edema.

Retinal Nerve Fiber Layer Thickness Measurement

Precise measurement of RNFL thickness is useful for evaluating patients with glaucoma, for distinguishing between patients with papilledema and crowded optic nerves, and for evaluating other neurodegenerative diseases. Computer image-processing algorithms have been developed to estimate RNFL thickness from both cube scans and circumpapillary OCT line scans acquired in cylindrical sections surrounding the optic disc.

In OCT, the RNFL appears as a highly backscattering layer at the vitreoretinal interface. Again, the challenge is to develop image-processing methods that are relatively insensitive to varying morphology and signal level in the images. As in the measurement of retinal thickness, the first step in image processing is boundary detection or segmentation. Figure 2-27 shows an example of a processed circumpapillary OCT image that has been segmented to detect RNFL thickness for a healthy patient, obtained

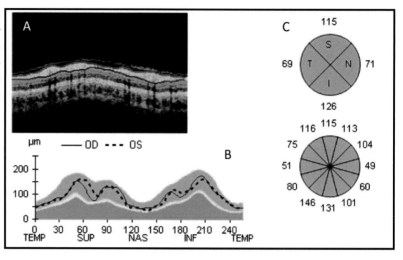

Figure 2-28. Optic Disc Cube 200 x 200 scan. (A) RNFL scan on 3.4-mm diameter circle. (B) RNFL thickness compared to a normative distribution. (C) RNFL global, quadrant, and clock hour thicknesses compared to a normative distribution (obtained with Cirrus HD-OCT).

with Spectralis HRA+OCT. The red lines in the image were produced automatically by the image-processing algorithm. The anterior boundary of the RNFL is assumed to lie at the vitreoretinal interface. The posterior boundary of the RNFL must occur between the vitreoretinal interface and boundary of the posterior retina. The most commonly used method to detect the posterior boundary of the RNFL starts with identifying the vitreoretinal interface followed by detection of the RPE photoreceptor layers as the second highly reflected layer. Then the boundary detection algorithm is moved backward to identify the point of increased signal intensity that is defined as the posterior boundary of the RNFL. Information from adjacent A-scans is also incorporated to assist boundary detection and to correct errors. The RNFL boundary detection algorithms are more sensitive to OCT image quality variations than the total retinal thickness measurement algorithms. Therefore, special care is required to ensure that the initial OCT images are of sufficient quality before accepting the results of automated RNFL measurements.

Nerve Fiber Layer Thickness Analysis

RNFL thickness can be analyzed and displayed in several complementary ways. Figure 2-28 shows the RNFL analysis from a 3.4-mm diameter circumpapillary OCT scan of a normal patient. The thickness measurements can be displayed as a graph of the RNFL thickness around the ONH compared to a normative population RNFL thickness distribution, shown in Figure 2-28B. Average values of global RNFL thickness, 4-quadrant RNFL thicknesses (ie, superior, inferior, nasal, temporal), and 12-clock hour RNFL thicknesses can be calculated and compared

to a normative distribution, shown in Figure 2-28C. These display conventions enable the graph of the RNFL thickness profile to be simplified and reduced to numerical values. The normative database accounts for the variation in RNFL thickness among normal patients in the population and may be used to assess the probability that a given RNFL thickness measurement is abnormal. Since normal patients lose RNFL as a function of age, this normative database is age adjusted. The normative values of RNFL thickness are represented by the different color codes, where green is within normal limits, yellow represents borderline, and red is outside normal limits. Extensive cross-sectional studies have been performed to develop criteria for diagnosing glaucoma based upon OCT measurements of RNFL thickness.[6,27-30,38-50] A detailed discussion of RNFL thickness and glaucoma is presented in Chapter 12.

Figure 2-29 shows an alternative RNFL thickness analysis obtained with RTVue-100. Figure 2-29A shows the segmented RNFL thickness from the 3.45-mm diameter circle scan. Figure 2-29B displays the thickness measurements around the circle compared to a normative distribution, and Figure 2-29C displays the sectoral thickness analysis. This RNFL thickness analysis reports 16 sectoral thicknesses, which are averaged to 6 larger sectors, and 2 hemisphere thickness values (Figure 2-29C).

Inner Retinal Complex Thickness Measurement and Analysis

Similar to the RNFL thickness measurement, inner layers of the macular retina can be segmented and measured and have shown to be potential indicators of glaucoma.[51,52] The inner retinal complex

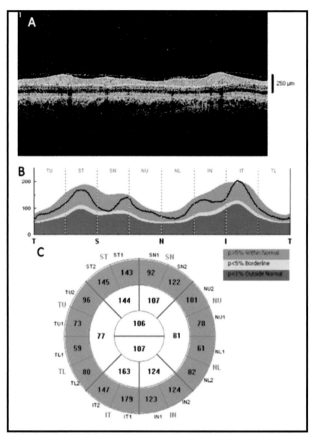

Figure 2-29. RNFL scan on 3.45-mm diameter circle. (A) Segmented B-scan on circle. (B) RNFL thickness compared to a normative distribution. (C) RNFL thickness in all sectors (obtained with RTVue-100).

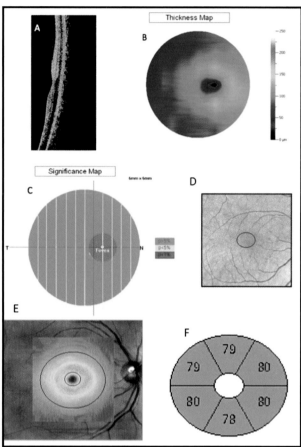

Figure 2-30. Inner retinal complex thickness analysis. (A) Vertical B-scan across macula. (B) GCC thickness map with bar scale. (C) GCC thickness significance map indicating an inner retinal complex thickness within normal limits. (D) En face macular scan. (E) Ganglion cell analysis GCL and IPL thickness. (F) Ganglion cell analysis summarized quantitative values. (A-C obtained with RTVue-100; D-F obtained with Cirrus.)

is defined as the combination of NFL, GCL, and IPL. The ganglion cell complex (GCC) scan reports the thickness of the inner retinal complex surrounding the macula. The GCC consists of 1 horizontal and 15 vertical B-scans over a 7-mm x 6-mm area. All B-scans included contain 933 A-scans and are spaced 0.5-mm apart as shown in Figure 2-30C. Figure 2-30A shows a vertical B-scan obtained from the GCC, and Figure 2-30B shows the thickness analysis as a topographic thickness map for a healthy patient. The thickness map shows a thicker inner retina in the macula surrounding the fovea. The significance map is entirely green, indicating the measured thickness values are all within the normal range. Parameters associated with the GCC scan include average, superior, and inferior GCC thicknesses; focal loss volume; and global loss volume. The focal loss volume is the sum of fractional deviations in regions with significant focal loss. The fractional deviation is calculated as a map of the GCC scanning area equal to the GCC thickness map, minus the normal reference map, divided by the normal reference map. Significant focal loss is defined as below the fifth percentile of a normal distribution of thickness values. The global loss volume is the sum of the fractional deviations in areas where fractional deviation is negative.[53]

A similar analysis is performed on the Cirrus HD-OCT, except that the macular NFL is not included in the segmentation of layers, which contains only the GCL and IPL (ganglion cell analysis). The rationale for including only these layers is that the axons overlying the GCL do not correspond to the cell bodies underneath; therefore, evaluation of structure-function correspondence will be confounded if the macular RNFL is included in this analysis. The inclusion or exclusion of the macular RNFL does not seem to affect glaucoma-discriminating ability, which remains no different than circumpapillary RNFL in comparing all people with glaucoma to healthy subjects. Figure 2-30D shows the Cirrus HD-OCT en face macular scan in a healthy person's eye. The purple circle, placed using an automated algorithm, represents the fovea. Figure 2-30E shows the GCL and IPL thickness using a pseudocolor scale (ganglion cell analysis), and Figure 2-30F shows the numerical summaries of the quantitative ganglion cell analysis.

Optic Nerve Head Analysis

Changes in the ONH are a well-established marker for glaucoma. Algorithms can be used to perform SD-OCT image analysis in order to assess the ONH and measure cup and disc parameters such as area and volume.[54,55] Optic disc topography measured by OCT has shown to be in agreement with other disc-measuring instruments.[44,56]

The ONH is typically imaged using cube scans or a combination of circle scans and radial scans at varying angular orientations, as shown previously in Figure 2-24. The boundary of the disc can be determined from each OCT image by the point at which the photoreceptor layer, RPE, and choriocapillaris terminate at the disc margin. The boundary point can be located automatically by image-processing algorithms. The disc diameter can be determined by measuring the distance between the disc boundaries on opposite sides of the disc. As shown in Figure 2-24B, the cup diameter can be measured by constructing a line parallel to and offset anteriorly by a standard amount to the line that connects the RPE/photoreceptor layer termination. Measurements from the multiple radial OCT images can be used to construct a 2D map of the ONH, as shown in Figure 2-24D. The disc area, cup area, neuroretinal rim area, and vertical and horizontal cup-to-disc ratios can be calculated.

Interpreting Optical Coherence Tomography Images of Retinal Pathologies

OCT enables cross-sectional and volumetric imaging of the retina with unprecedented resolution and provides a direct visualization of retinal pathology. On OCT images, pathologies such as macular hole, vitreomacular traction, and accumulation of subretinal fluid can often appear as prominent structural alterations. Macular disease can also produce abnormalities that change the optical properties of the retina, such as edema, hemorrhage, or drusen. Disease can also result in retinal atrophy, such as loss of the RNFL in glaucoma or atrophy of internal retinal layers in macular dystrophies. Many diseases may involve combinations of these alterations.

As discussed previously, OCT imaging can be used in conjunction with image-processing algorithms to perform quantitative measurements of retinal architecture. This approach, called *morphometry*, provides an objective measure for diagnosing disease, tracking disease progression, and evaluating response to therapy. The unprecedented resolution and high speed of SD-OCT imaging enables excellent reproducibility of morphometric measurements and sensitivity to small changes in retinal architecture. In this section, we present an overview of how to interpret OCT images of retinal pathologies.

General Features Associated With Pathology

Many retinal diseases manifest as major structural disruptions of the normal retinal architecture. For example, changes in the morphology of the fovea in macular hole, vitreomacular traction, and retinal detachment are often indicative of disease. Steepening of the foveal contour is commonly associated with vitreomacular traction and macular pseudoholes or lamellar holes. Loss or flattening of the foveal contour may occur with impending macular holes, foveal edema, or foveal retinal detachments. OCT can distinguish between various stages of macular holes, pseudoholes, and lamellar holes.[57,58] OCT is also able to image the various stages of macular hole formation. Impending macular holes, for example, can be identified by thickening of the fovea with the formation of cystic spaces and disruption between the inner retina and photoreceptor layer. Vitreomacular traction can be assessed by visualizing the vitreal detachment and its disruption of retinal architecture in the fovea. Surgically repaired macular holes often have varying morphologies that can be shown on OCT images.[58-61]

Retinal thickness is an important consideration in the assessment of many macular diseases. Retinal thickness may be increased with edema, vitreomacular traction, retinal detachment, retinoschisis, and retinal vascular occlusion. The accumulation of intraretinal fluid leads both to increased retinal thickness as well as change in the scattering properties of the tissue. It is especially important to characterize retinal thickening in the fovea, where edema can have

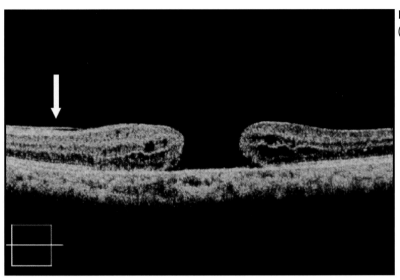

Figure 2-31. Full-thickness macular hole (obtained with Cirrus HD-OCT).

a profound effect on visual acuity. The high axial image resolution of OCT, combined with its ability to clearly identify the anterior and posterior boundaries of the retina, make OCT well suited for the quantitative measurement of retinal thicknesses.[34,36,62-64] Retinal edema may be further characterized by direct visualization of intraretinal cystic spaces or traction from the posterior hyaloid or an ERM.

Retinal abnormalities can also be associated with changes in optical properties that can be detected in OCT images. Backscattering may increase with inflammation or infiltrate into layers of the retina or choroid, fibrosis (such as in a disciform or other scar), hard exudate, and hemorrhage. Both hard exudate and hemorrhage are highly backscattering while producing pronounced shadowing of deeper retinal structures. Blood vessels, for example, are most readily identified by their shadowing effects upon deeper structures. The distinction between blood, serous fluid, and exudate may also be made based on backscattering. Serous fluid, which contains few cells, is optically transparent, so it is clearly recognizable on OCT images as a region devoid of backscattering, in contrast to blood, which exhibits enhanced reflectivity and increased attenuation of the incident light. Cloudy subretinal exudate typically has an intermediate appearance between blood and serous fluid on OCT images. Decreased backscattering may be caused by retinal edema, in which fluid accumulation leads to a decreased density of tissue and cyst formation, with a corresponding reduction in the backscattering. Alterations in cellular structure, such as hypopigmentation of the RPE, may also result in reduced backscattering.

The intensity of the OCT image is determined by both the feature being imaged and the scattering and absorption characteristics of the overlying tissue. Thus, care is required in interpreting OCT images because the brightness of various features may be affected by abnormalities in the cornea, aqueous, lens, vitreous, as well as anterior retinal layers, which can produce shadowing. Morphological causes of reduced backscattering must be distinguished from alterations in the incident light caused by dense cataracts, cloudy media, astigmatism, poorly centered intraocular lens implants, or poor alignment of the OCT instrument while imaging. Abnormalities in the intervening structures typically cause a diffuse decrease in intensity throughout the OCT image in all retinal layers. Focal decreases in backscattering may be caused by shadowing from hyperreflective tissues, such as hemorrhage, hard exudate, or a detached RPE.

Macular Holes

OCT imaging can provide important diagnostic information on pathologies such as macular hole and is a powerful adjunct to fundus examination or fluorescein angiography for the staging of macular holes.[36,57,58] OCT can differentiate macular holes from partial-thickness lamellar holes or pseudo-holes.[65] Figure 2-31 shows an OCT image of a full-thickness macular hole. The full-thickness macular hole is characterized by a loss of the normal foveal contour and disruption of the normal retinal organization extending throughout the full thickness of the retina. Intraretinal edema and cystic changes are seen adjacent to the hole. The RPE is intact in the base of the hole, and the adjacent retina has

Figure 2-32. Macular pseudohole with ERM (obtained with Cirrus HD-OCT).

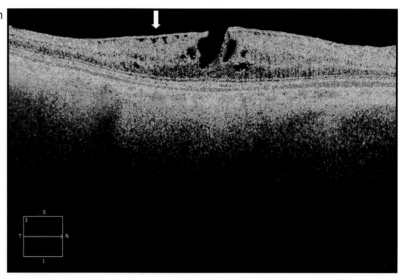

Figure 2-33. Lamellar or partial-thickness macular hole (obtained with Cirrus HD-OCT).

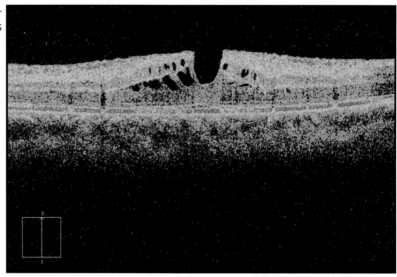

the appearance of being lifted away from the RPE. Cystic changes are present and appear in the INL and ONL. An ERM is shown producing traction on the left side of the image, indicated by the arrow.

Figure 2-32 shows a macular pseudohole with an ERM. There is a disruption of the inner retina in the area of the hole with adjacent separation of the retina between the OPL and ONL. However, the ONL and IS and OS of the photoreceptors are intact. Müller cells are seen spanning the separation in retinal layers. The ERM is visible as a thin, highly backscattering line between the vitreous and RNFL, as indicated by the arrow. The ERM is producing traction on the inner retina with a wavy appearance of the inner retina and the formation of small cystic spaces in the RNFL.

Figure 2-33 shows a lamellar or partial-thickness macular hole. A partial-thickness hole is visible centrally, with the photoreceptor layer appearing largely intact in the region of the hole. There is a separation between the OPL and the ONL. The retina adjacent to the hole appears normal, with all major retinal layers intact.

OCT can be used to stage macular holes based upon their characteristic cross-sectional appearance, and it has provided information on the pathogenesis of macular hole development.[57,58] OCT imaging can also provide objective, quantitative information about a macular hole, including the diameter of the hole, identification of vitreomacular traction strands, the extent of intraretinal cystic edema, and the extent of surrounding subretinal fluid accumulation. OCT imaging performed pre- and postoperatively can be used to assess the effectiveness of surgical treatment.[60,62,65-68]

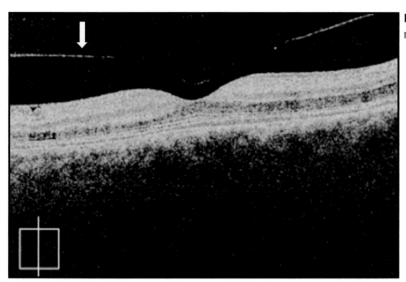

Figure 2-34. Posterior vitreous detachment (obtained with Cirrus HD-OCT).

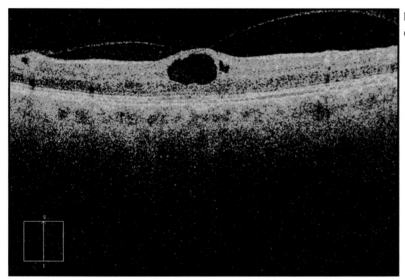

Figure 2-35. Vitreomacular traction syndrome (obtained with Cirrus HD-OCT).

Vitreous and Vitreoretinal Interface Abnormalities

OCT can provide structural information on the vitreous and vitreoretinal interface.[57,65,69-72] The normal vitreous is optically transparent and, therefore, not visible in OCT imaging. However, the vitreoretinal interface can be seen in OCT images as a high-contrast boundary between the vitreous and retina. Pathologies where the vitreous has inflammatory infiltrate, vitreous condensations, or hemorrhage result in increased optical scattering and are visible in the OCT image.

The posterior hyaloid is normally indistinguishable from the superficial retina on the OCT image, but it becomes visible when the posterior vitreous is detached. Figure 2-34 shows an example of a posterior vitreous detachment, with the hyaloid visible as a thin, weakly reflecting surface located a few-hundred microns above the retina. OCT can often detect the initial, partial detachment of posterior vitreous more accurately than biomicroscopy. When present, an operculum or pseudo-operculum can be visualized as a focal, thin area of backscatter anterior to the retinal surface. A complete posterior vitreous detachment often may not appear on an OCT image if it is more than 1 or 2 mm from the retina.

Figure 2-35 shows an example of vitreomacular traction syndrome. The vitreous is detached peripheral to the fovea and is exerting foveal traction, causing a separation between the ONL and the OPL.

Figure 2-36. ERM (obtained with Cirrus HD-OCT).

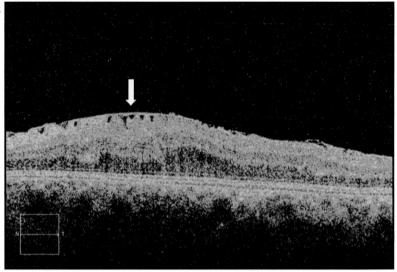

Figure 2-37. Central serous chorioretinopathy (obtained with Cirrus HD-OCT).

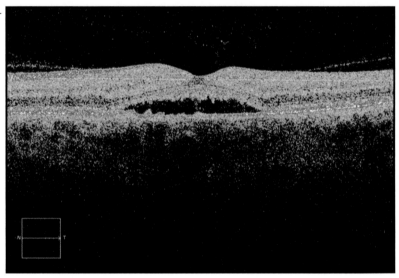

As seen in Figure 2-36, OCT can also be used to visualize ERMs.[69,71,73] An ERM that is separated from the retina can be distinguished from the posterior hyaloid based on the ERM's higher reflectivity, greater thickness, and differences in contour. An ERM in contact with the retina usually has a flatter contour than a detached posterior hyaloid, indicating greater tension. Structural deformation of the retina and alteration of the normal foveal contour can also be present. OCT can be used also to assess the outcome of surgical peeling of ERM.[69,71,74]

Subretinal Fluid, Hemorrhage, and Fibrovascular Proliferation

OCT is extremely useful for evaluating detachments of the neurosensory retina and RPE.[65,75]

Figure 2-37 shows an example of an OCT image of central serous chorioretinopathy. The OCT image shows a neurosensory retinal detachment with a shallow elevation of the retina. Subretinal fluid is present as an optically clear space between the retina and RPE. The normal retinal architectural morphology is preserved in the area of the detachment with all retinal layers present and intact. The photoreceptor layer is thicker than normal with increased backscattering, possibly indicative of a disruption in normal photoreceptor metabolism. The OCT image shows a well-defined boundary between the retina and subretinal fluid. The RPE and choriocapillaris are visible as a highly scattering layer, and the RPE is in contact with the choriocapillaris. OCT imaging is sensitive to small collections of subretinal fluid, which may be difficult to visualize

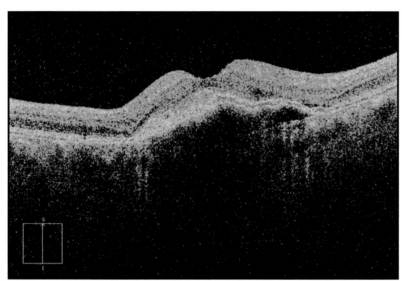

Figure 2-38. RPE detachment (obtained with Cirrus HD-OCT).

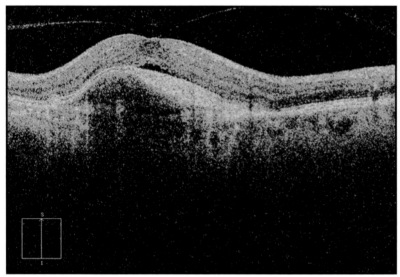

Figure 2-39. RPE detachment (obtained with Cirrus HD-OCT).

with ophthalmoscopy or biomicroscopy, and can also longitudinally track the resolution of subretinal fluid upon treatment.

Figure 2-38 shows an example of a retinal pigment epithelial detachment (PED), which has distinctive features on OCT. The RPE is visible as a thin, highly scattering band attached posteriorly to the outer retina. Although there is distortion of the normal retinal contour, the retinal architectural morphology is preserved, and all retinal layers are present and intact. The detached RPE exhibits increased backscattering, perhaps due to the refractive index difference between serous fluid and the choriocapillaris, or due to morphological changes in the RPE itself. The increased backscattering from the RPE produces shadowing of the choroid below the detachment. If an RPE tear is present, focal interruptions of the RPE can be detected.[76] The PED tends to have a pleated or tent profile, rather than the dome-shaped profile associated with neurosensory retinal detachment, and the retracted RPE exhibits increased backscattering. The bare choroid also exhibits increased backscattering from choroidal vessels and appears brighter than normal as a result of reduced shadowing because the RPE is absent. Figure 2-39 also shows a RPE detachment with a posterior vitreous detachment.

The increased reflectivity from the photoreceptors in a neurosensory detachment may mimic the high reflectivity from the pigment epithelium, but usually it does not produce significant shadowing of the RPE and choroid. Thus, the differentiation

Figure 2-40. Subretinal hemorrhage with cystoid edema (obtained with Cirrus HD-OCT).

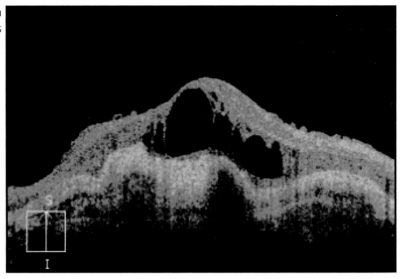

between neurosensory retinal detachment and PED often relies upon assessing the strength of the backscattering below the serous fluid collection and evaluating the angle of the detachment. OCT images of neurosensory detachments may occasionally be confused with severe retinal edema, since, in many cases, the fluid accumulation and reduced backscattering that occur with edema are preferentially seen in the outer retinal layers. In these cases, it is important to identify a smooth and continuous fluid-retina boundary to establish the diagnosis of a sensory retinal detachment. OCT imaging can also distinguish retinoschisis from retinal detachment as a splitting between the layers of the neuroretina.[77-79]

Figure 2-40 shows an example of a subretinal hemorrhage with cystoid edema. OCT images of hemorrhagic detachments of the RPE have characteristics similar to a serous RPE detachment, but they can be differentiated by the presence of optical backscattering arising from blood directly beneath the detached RPE. In this case, the blood usually appears moderately, rather than highly, backscattering because of the attenuation of the incident light through the detached RPE. The image penetration through both the detached RPE and hemorrhage is usually less than 100 μm. Similarly, in cases of hemorrhage into the vitreous, the attenuation of incident light depends on the thickness of the scattering medium. Thin hemorrhages appear as thin, highly reflective bands that have little effect on the underlying tissue. Thick hemorrhages, however, completely attenuate the incident light after more than approximately 200 μm and produce a strong shadowing of underlying structures.

Macular Edema

OCT imaging can be particularly useful in evaluating and quantifying macular edema. The ability to both image and quantitatively measure changes in retinal thickness is especially helpful in assessing and tracking patients with macular edema from diabetic retinopathy or for screening and monitoring patients with macular edema after cataract surgery. Figure 2-41 shows an example of an OCT image of cystoid macular edema. The normal foveal contour is absent, and the retinal thickness is increased to 734 μm in the fovea. Large cystic structures in the nuclear layers are present. OCT imaging can clearly identify edema as well as concomitant pathologies such as cysts, lamellar macular holes, exudate, and neovascularization. OCT measurements of changes in central foveal thickness correlate with visual acuity changes.[34,80,81]

Figure 2-42 shows an example of an OCT image of edema due to a central retinal vein occlusion. Pronounced retinal edema is observed centrally disrupting the normal foveal contour. Cystoid changes are present and can be seen in the INL and ONL. Müller cells are seen spanning the layers of the retina. In venous occlusive diseases, OCT is especially useful in quantitatively monitoring the development of macular edema and resolution following treatment. OCT imaging can identify macular thickening, cyst formation, lamellar macular holes, subretinal fluid accumulation, and papilledema. Retinal artery obstruction is associated with acute macular edema followed by retinal atrophy. These changes in morphology can be visualized by OCT. As noted previously, OCT imaging can be used to quantitatively assess retinal thickness, thus providing an objective assessment of disease progression or resolution.[65,80,82,83]

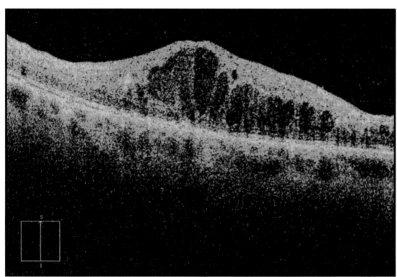

Figure 2-41. Cystoid macular edema (obtained with Cirrus HD-OCT).

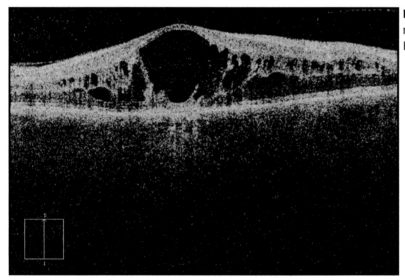

Figure 2-42. Edema due to a central retinal vein occlusion (obtained with Cirrus HD-OCT).

Retinal Pigment Epithelium and Choriocapillaris

OCT imaging can be used to assess abnormalities in the RPE that are associated with disease.[36,84,85] The RPE and choriocapillaris are usually not separately resolvable on OCT images, and they appear as a thin, highly backscattering band at the posterior boundary of the retina. The junction between the photoreceptor IS and OS also produces a thin, highly reflective band that is anterior to the RPE and choroid. These features define the posterior boundary of the neurosensory retina and the photoreceptor OS on OCT images. Alterations in these features provide useful information on chorioretinal pathologies such as age-related macular degeneration and choroidal neovascularization.

Hyperpigmentation of the RPE leads to increased reflectivity, mild thickening of the posterior reflective boundary, and concomitant shadowing of the backscattering from the choroid. Detachments of the RPE also produce shadowing of the choroid, as discussed previously. Disciform scars and other fibroses appear as a severely thickened posterior reflection, due to the high reflectivity and extension of fibrotic structures into the retina. Hypopigmentation or pigment epithelial atrophy results in decreased reflection and an associated window defect, thus enabling increased penetration of the OCT beam to the choroid and increased signals from the deeper layers.

Figure 2-43 shows an example of pigmentary abnormalities resulting from nonexudative age-related macular degeneration. Irregularities in the

Figure 2-43. Nonexudative age-related macular degeneration (obtained with Cirrus HD-OCT).

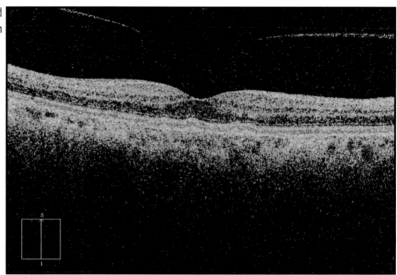

Figure 2-44. Choroidal neovascularization (obtained with Cirrus HD-OCT).

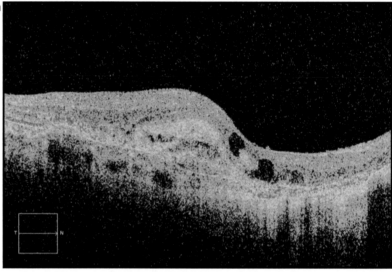

RPE and the IS and OS of the photoreceptors can be observed. The RPE and choriocapillaris have a roughened and disrupted appearance with evidence of disruption or irregularity in the OS of the photoreceptors. The inner retinal layers appear to have normal architectural morphology at this stage in the disease. A posterior vitreous detachment is also shown.

Figure 2-44 shows an example of choroidal neovascularization. There is a disruption of the RPE, the choriocapillaris, and photoreceptor OS. The ingrowth of new blood vessels through Bruch's membrane results in a fragmented and thickened appearance of the RPE, choriocapillaris, and photoreceptor OS. There is edema of the overlying retina due to intraretinal or subretinal fluid leakage from the neovascularization. This is manifest as a thickening and deviation from the normal retinal contour with an increase in thickness of the layers of the retina. In some cases, the site of penetration of the choroidal neovascularization through the RPE layer can be detected as a break in the continuous signal normally occurring in this layer. In cases of chronic edema, there can be a loss of contrast between the layers of the retina, resulting in a smeared-out and homogenous appearance.

Figure 2-45A shows an example of drusen. Drusen are visible as an apparent modulation or waviness in the thin, highly backreflecting and backscattering bands from the boundary of the photoreceptor IS and OS and the RPE and choroid. This is consistent with accumulation of material within or

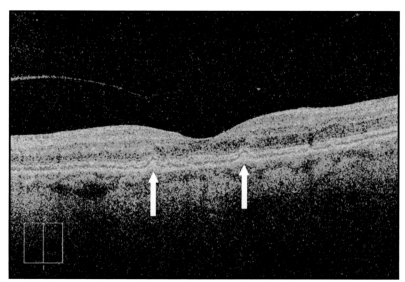

Figure 2-45A. Drusen (obtained with Cirrus HD-OCT).

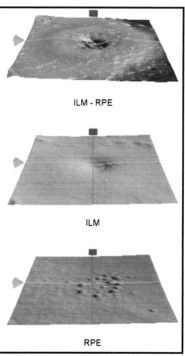

Figure 2-45B. Layers of macular cube 200 x 200 scan. (Top) Retinal thickness. (Middle) ILM thickness. (Bottom) RPE thickness showing drusen in the cube scan area (obtained with Cirrus HD-OCT).

beneath Bruch's membrane. The elevated appearance of the RPE appears similar to a serous PED. However, drusen have shallow margins and lower backscattering with less shadowing. SD-OCT segmentation analysis allows 3D visualization of selected layers of the retina. Figure 2-45B shows the total retinal, ILM, and RPE thicknesses, where the size and location of the drusen are clearly shown in the RPE layer.

Atrophy of the Retinal Nerve Fiber Layer and Retina: Glaucoma and Dystrophy

The ability of OCT to visualize and quantitatively measure retinal microstructure makes it a powerful tool for diagnosing and tracking neurodegenerative diseases such as glaucoma. Alterations in the thickness of the RNFL have been shown to be an important diagnostic of glaucoma and a measure of disease progression.[6,27,28] The RNFL appears in OCT images as a distinct, highly backscattering layer in the superficial retina. As discussed previously, RNFL thickness may be assessed at individual points on a cylindrical or linear tomogram in the peripapillary region or sampled from a high-density scan. Computer image-processing algorithms can be used to evaluate retinal, inner retinal complex, and RNFL thicknesses. Figure 2-46A shows a circumpapillary OCT image around the optic disc from a patient with glaucoma. Corresponding measurements of the RNFL compared to a normative distribution are shown in Figure 2-46B for the thickness profile

along the scan. Figure 2-46C also shows the global, quadrant, and clock hour RNFL thickness measurements compared to a normative distribution. Average global RNFL thickness for this patient is considered outside normal limits, as indicated by the red background, with most damage occurring superiorly, temporally, and inferiorly. A small portion of circumpapillary RNFL thickness remains within normal limits in clock hours 8 and 9. The use of automated algorithms greatly facilitates the interpretation of OCT images.

OCT images through the optic disc are useful for assessing disc and cup parameters and for evaluating glaucoma. Figure 2-47 shows an OCT image of the optic disc for the same patient shown in Figure 2-46. Cupping and global damage to the tissue surrounding the disc is evident in the tomogram and thickness analysis. This analysis may be compared with the normal image and analysis of the optic disc in Figure 2-24. As described previously, automated algorithms can also be applied to OCT images of the ONH in order to perform quantitative measurements of disc parameters.

Figure 2-46. (A) Circumpapillary tomography of glaucomatous patient. (B) RNFL thickness profile compared to a normative distribution. (C) Global, quadrant, and clock hour RNFL thicknesses compared to a normative distribution (obtained with Cirrus HD-OCT).

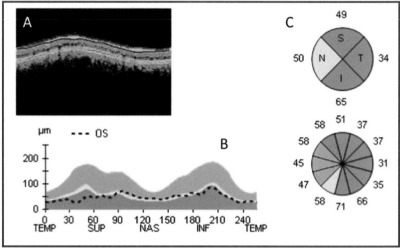

Figure 2-47. ONH analysis of glaucoma patient (obtained with RTVue-100).

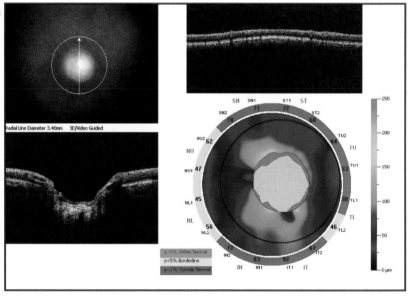

OCT images can also be assessed longitudinally to offer glaucoma progression assessment. Different commercially available SD-OCT systems have their own methods of presenting the RNFL, ONH, and GCC structural changes for a patient over a follow-up period. An eye is defined as progressing when the difference between consequent visits exceeds the inherent measurement error of the device. Other devices define progression when the rate of measurement change exceeds the rate found in the general population. Figure 2-48 shows a glaucoma patient who has been listed as a possible progressor by all 3 methods of progression assessment. This progression analysis was obtained with Cirrus HD-OCT's Guided Progression Analysis software, which uses 2 visits as baseline visits and registers all follow-up visits to these first 2 visits. The Cirrus Guided Progression Analysis determines if the patient is progressing by 3 methods. At the top left of the printout, the RNFL thickness maps are assessed to determine if change has occurred within the cube scan. Here change is reported as a color-coded cluster: yellow to indicate change that would be observed in less than 5% of the normal population and red to indicate thinning that appears in less than 1%. The second method uses the RNFL thickness profiles, where the most recent visit is compared to the baseline visit. Color coding is used once again to indicate if change occurred on the RNFL thickness profile. The third method determines if progression has occurred using average RNFL thickness measured on the 3.4-mm diameter circle and plotting

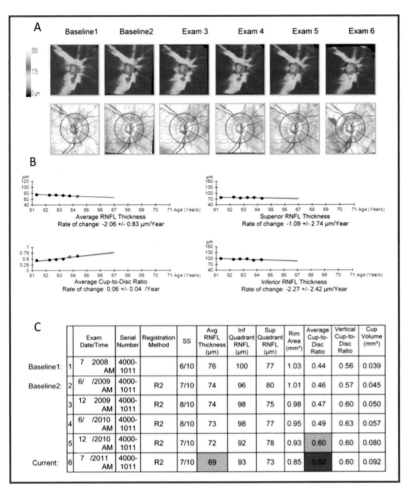

Figure 2-48. Guided Progression Analysis for assessment of glaucomatous RNFL change (obtained with Cirrus HD-OCT).

	Exam Date/Time	Serial Number	Registration Method	SS	Avg RNFL Thickness (µm)	Inf Quadrant RNFL (µm)	Sup Quadrant RNFL (µm)	Rim Area (mm²)	Average Cup-to-Disc Ratio	Vertical Cup-to-Disc Ratio	Cup Volume (mm³)
Baseline1: 1	7 2008 AM	4000-1011		6/10	76	100	77	1.03	0.44	0.56	0.039
Baseline2: 2	6/ /2009 AM	4000-1011	R2	7/10	74	96	80	1.01	0.46	0.57	0.045
3	12 2009 AM	4000-1011	R2	8/10	74	98	75	0.98	0.47	0.60	0.050
4	6/ /2010 AM	4000-1011	R2	8/10	73	98	77	0.95	0.49	0.63	0.057
5	12 /2010 AM	4000-1011	R2	7/10	72	92	78	0.93	0.60	0.60	0.080
Current: 6	7 /2011 AM	4000-1011	R2	7/10	69	93	73	0.85	0.62	0.60	0.092

this measurement with age to determine if a significant rate of change has occurred. Figure 2-48 shows that while the average and inferior RNFL thicknesses remain stable throughout the follow-up, the superior region shows thinning that exceeds the rate in the general population. The results of the 3 progression tests can be seen in the lower right summary panel of the printout. Glaucoma progression cases will be further described in the glaucoma section of this book.

Since OCT can provide detailed images of retinal layers, it can be applied to a wide range of other retinal diseases that are associated with atrophy of the retina. Figure 2-49 shows an example of OCT imaging of the normal retina in the macular region compared to a macular scan obtained from a patient with retinitis pigmentosa. Retinitis pigmentosa is evident as abnormal thinning of the substantial photoreceptor layer outside the fovea and manifests as a reduction in the thickness of the ONL when compared to the normal retina shown in Figure 2-49A. Although many degenerative retinal disorders do not yet have

effective treatments, OCT may prove useful in diagnosis and clinical research because it enables direct visualization and measurement of changes in retinal architecture that would be useful in elucidating disease pathogenesis or assessing future therapies.

The ability of OCT to perform quantitative measurements of retinal morphology, or morphometry, is especially powerful because it provides a means for comparing imaging measurements to the normal population in order to assess the probability of a suspected diagnosis. Morphometry can also provide an objective measurement of disease progression and the efficacy of treatment.

Quality, Artifacts, and Errors in Optical Coherence Tomography Images

In order to realize the full diagnostic potential of OCT imaging and to avoid diagnostic errors, high-

Figure 2-49A. Normal macula (obtained with Cirrus HD-OCT).

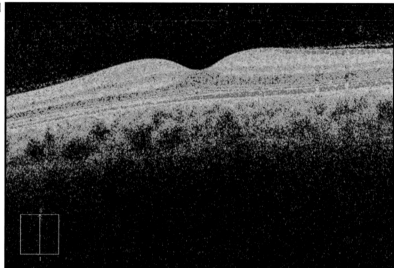

Figure 2-49B. Retinitis pigmentosa (obtained with Cirrus HD-OCT).

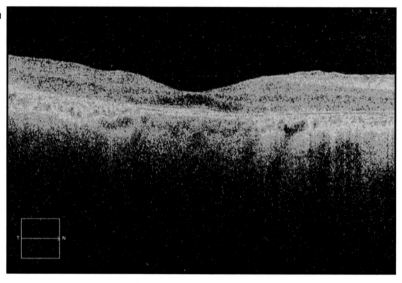

quality OCT images are required. Since optical back-reflection and backscattering from retinal structures are very weak, reduction in the signal level of images can occur as the result of operator error during imaging. Although OCT imaging can be performed in patients with ocular opacities, care is required to ensure that images have sufficient quality. Signal to noise, or the brightness of retinal features when compared to background noise, is an important indicator of OCT image quality. SD-OCT has been shown to have a greater signal to noise when compared to TD-OCT.[86] Each SD-OCT device has its own manufacturer-recommended level of signal quality for an acceptable scan. These prescribed parameter values differ between devices because each uses a different algorithm to measure and evaluate signal qual-

ity. If the appropriate signal quality is not reached, the scan is susceptible to artifacts, segmentation error, and algorithm failure. Figure 2-49A shows an example of a normal OCT image. Figure 2-50 shows an OCT image with a low signal. The image has a washed-out and dim appearance, with loss of signal and reduced dynamic range. Structures such as the low backscattering GCL and the INL and ONL of the retina have a blue-black appearance in false-color images, indicating that their signal level is close to the background noise level. If there is sufficient loss of signal, then even the higher scattering layers such as the RPE, NFL, and plexiform layers can have reduced intensities. Although scattering from cataracts produces a reduction in image intensity, it usually does not degrade image quality, except

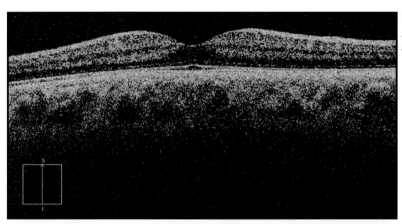

Figure 2-50. Scan with low signal creating a washed-out appearance (obtained with Cirrus HD-OCT).

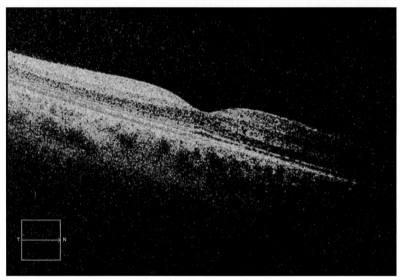

Figure 2-51. Scan with vignetting due to iris (obtained with Cirrus HD-OCT).

in cases of severe opacity. However, care must be taken with these patients, and careful imaging techniques must be used to ensure that images have sufficient signal levels.

Figure 2-51 shows an example of an OCT image that has vignetting. Vignetting occurs when the OCT imaging beam is blocked by the iris during a portion of the beam scan and is characterized by loss of signal over one of the sides of the OCT image. This problem is the result of improper alignment of the OCT imaging beam, which should be centered along the axis of the eye during the imaging procedure. The OCT instrument is designed so that the OCT imaging beam pivots about the pupil when the beam is scanned on the retina. However, the instrument must be positioned at the correct distance from the eye in order for this beam pivot point to coincide with the pupil. Correct registration of the circle scan is also important in circumpapillary scans. For volumetric scans where the circle is sampled from a cube

of data, the circle can be repositioned post-scan to ensure centration of the optic disc. Circumpapillary circle scans, however, must be positioned centrally to the optic disc because horizontal and vertical deviations from correct circle placement can substantially affect RNFL thickness measurements.[87]

Figure 2-52A shows an OCT image with unstable patient fixation. The OCT image exhibits sharp discontinuity of retinal features that are associated with changes in the patient's fixation that occur during the middle of the OCT scan. The SD-OCT en face image (Figure 2-52B) perhaps more clearly shows discontinuities of the blood vessels that can be noted by the operator and the scan repeated, if necessary. The SD-OCT retinal thickness analysis shown overlaying the LSO image (Figure 2-52C) shows errors in the retinal thickness measurements but no discontinuities in the blood vessels on the LSO image because it was acquired once the scan was completed. Special care must be exercised in imaging

Figure 2-52A. Scan with eye movement creating discontinuities in the retinal features (obtained with Cirrus HD-OCT).

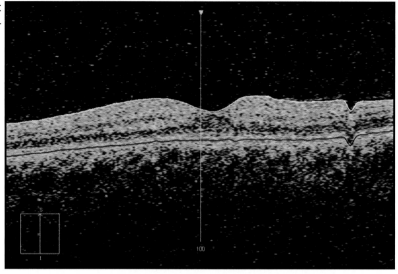

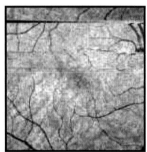

Figure 2-52B. En face image of scan with eye movement creating discontinuities in the retinal features (obtained with Cirrus HD-OCT).

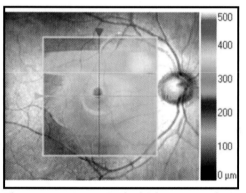

Figure 2-52C. Retinal thickness analysis overlaid on LSO image from scan with eye movement (obtained with Cirrus HD-OCT).

patients with compromised central vision who have difficulty in maintaining fixation or in patients who have reduced compliance. Post-processing and image-registration algorithms, however, are making it possible to match the en face to a fundus image to correct the scan for motion artifacts.[88]

OCT imaging is powerful because a wide range of image-processing algorithms can be used to obtain quantitative information from OCT images. However, care is required to ensure that the initial image data are of sufficient quality before these image-processing and measurement algorithms are applied. Even the most robust methods for image processing will generate incorrect measurements if the initial image is of low quality. Figure 2-53 shows an example of a healthy patient's RNFL measurement error occurring on a circumpapillary OCT

image that has a low signal level. The algorithm fails to detect the correct RNFL boundary for the image and results in an anomalously thin measurement. Mean global RNFL thickness and the superior quadrant RNFL thickness are both reported outside normal limits, with borderline regions inferonasally. Generally, it is more difficult to measure the RNFL than the overall retinal thickness because the RNFL measurement depends upon reliable detection of the posterior boundary of the RNFL, which has lower contrast than the anterior or posterior retinal boundaries. The performance of the algorithms can be checked by a visual inspection of the boundaries to confirm that the software-drawn boundary lines match the boundaries in the OCT image.

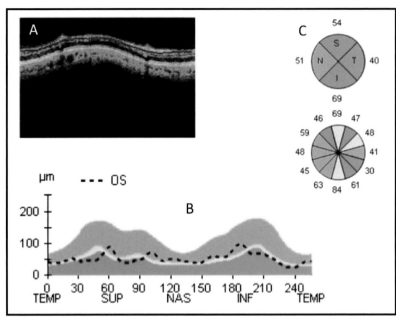

Figure 2-53. RNFL thickness measurement error for a healthy patient. (A) Low signal quality shown in circumpapillary scan. (B) RNFL profile thickness measurement error compared to a normative distribution. (C) RNFL global, quadrant, and clock hour thickness measurement error compared to a normative distribution.

Conclusion

This chapter described the interpretation of normal SD-OCT images, as well as provided the basic principles of interpreting SD-OCT images of retinal pathology. OCT enables cross-sectional as well as volumetric imaging of the retina at unprecedented resolutions, thus enabling the visualization of gross retinal features such as retinal thickness, as well as fine details such as individual retinal layers. The ability to detect abnormalities in retinal architecture can be a powerful and definitive diagnostic tool for many retinal diseases. Automated image-processing techniques enable quantitative measurements of retinal morphology that can be compared with a normative database in order to enhance diagnostic performance. SD-OCT provides a powerful tool to diagnose disease, track disease progression, and monitor the efficacy of treatments. In this context, SD-OCT may be the most powerful and definitive single diagnostic device that can be used in ophthalmology.

References

1. Huang D, Swanson EA, Lin CP, et al. Optical coherence tomography. *Science.* 1991;254(5035):1178-1181.
2. Hee MR, Izatt JA, Swanson EA, et al. Optical coherence tomography of the human retina. *Arch Ophthalmol.* 1995;113(3):325-332.
3. Izatt JA, Hee MR, Swanson EA, et al. Micrometer-scale resolution imaging of the anterior eye in vivo with optical coherence tomography. *Arch Ophthalmol.* 1994;112(12):1584-1589.
4. Puliafito CA, Hee MR, Lin CP, et al. Imaging of macular diseases with optical coherence tomography. *Ophthalmology.* 1995;102(2):217-229.
5. Fujimoto JG, Pitris C, Boppart SA, Brezinski ME. Optical coherence tomography: an emerging technology for biomedical imaging and optical biopsy. *Neoplasia.* 2000; 2(1-2):9-25.
6. Schuman JS. Spectral domain optical coherence tomography for glaucoma (an AOS thesis). *Trans Am Ophthalmol Soc.* 2008;106:426-458.
7. Wojtkowski M, Srinivasan V, Fujimoto JG, et al. Three-dimensional retinal imaging with high-speed ultrahigh-resolution optical coherence tomography. *Ophthalmology.* 2005;112(10):1734-1746.
8. Wojtkowski M, Bajraszewski T, Gorczynska I, et al. Ophthalmic imaging by spectral optical coherence tomography. *Am J Ophthalmol.* 2004;138(3):412-419.
9. Helb HM, Issa PC, Fleckenstein M, et al. Clinical evaluation of simultaneous confocal scanning laser ophthalmoscopy imaging combined with high-resolution, spectral-domain optical coherence tomography. *Acta Ophthalmol.* 2010;88:842-849.
10. Patterson M, Chance B, Wilson B. Time resolved reflectance and transmittance for the non-invasive measurement of tissue optical properties. *Appl Opt.* 1989;28(12):2331-2336.
11. Flock ST, Wilson BC, Patterson MS. Monte Carlo modeling of light propagation in highly scattering tissues—II: comparison with measurements in phantoms. *IEEE Trans Biomed Eng.* 1989;36(12):1169-1173.
12. Flock ST, Patterson MS, Wilson BC, Wyman DR. Monte Carlo modeling of light propagation in highly scattering tissue—I: model predictions and comparison with diffusion theory. *IEEE Trans Biomed Eng.* 1989;36(12):1162-1168.
13. Cheong WF, Prahl SA, Welch AJ. A review of the optical properties of biological tissues. *IEEE J Quantum Electron.* 1990;26(12):2166-2185.
14. Fujimoto JG, Brezinski ME, Tearney GJ, et al. Optical biopsy and imaging using optical coherence tomography. *Nat Med.* 1995;1(9):970-972.

15. Schmitt JM, Knuttel A, Yadlowsky M, Eckhaus MA. Optical-coherence tomography of a dense tissue: statistics of attenuation and backscattering. *Phys Med Biol.* 1994;39(10):1705-1720.

16. Hogan H, Alvarado JA, Weddell JE. *Histology of the Human Eye: An Atlas and Textbook.* Philadelphia, PA: WB Saunders; 1971.

17. Gass JDM. *Stereoscopic Atlas of Macular Diseases: Diagnosis and Treatment.* 3rd ed. Vol 1. St. Louis, MO: CV Mosby; 1987.

18. Krebs W, Krebs I. *Primate Retina and Choroid: Atlas of Fine Structure in Man and Monkey.* New York, NY: Springer Verlag; 1991.

19. Spalton DJ, Hunter PA. *Atlas of Clinical Ophthalmology.* 2nd ed. St. Loius, MO: Mosby; 1994.

20. Toth CA, Narayan DG, Boppart SA, et al. A comparison of retinal morphology viewed by optical coherence tomography and by light microscopy. *Arch Ophthalmol.* 1997;115(11):1425-1428.

21. Huang Y, Cideciyan AV, Papastergiou GI, et al. Relation of optical coherence tomography to microanatomy in normal and rd chickens. *Invest Ophthalmol Vis Sci.* 1998;39(12):2405-2416.

22. Li Q, Timmers AM, Hunter K, et al. Noninvasive imaging by optical coherence tomography to monitor retinal degeneration in the mouse. *Invest Ophthalmol Vis Sci.* 2001;42(12):2981-2989.

23. Drexler W, Morgner U, Kartner FX, et al. In vivo ultra-high-resolution optical coherence tomography. *Opt Lett.* 1999;24(17):1221-1223.

24. Drexler W, Sattmann H, Hermann B, et al. Enhanced visualization of macular pathology with the use of ultrahigh-resolution optical coherence tomography. *Arch Ophthalmol.* 2003;121(5):695-706.

25. Sidman RL. The structure and concentration of solids in photoreceptor cells studied by refractometry and interference microscopy. *J Biophys Biochem Cytol.* 1957;3(1):15-30.

26. Schuman JS, Hee MR, Arya AV, et al. Optical coherence tomography: a new tool for glaucoma diagnosis. *Curr Opin Ophthalmol.* 1995;6(2):89-95.

27. Schuman JS, Hee MR, Puliafito CA, et al. Quantification of nerve fiber layer thickness in normal and glaucomatous eyes using optical coherence tomography. *Arch Ophthalmol.* 1995;113(5):586-596.

28. Schuman JS, Pedut-Kloizman T, Hertzmark E, et al. Reproducibility of nerve fiber layer thickness measurements using optical coherence tomography. *Ophthalmology.* 1996;103(11):1889-1898.

29. Wollstein G, Paunescu LA, Ko TH, et al. Ultrahigh-resolution optical coherence tomography in glaucoma. *Ophthalmology.* 2005;112(2):229-237.

30. Kim JS, Ishikawa H, Gabriele ML, et al. Retinal nerve fiber layer thickness measurement comparability between time domain optical coherence tomography (OCT) and spectral domain OCT. *Invest Ophthalmol Vis Sci.* 2010;51(2):896-902.

31. Radhakrishnan S, Rollins AM, Roth JE, et al. Real-time optical coherence tomography of the anterior segment at 1310 nm. *Arch Ophthalmol.* 2001;119(8):1179-1185.

32. Sarunic MV, Asrani S, Izatt JA. Imaging the ocular anterior segment with real-time, full-range Fourier-domain optical coherence tomography. *Arch Ophthalmol.* 2008;126(4):537-542.

33. Brezinski ME, Tearney GJ, Bouma BE, et al. Optical coherence tomography for optical biopsy. Properties and demonstration of vascular pathology. *Circulation.* 1996;93(6):1206-1213.

34. Hee MR, Puliafito CA, Duker JS, et al. Topography of diabetic macular edema with optical coherence tomography. *Ophthalmology.* 1998;105(2):360-370.

35. Mujat M, Chan R, Cense B, et al. Retinal nerve fiber layer thickness map determined from optical coherence tomography images. *Opt Express.* 2005;13(23):9480-9491.

36. Srinivasan VJ, Wojtkowski M, Witkin AJ, et al. High-definition and 3-dimensional imaging of macular pathologies with high-speed ultrahigh-resolution optical coherence tomography. *Ophthalmology.* 2006;113(11):2054.e1-14.

37. Ishikawa H, Kim J, Friberg TR, et al. Three-dimensional optical coherence tomography (3D-OCT) image enhancement with segmentation-free contour modeling C-mode. *Invest Ophthalmol Vis Sci.* 2009;50(3):1344-1349.

38. Sung KR, Kim DY, Park SB, Kook MS. Comparison of retinal nerve fiber layer thickness measured by Cirrus HD and Stratus optical coherence tomography. *Ophthalmology.* 2009;116(7):1264-1270, 70.e1.

39. Chang RT, Knight OJ, Feuer WJ, Budenz DL. Sensitivity and specificity of time-domain versus spectral-domain optical coherence tomography in diagnosing early to moderate glaucoma. *Ophthalmology.* 2009;116(12):2294-2299.

40. Leung CK, Cheung CY, Weinreb RN, et al. Retinal nerve fiber layer imaging with spectral-domain optical coherence tomography: a variability and diagnostic performance study. *Ophthalmology.* 2009;116(7):1257-1263, 63.e1-2.

41. Blumenthal EZ, Williams JM, Weinreb RN, Girkin CA, Berry CC, Zangwill LM. Reproducibility of nerve fiber layer thickness measurements by use of optical coherence tomography. *Ophthalmology.* 2000;107(12):2278-2282.

42. Bowd C, Weinreb RN, Williams JM, Zangwill LM. The retinal nerve fiber layer thickness in ocular hypertensive, normal, and glaucomatous eyes with optical coherence tomography. *Arch Ophthalmol.* 2000;118(1):22-26.

43. Zangwill LM, Williams J, Berry CC, Knauer S, Weinreb RN. A comparison of optical coherence tomography and retinal nerve fiber layer photography for detection of nerve fiber layer damage in glaucoma. *Ophthalmology.* 2000;107(7):1309-1315.

44. Zangwill LM, Bowd C, Berry CC, et al. Discriminating between normal and glaucomatous eyes using the Heidelberg Retina Tomograph, GDx Nerve Fiber Analyzer, and Optical Coherence Tomograph. *Arch Ophthalmol.* 2001;119(7):985-993.

45. Bowd C, Zangwill LM, Berry CC, et al. Detecting early glaucoma by assessment of retinal nerve fiber layer thickness and visual function. *Invest Ophthalmol Vis Sci.* 2001;42(9):1993-2003.

46. Bowd C, Zangwill LM, Blumenthal EZ, et al. Imaging of the optic disc and retinal nerve fiber layer: the effects of age, optic disc area, refractive error, and gender. *J Opt Soc Am A Opt Image Sci Vis.* 2002;19(1):197-207.

47. Williams ZY, Schuman JS, Gamell L, et al. Optical coherence tomography measurement of nerve fiber layer thickness and the likelihood of a visual field defect. *Am J Ophthalmol.* 2002;134(4):538-546.

48. Aydin A, Wollstein G, Price LL, Fujimoto JG, Schuman JS. Optical coherence tomography assessment of retinal nerve fiber layer thickness changes after glaucoma surgery. *Ophthalmology.* 2003;110(8):1506-1511.

49. Guedes V, Schuman JS, Hertzmark E, et al. Optical coherence tomography measurement of macular and nerve fiber layer thickness in normal and glaucomatous human eyes. *Ophthalmology.* 2003;110(1):177-189.

50. Gonzalez-Garcia AO, Vizzeri G, Bowd C, Medeiros FA, Zangwill LM, Weinreb RN. Reproducibility of RTVue retinal nerve fiber layer thickness and optic disc measurements and agreement with Stratus optical coherence tomography measurements. *Am J Ophthalmol.* 2009;147(6):1067-74, 74.e1.

51. Ishikawa H, Stein DM, Wollstein G, Beaton S, Fujimoto JG, Schuman JS. Macular segmentation with optical coherence tomography. *Invest Ophthalmol Vis Sci.* 2005;46(6):2012-2017.

52. Tan O, Li G, Lu AT, Varma R, Huang D. Mapping of macular substructures with optical coherence tomography for glaucoma diagnosis. *Ophthalmology*. 2008;115(6):949-956.

53. Tan O, Chopra V, Lu AT, et al. Detection of macular ganglion cell loss in glaucoma by Fourier-domain optical coherence tomography. *Ophthalmology*. 2009;116(12):2305-2314.e1-2.

54. Chen TC. Spectral domain optical coherence tomography in glaucoma: qualitative and quantitative analysis of the optic nerve head and retinal nerve fiber layer (an AOS thesis). *Trans Am Ophthalmol Soc*. 2009;107:254-281.

55. Nassif N, Cense B, Park B, et al. In vivo high-resolution video-rate spectral-domain optical coherence tomography of the human retina and optic nerve. *Opt Express*. 2004;12(3):367-376.

56. Schuman JS, Wollstein G, Farra T, et al. Comparison of optic nerve head measurements obtained by optical coherence tomography and confocal scanning laser ophthalmoscopy. *Am J Ophthalmol*. 2003;135(4):504-512.

57. Hee MR, Puliafito CA, Wong C, et al. Optical coherence tomography of macular holes. *Ophthalmology*. 1995;102(5):748-756.

58. Gaudric A, Haouchine B, Massin P, Paques M, Blain P, Erginay A. Macular hole formation: new data provided by optical coherence tomography. *Arch Ophthalmol*. 1999;117(6):744-751.

59. Takahashi H, Kishi S. Optical coherence tomography images of spontaneous macular hole closure. *Am J Ophthalmol*. 1999;128(4):519-520.

60. Takahashi H, Kishi S. Tomographic features of a lamellar macular hole formation and a lamellar hole that progressed to a full-thickness macular hole. *Am J Ophthalmol*. 2000;130(5):677-679.

61. Takahashi H, Kishi S. Tomographic features of early macular hole closure after vitreous surgery. *Am J Ophthalmol*. 2000;130(2):192-196.

62. Massin P, Vicaut E, Haouchine B, Erginay A, Paques M, Gaudric A. Reproducibility of retinal mapping using optical coherence tomography. *Arch Ophthalmol*. 2001;119(8):1135-1142.

63. Polito A, Shah SM, Haller JA, et al. Comparison between retinal thickness analyzer and optical coherence tomography for assessment of foveal thickness in eyes with macular disease. *Am J Ophthalmol*. 2002;134(2):240-251.

64. Strom C, Sander B, Larsen N, Larsen M, Lund-Andersen H. Diabetic macular edema assessed with optical coherence tomography and stereo fundus photography. *Invest Ophthalmol Vis Sci*. 2002;43(1):241-245.

65. Schmidt-Erfurth U, Leitgeb RA, Michels S, et al. Three-dimensional ultrahigh-resolution optical coherence tomography of macular diseases. *Invest Ophthalmol Vis Sci*. 2005;46(9):3393-3402.

66. Imai M, Iijima H, Gotoh T, Tsukahara S. Optical coherence tomography of successfully repaired idiopathic macular holes. *Am J Ophthalmol*. 1999;128(5):621-627.

67. Mikajiri K, Okada AA, Ohji M, et al. Analysis of vitrectomy for idiopathic macular hole by optical coherence tomography. *Am J Ophthalmol*. 1999;128(5):655-657.

68. Ip MS, Baker BJ, Duker JS, et al. Anatomical outcomes of surgery for idiopathic macular hole as determined by optical coherence tomography. *Arch Ophthalmol*. 2002;120(1):29-35.

69. Wilkins JR, Puliafito CA, Hee MR, et al. Characterization of epiretinal membranes using optical coherence tomography. *Ophthalmology*. 1996;103(12):2142-2151.

70. Munuera JM, Garcia-Layana A, Maldonado MJ, Aliseda D, Moreno-Montanes J. Optical coherence tomography in successful surgery of vitreomacular traction syndrome. *Arch Ophthalmol*. 1998;116(10):1388-1389.

71. Azzolini C, Patelli F, Codenotti M, Pierro L, Brancato R. Optical coherence tomography in idiopathic epiretinal macular membrane surgery. *Eur J Ophthalmol*. 1999;9(3):206-211.

72. Gallemore RP, Jumper JM, McCuen BW 2nd, Jaffe GJ, Postel EA, Toth CA. Diagnosis of vitreoretinal adhesions in macular disease with optical coherence tomography. *Retina*. 2000;20(2):115-120.

73. Koizumi H, Spaide RF, Fisher YL, Freund KB, Klancnik JM Jr, Yannuzzi LA. Three-dimensional evaluation of vitreomacular traction and epiretinal membrane using spectral-domain optical coherence tomography. *Am J Ophthalmol*. 2008;145(3):509-517.

74. Massin P, Allouch C, Haouchine B, et al. Optical coherence tomography of idiopathic macular epiretinal membranes before and after surgery. *Am J Ophthalmol*. 2000;130(6):732-739.

75. Hee MR, Puliafito CA, Wong C, et al. Optical coherence tomography of central serous chorioretinopathy. *Am J Ophthalmol*. 1995;120(1):65-74.

76. Giovannini A, Amato G, Mariotti C, Scassellati-Sforzolini B. Optical coherence tomography in the assessment of retinal pigment epithelial tear. *Retina*. 2000;20(1):37-40.

77. Azzolini C, Pierro L, Codenotti M, Brancato R. OCT images and surgery of juvenile macular retinoschisis. *Eur J Ophthalmol*. 1997;7(2):196-200.

78. Ip M, Garza-Karren C, Duker JS, et al. Differentiation of degenerative retinoschisis from retinal detachment using optical coherence tomography. *Ophthalmology*. 1999;106(3):600-605.

79. Takano M, Kishi S. Foveal retinoschisis and retinal detachment in severely myopic eyes with posterior staphyloma. *Am J Ophthalmol*. 1999;128(4):472-476.

80. Hee MR, Puliafito CA, Wong C, et al. Quantitative assessment of macular edema with optical coherence tomography. *Arch Ophthalmol*. 1995;113(8):1019-1029.

81. Witkin AJ, Ko TH, Fujimoto JG, et al. Ultra-high resolution optical coherence tomography assessment of photoreceptors in retinitis pigmentosa and related diseases. *Am J Ophthalmol*. 2006;142(6):945-952.

82. Otani T, Kishi S, Maruyama Y. Patterns of diabetic macular edema with optical coherence tomography. *Am J Ophthalmol*. 1999;127(6):688-693.

83. Rivellese M, George A, Sulkes D, Reichel E, Puliafito C. Optical coherence tomography after laser photocoagulation for clinically significant macular edema. *Ophthalmic Surg Lasers*. 2000;31(3):192-197.

84. Hee MR, Baumal CR, Puliafito CA, et al. Optical coherence tomography of age-related macular degeneration and choroidal neovascularization. *Ophthalmology*. 1996;103(8):1260-1270.

85. Giovannini A, Amato GP, Mariotti C, Scassellati-Sforzolini B. OCT imaging of choroidal neovascularisation and its role in the determination of patients' eligibility for surgery. *Br J Ophthalmol*. 1999;83(4):438-442.

86. De Boer JF, Cense B, Park BH, Pierce MC, Tearney GJ, Bouma BE. Improved signal-to-noise ratio in spectral-domain compared with time-domain optical coherence tomography. *Opt Lett*. 2003;28(21):2067-2069.

87. Gabriele ML, Ishikawa H, Wollstein G, et al. Optical coherence tomography scan circle location and mean retinal nerve fiber layer measurement variability. *Invest Ophthalmol Vis Sci*. 2008;49(6):2315-2321.

88. Ricco S, Chen M, Ishikawa H, et al. *Correcting motion artifacts in retinal spectral domain optical coherence tomography via image registration*. Proceedings of the 12th International Conference on Medical Image Computing and Computer-Assisted Intervention. Berlin, Germany: Springer Verlag; 2009.

Section II

Optical Coherence Tomography in Retinal Diseases

Chapter 3

Vitreoretinal Interface Disorders

Heeral R. Shah, MD; Elias C. Mavrofrides, MD;

Adam H. Rogers, MD; Steven N. Truong, MD, FACS;

Carmen A. Puliafito, MD, MBA; James G. Fujimoto, PhD; and Jay S. Duker, MD

- Idiopathic Epiretinal Membrane
- Vitreomacular Traction Syndrome
- Idiopathic Macular Hole

Abnormalities of the vitreoretinal interface are involved in the pathogenesis of several macular conditions. In idiopathic epiretinal membrane (ERM) formation, a layer of abnormal tissue develops on the surface of the retina usually following posterior vitreous detachment. Contraction of this membrane can result in retinal distortion and/or vascular leakage with associated vision loss. In other conditions, such as vitreomacular traction syndrome or idiopathic macular hole, there are abnormal attachments between the vitreous and retina. The resulting traction exerted on the retina causes alterations in retinal anatomy and subsequent loss of vision.

Optical coherence tomography (OCT) has become a powerful tool in the evaluation of these conditions. The vitreoretinal changes that characterize these conditions are often subtle and difficult to distinguish on biomicroscopic examination. By providing a high-resolution cross-sectional image of the retina and vitreoretinal interface, OCT can provide valuable information not visible on biomicroscopy. In addition, OCT can provide a more objective means to monitor the natural history and therapeutic response of these conditions.

Idiopathic Epiretinal Membrane

Idiopathic ERMs occur in approximately 6% of patients over the age of 60 with the incidence increasing with age.[1] Symptoms vary from minimal to severe depending on the location, density, and contraction of the membrane. On slit-lamp biomicroscopy, a mild ERM appears as a glistening layer on the retinal surface. Denser membranes may be seen as a gray sheet overlying the retina. Contraction of these membranes can result in retinal distortion, often affecting the course of adjacent retinal vessels. Traction on the vessels may also cause increased permeability and associated retinal edema. Fluorescein angiography highlights the retinal vascular distortion and leakage.

OCT has become a useful diagnostic technique in evaluating ERMs. ERMs are visible on the OCT image as a highly reflective layer on the inner retinal surface. In most patients, the membrane is globally adherent to the retina. In approximately 25% of patients, the membrane is separated from the inner retina, enhancing visibility.[2] In this situation, the ERM must be distinguished from a detached posterior hyaloid face, which can also appear as a reflective band above the retinal surface. The posterior hyaloid usually has a thin, patchy reflection compared to the denser reflection of an ERM. Additionally, the degree of separation from the inner retina is usually greater for the posterior hyaloid.

Schuman JS, Puliafito CA, Fujimoto JG, Duker JS, eds.
Optical Coherence Tomography of Ocular Diseases,
Third Edition (pp 69-110).
© 2013 SLACK Incorporated.

By providing qualitative and quantitative information about retinal anatomy, OCT can identify factors contributing to vision loss in patients with ERMs. Quantitative measurements of membrane thickness and reflectivity can be used to establish the degree of membrane opacity. Loss of the normal foveal contour is an early sign of retinal distortion from mild membrane formation. More advanced membranes can result in variable retinal thickening that can be quantified on the OCT image. Studies have shown that OCT measurements of retinal thickness correlate with visual acuity in patients with ERMs.[3,4]

ERMs also frequently cause retinal distortion that creates a pseudohole appearance. OCT can effectively distinguish macular pseudohole from lesions that may appear similar on clinical exam. ERM with macular pseudohole displays a steep foveal pit contour with thickening of the macular edges on the OCT image. Although this may simulate a full-thickness hole, the presence of retinal tissue at the base of the pit establishes this as a pseudohole.

Many studies have attempted to establish prognostic indicators of operative success after ERM surgery.[2,4-7] Potential indicators include preoperative vision, duration of symptoms, membrane location, membrane thickness, pseudohole formation, retinal thickness, and cystoid macular edema (CME). Studies have been able to establish some predictive significance of preoperative vision and duration of symptoms. Since studies investigating the other characteristics have relied on subjective assessments, the results are controversial. Quantitative measurement with OCT may provide a new means for investigating the significance of these factors.

Preoperative OCT imaging can also help direct the operative approach. In cases with separation between the membrane and retina, the surgeon may be directed to these areas to initiate membrane peeling. When the membrane is globally attached to the inner retina, the surgeon may anticipate more difficulty peeling the membrane. The surgeon may also proceed with particular caution when extensive intraretinal edema leaves a thin, friable inner retinal layer beneath the membrane.

Postoperative OCT imaging can be used to document surgical response. The completeness of ERM removal can often be assessed by comparing pre- and postoperative images. Recent studies have used OCT measurements to monitor changes in retinal thickness after surgery. These studies have shown that retinal thickness decreases following successful ERM peeling.[3,4] Azzolini and others have shown a correlation between this decrease in retinal thickness and improved visual acuity after surgery.[3]

Vitreomacular Traction Syndrome

Vitreomacular traction syndrome refers to conditions in which retinal changes develop from incomplete posterior vitreous detachment with persistent vitreous adhesion to the macula. A broad area of vitreous attachment around the optic nerve and macula is often seen ophthalmoscopically. In rare cases, thin vitreous strands attaching to the fovea may be identified.[8] Traction on the retina frequently causes retinal distortion and subsequent CME. These changes result in central vision loss and metamorphopsia.

Although the vitreous attachment to the macula usually appears broad on clinical exam, OCT typically shows a perifoveal vitreous detachment with focal adhesion to the fovea. This configuration appears identical to the vitreous attachment identified in idiopathic macular hole. Why some patients with this progress toward CME (vitreomacular traction syndrome) while others develop macular holes remains unclear. Variations in the location, density, and diameter of the vitreoretinal adhesion may explain these differences. Qualitative and quantitative studies using OCT imaging may clarify this issue in the future.

As with other vitreoretinal interface abnormalities, OCT is extremely useful in monitoring the progression of patients with vitreomacular traction syndrome. Spontaneous resolution of vitreoretinal traction with normalization of the retinal contour has been documented with OCT.[9,10] On the other hand, persistent traction can lead to progressive retinal edema and thickening. Quantifying such changes with OCT can be valuable in determining the need and/or timing of surgical intervention. After surgery, OCT can be used to evaluate the anatomic response. Cases in the literature have documented improved retinal anatomy in association with increased visual acuity following vitrectomy surgery.[11,12]

Idiopathic Macular Hole

Idiopathic macular holes typically occur in the sixth to seventh decade of life with a 2:1 female preponderance. Symptoms include decreased visual acuity, metamorphopsia, and central scotoma. Bilateral involvement occurs in 15% to 20% of patients.

Lesions that can ophthalmoscopically resemble various stages of macular hole development are relatively common.[13] These lesions include ERM with pseudohole, lamellar hole, macular cysts, and foveal detachment. OCT imaging can effectively distinguish between these conditions. Full-thickness macular holes show complete loss of retinal tissue in the fovea extending to the retinal pigment epithelium (RPE) layer. In contrast, ERM with pseudohole shows a steepened foveal pit contour with persistent retinal tissue at the base of the pit. Lamellar holes show partial-thickness loss or separation of retinal tissue with a thin layer of persistent outer retina above the RPE. Macular cysts are identified by clear, signal-free areas that are within the retina. A similar clear space under the fovea characterizes a foveal detachment.

Gass has most completely described the stages of macular hole formation based on biomicroscopic findings.[14] In describing these stages, he emphasized the role of vitreomacular traction in macular hole development. A Stage 1 impending hole is characterized by a foveal detachment that is seen as a yellow spot or ring in the fovea. Approximately half of the impending holes will resolve spontaneously at the time of posterior vitreous detachment, while half will progress to more advanced stages. Stage 2 macular holes have a full-thickness dehiscence of the retina that measures less than 400 μm. A small dehiscence may not be visible biomicroscopically. Stage 3 holes develop with further enlargement of the hole to greater than 400 μm. Stage 4 holes are characterized by complete posterior vitreous detachment regardless of hole size.

OCT has enhanced our understanding of the pathogenesis of macular holes. OCT imaging of the vitreoretinal interface has confirmed the role of vitreomacular traction in macular hole development. Hee and associates were the first to identify a perifoveal vitreous detachment with persistent vitreous traction on the fovea in the fellow eye of patients with unilateral macular hole.[13] Although this configuration was clearly identified on OCT, these changes could not be seen biomicroscopically.

Several subsequent studies looking at fellow eyes have confirmed the importance of this configuration in hole development.[15-19] Some patients maintain a normal visual acuity and foveal contour despite this abnormal foveal attachment. In other patients, progressive traction results in retinal distortion and Stage 1 impending hole formation. Spaide et al have shown that the diameter of vitreous attachment measured on OCT may correlate with the changes induced in foveal anatomy.[20] In this study, narrow attachments were more likely to induce foveal changes than broader attachments. As a result, OCT may become important in identifying patients at increased risk for hole formation.

The anatomic changes identified on OCT have also been correlated with the various stages of macular hole formation. Some patients with persistent foveal traction have developed foveal detachment consistent with a Stage 1 impending hole as described by Gass.[14] Several studies have subsequently shown the development of a pseudocyst as the initial stage of macular hole formation.[15,17,18] This appears as a minimally reflective cavity within the fovea beneath the area of persistent vitreal attachment. Spontaneous resolution of these changes has been documented on OCT with complete detachment of the vitreous. Enlargement of this pseudocyst with loss of the outer retinal layers and dehiscence of the inner retinal layers characterizes progression to a Stage 2 hole. An operculum with vitreous attachment may remain connected to one edge of the hole. Stage 3 holes show further enlargement of the full-thickness defect with variable amounts of subretinal and intraretinal edema at the edges of the hole. An operculum may still be visualized but is now completely separated and suspended above the hole. Because the vitreous has completely detached from the optic nerve and macula, Stage 4 macular holes show large full-thickness defects in the retina without visualization of the posterior hyaloid.

Vitrectomy surgery has become an effective treatment in achieving anatomic closure and improved visual acuity in patients with full-thickness macular holes. One of the quickly expanding roles for OCT is in the perioperative assessment of macular hole patients. Postoperative anatomic changes can be documented with OCT. The fovea can demonstrate 1 of 4 distinct patterns after macular hole surgery: open, closed, thin, and foveolar detachment.[21] Closed holes have reapproximation of the hole edges with a relatively normal foveal contour and thickness. Thin cases will have closure of the hole but a central foveal thickness of less than 100 μm. In foveolar detachment, the reapproximated edges of the hole remain detached from the underlying RPE. Over time, the subretinal fluid may be resorbed with resolution of the detachment. These anatomic changes on OCT often correlate with visual improvement, providing useful information about the patient's response to surgery. A recent study demonstrated that vitrectomy surgery with membrane peel can significantly improve visual acuity and central foveal thickness in patients with vitreomacular traction syndrome. Furthermore, eyes with lamellar holes had worse visual results, while those with CME or perifoveal vitreomacular traction syndrome had better visual outcomes.

Quantitative information about the macular hole can also be obtained from the OCT tomogram. Measurements of minimum hole diameter, base diameter, and retinal edge thickness may be useful in predicting surgical success. Ip and associates were the first to show that preoperative minimum hole diameter determined by OCT has prognostic significance for postoperative success.[22] Macular holes less than 400 μm on OCT had a significantly higher rate of anatomic closure compared to larger holes. There was also a trend for greater visual improvement in patients with smaller holes. Ullrich has subsequently shown that both preoperative minimum hole diameter and base diameter are prognostic factors for visual outcome and anatomic success.[23] The preoperative base diameter, which can only be measured by OCT, showed the strongest correlation with these outcomes.[24]

References

1. Pearstone AD. The incidence of idiopathic preretinal macular gliosis. *Ann Ophthalmol.* 1985;17:378.
2. Wilkins JR, Puliafito CA, Hee MR, et al. Characterization of epiretinal membranes using optical coherence tomography. *Ophthalmology.* 1996;103:2142-2151.
3. Azzolini C, Patelli F, Codenotti M, Pierro L, Brancato R. Optical coherence tomography in idiopathic epiretinal membrane surgery. *Eur J Ophthalmol.* 1999;9:206-211.
4. Massin P, Allouch C, Haouchine B, et al. Optical coherence tomography of idiopathic epiretinal membrane before and after surgery. *Am J Ophthalmol.* 2000;130:732-739.
5. Trese MT, Chandler DB, Machemer R. Macular pucker I. Prognostic criteria. *Graefes Arch Clin Exp Ophthalmol.* 1983;221:12-15.
6. Rice TA, De Bustros S, Michels RG, et al. Prognostic factors in vitrectomy for epiretinal membranes of the macula. *Ophthalmology.* 1986;93:602-610.
7. Pesin SR, Olk RJ, Grand MG, et al. Vitrectomy for premacular fibroplasias. Prognostic factors, long-term follow-up, and time course of visual improvement. *Ophthalmology.* 1991;98:1109-1114.
8. Smiddy WE, Michels RG, Glaser BM, De Bustros S. Vitrectomy for macular traction caused by incomplete vitreous separation. *Arch Ophthalmol.* 1988;106:624-628.
9. Sulkes DJ, Ip MS, Baumal CR, Wu HK, Puliafito CA. Spontaneous resolution of vitreomacular traction documented by optical coherence tomography. *Arch Ophthalmol.* 2000;118:286-287.
10. Kusaka S, Saito Y, Okada AA, et al. Optical coherence tomography in spontaneously resolving vitreomacular traction syndrome. *Ophthalmologica.* 2001;215:139-141.
11. Munuera JM, Garcia-Layana A, Maldonado MJ, et al. Optical coherence tomography of successful surgery of vitreomacular traction syndrome. *Arch Ophthalmol.* 1998;116:1388-1389.
12. Uchino E, Uemura A, Doi N, Ohba N. Postsurgical evaluation of idiopathic vitreomacular traction syndrome by optical coherence tomography. *Am J Ophthalmol.* 2001;132:122-123.
13. Hee MR, Puliafito CA, Wong C, et al. Optical coherence tomography of macular holes. *Ophthalmology.* 1995;102:748-756.
14. Gass JDM. Reappraisal of biomicroscopic classification of stages of development of macular hole. *Arch Ophthalmol.* 1995;119:752-759.
15. Gaudric A, Haouchine B, Massin P, Paques M, Blain P, Erginay A. Macular hole formation. *Arch Ophthalmol.* 1999;117:744-751.
16. Spiritus A, Dralands L, Stalmans I, Spileers W. OCT studies of fellow eyes of macular holes. *Bull Soc Belge Ophthalmol.* 2000;275:81-84.
17. Azzolini C, Patelli F, Brancato R. Correlation between optical coherence tomography data and biomicroscopic interpretation of idiopathic macular hole. *Am J Ophthalmol.* 2001;132:348-355.
18. Haouchine B, Massin P, Gaudric A. Foveal pseudocyst as the first step in macular hole formation. *Ophthalmology.* 2001;108:15-22.
19. Tanner V, Chauhan S, Jackson TL, Williamson TH. Optical coherence tomography of the vitreoretinal interface in macular hole formation. *Br J Ophthalmol.* 2001;85:1092-1097.
20. Spaide RF, Wong D, Fisher Y, Goldbaum M. Correlation of vitreous attachment and foveal deformation in early macular hole states. *Am J Ophthalmol.* 2002;133:226-229.
21. Desai VN, Hee MR, Puliafito CA. Optical coherence tomography of macular holes. In: Madreperla SA, McCuen BW, eds. *Macular Hole.* Boston, MA: Butterworth-Heinemann; 1999:37-47.
22. Ip MS, Baker BJ, Duker JS, et al. Anatomical outcomes of surgery for idiopathic macular hole as determined by optical coherence tomography. *Arch Ophthalmol.* 2002;120:29-35.
23. Ullrich S, Haritoglou C, Gass C, Schaumberger M, Ulbig MW, Kampik A. Macular hole size as a prognostic factor in macular hole surgery. *Br J Ophthalmol.* 2002;86:390-393.
24. Witkin AJ, Patron ME, Castro LC, Reichel E, Rogers AH, Baumal CR, Duker JS. Anatomic and visual outcomes of vitrectoy for vitreomacular traction syndrome. *Ophthalmic Surg Lasers Imaging.* 2010;41(4):425-431.

Index to Cases

Case 3-1. Idiopathic Epiretinal Membrane

Clinical Summary

A 60-year-old female presents with complaints of distortion in each eye for 1 year. Visual acuity measures 20/40 in the right eye and 20/50 in the left eye. Dilated fundus examination of the right eye shows an ERM in the central macula with retinal striae (A). Fundus examination of the left eye shows a slightly more prominent ERM in the central macula with striae and macular thickening (B).

Optical Coherence Tomography

Horizontal OCT scan (C) through the right eye shows a hyperreflective linear structure at the retinal surface, consistent with an ERM with macular thickening. The membrane is absent nasal to the fovea. Central foveal thickness measures 398 μm (D). The ILM-RPE map (E) demonstrates the area of thickening, with striae present at the edges. Horizontal OCT scan (F) through the left eye shows a prominent hyperreflective ERM. Hyporeflective spaces at the retinal surface beneath the membrane suggest an increase in traction, resulting in retinal striae. Central foveal thickness is 390 μm (G). The ILM-RPE map (H) similarly illustrates the region of thickening and focal areas of traction.

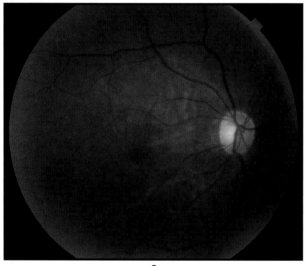

A

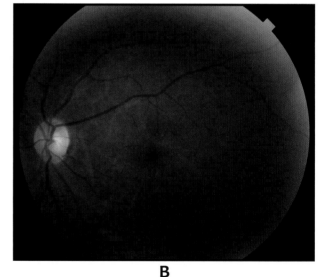

B

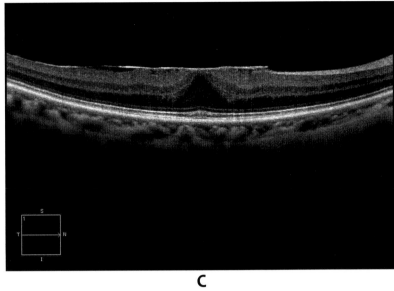

C

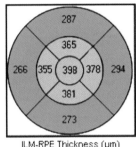

ILM-RPE Thickness (µm)

D

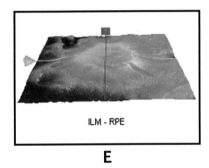

ILM - RPE

E

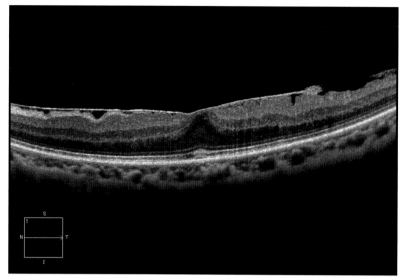

F

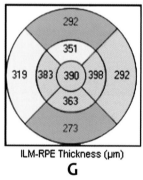

ILM-RPE Thickness (µm)

G

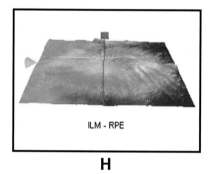

ILM - RPE

H

Case 3-2. Dense Epiretinal Membrane With Extensive Macular Edema

Clinical Summary

A 60-year-old male complains of worsening vision in the right eye over the past year. He has not noticed any improvement after cataract extraction 2 months ago. His visual acuity in this eye is 20/100. On dilated fundus examination (A), there is evidence of a dense ERM that has resulted in retinal distortion and pseudohole formation. There is extensive intraretinal edema in the area of this membrane. Fluorescein angiography (B) shows a large area of hyperfluorescent leakage extending from the fovea to the superior temporal arcade.

Optical Coherence Tomography

The OCT scan (C) is offset slightly to include more of the superior macula. This scan shows persistent attachment of the vitreous to the fovea. The detached portions of the posterior vitreous appear as discrete bands above the surface of the retina. At the fovea, there is a relatively broad attachment of the vitreous to the inner retinal layers. The ERM is best identified superior to the fovea, where there is a small amount of separation between the highly reflective membrane and the inner retinal surface. There is extensive fluid accumulation within the retina with the development of large intraretinal cysts. The retinal thickness is greatly increased throughout the macular region with the fovea measuring 731 µm.

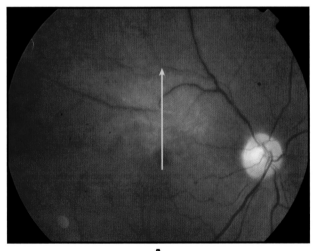

A

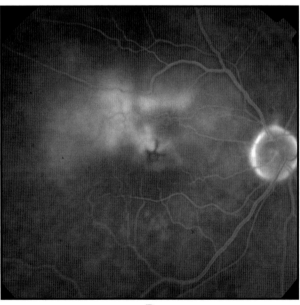

B

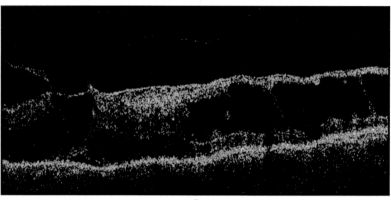

C

Case 3-3A. Vitreomacular Traction

Clinical Summary

An 85-year-old female presents with a mild decline in vision in the left eye and distortion. Her visual acuity measures 20/100. Dilated fundus examination reveals a small, yellow foveal cyst and ERM temporal to the fovea (A, B).

Optical Coherence Tomography

A horizontal OCT scan (C) demonstrates 2 hyper-reflective linear densities—one on the surface of the retina temporal to the fovea and the second in the vitreous inserting into the foveal region. This may represent delaminated posterior hyaloid face, with the partially detached component exerting traction at the fovea. A faint linear density is also visible nasal to the fovea in the vitreous, also inserting at the retina. Loss of foveal contour with thickening of the retina is evident, along with an intraretinal cyst. Another cut demonstrates displacement of intraretinal tissue (D). Central foveal thickness is 442 µm (E). The ILM-RPE map (F) and ILM map (G) reveal the retinal and ILM contour, respectively.

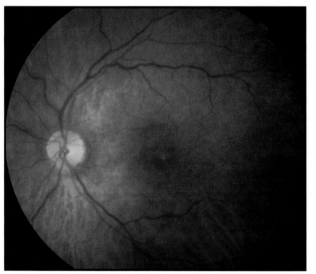

A

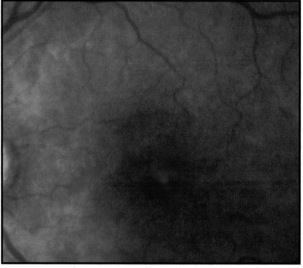

B

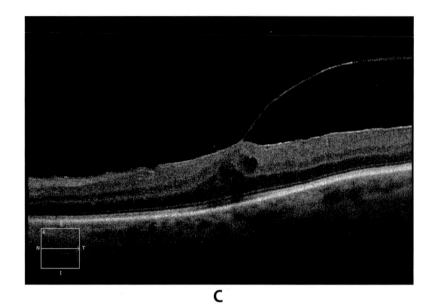

C

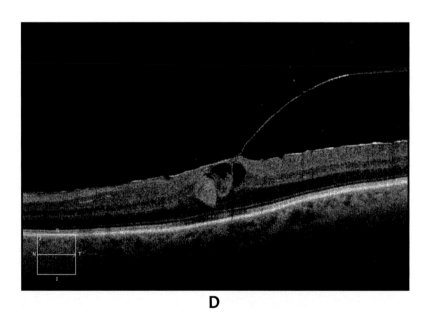

D

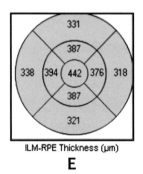

ILM-RPE Thickness (μm)

E

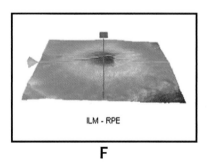

ILM - RPE

F

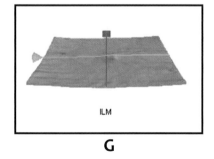

ILM

G

Case 3-3B. Vitreomacular Traction

Clinical Summary

A 69-year-old female presents complaining of several years of distortion in the right eye. Visual acuity measures 20/100. Dilated fundus exam reveals a dense ERM with macular edema and 300-µm foveal cyst (A).

Optical Coherence Tomography

A horizontal OCT scan (B) reveals a hyperreflective linear density originating from the vitreous cavity, inserting at a focal point on the retina, and running along the surface of the retina. This suggests a taut posterior hyaloid face with significant focal traction temporal to the fovea, leading to an irregular retinal surface. Hyporeflective spaces are present within the inner and outer retinal layers, suggestive of macular edema. The ILM map (C) better demonstrates the extent of traction present. Central foveal thickness is 1044 µm (D). The ILM-RPE overlay demonstrates the contour (E).

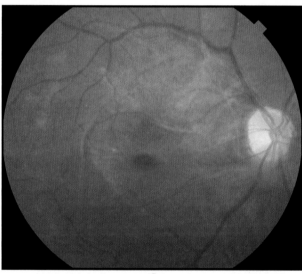

A

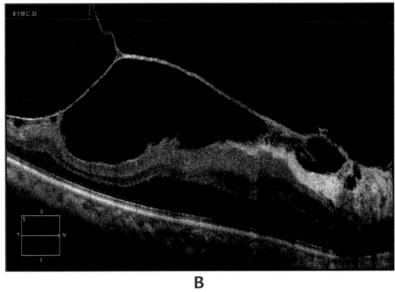

B

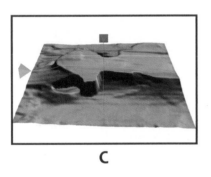

C

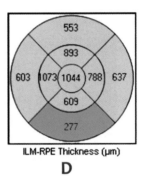

ILM-RPE Thickness (µm)

D

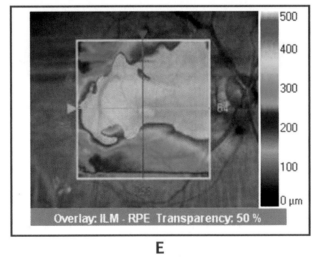

Overlay: ILM - RPE Transparency: 50 %

E

Case 3-4. Vitreomacular Traction RTVue-100

Clinical Summary

A 66-year-old female presents for follow-up after a pars plana vitrectomy in the right eye for vitreomacular traction syndrome. She denies any visual changes in the left eye. Visual acuity in the left eye is 20/70. Dilated fundus exam of the left eye (A) reveals faint vitreomacular traction.

Optical Coherence Tomography

Horizontal OCT scan (B) along the superior macula reveals a hyperreflective line along the surface of the retina, which splits into 2 lines, suggestive of schisis of the posterior hyaloid. The 3D thickness map (C) illustrates the retinal contour in this area. Central foveal thickness is 285 µm (D).

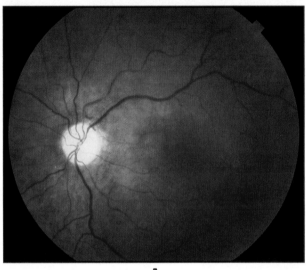

A

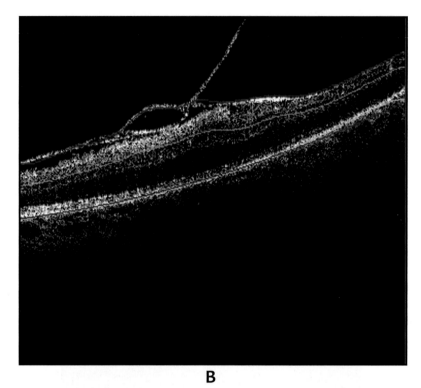

B

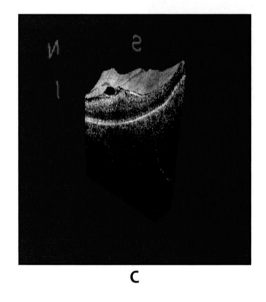

C

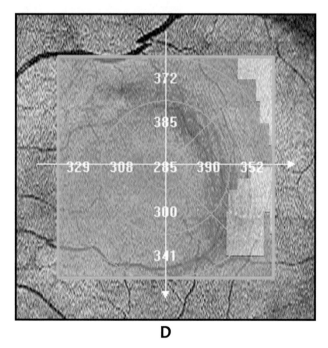

D

Case 3-5. *Vitreomacular Traction and Epiretinal Membrane Successfully Treated With Vitrectomy Surgery*

Clinical Summary

A 67 year old notes a progressive decrease in vision of the left eye over the past 6 months. The visual acuity in this eye is 20/200. Fundus examination (A) demonstrates macular edema and retinal folds associated with a glistening ERM. Pars plana vitrectomy with membrane peeling is performed. Three months postoperatively, the macular edema resolved with improvement in visual acuity to 20/40.

Optical Coherence Tomography

Preoperative OCT (B) defines vitreomacular traction with attachment of the posterior hyaloid (2 low reflective lines in the vitreous cavity) directly to the fovea. The tractional forces from the vitreous lead to the formation of cystoid macular edema, visible as the large, hyporeflective, black circular spaces in the fovea. Increased linear reflectivity along the anterior retina represents ERM formation. Central foveal thickness measures 415 µm. Postoperative OCT (C) demonstrates relief of the vitreomacular traction with removal of the ERM, resulting in a normal foveal contour. Foveal thickness measures 235 µm.

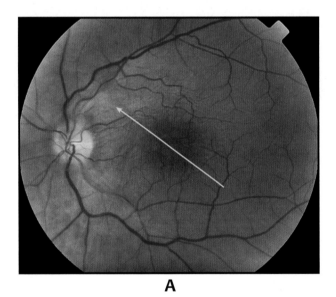

A

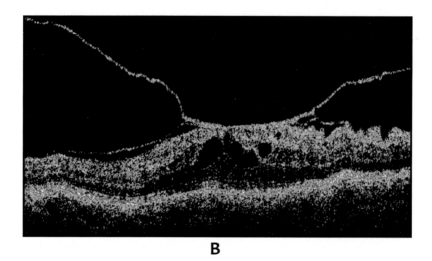

B

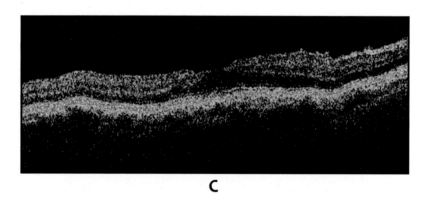

C

Case 3-6. Evolution of Vitreomacular Traction to Full-Thickness Macular Hole

Clinical Summary

A 67-year-old female presents with complaints of mild distortion in central vision in the right eye while reading. Visual acuity is 20/25 in each eye. Dilated fundus exam of the right eye (A) reveals a small, yellow cyst within the fovea and fine macular drusen.

Optical Coherence Tomography

Horizontal OCT scan of the right eye (B) reveals a hyperreflective line in the vitreous with focal attachment to the fovea. A hyporeflective space within the retina suggests fluid accumulation due to traction. The ILM-RPE map (C) and ILM map (D) demonstrate the focal area of attachment.

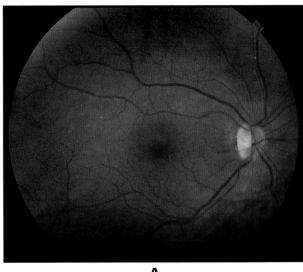

A

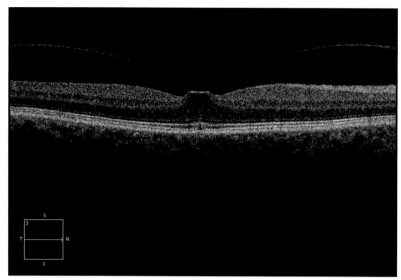

B

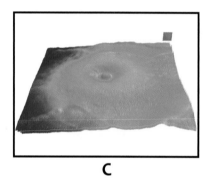

C

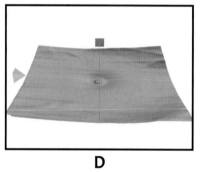

D

Case 3-6. Evolution of Vitreomacular Traction to Full-Thickness Macular Hole (continued)

Follow-Up

Six months later, she returns with complaints of a decline in vision. Visual acuity in the right eye is 20/50. Fundus exam reveals a small full-thickness macular hole (E). Horizontal OCT scan (F) demonstrates a small, full-thickness retinal defect. A hyperreflective line attached to larger hyperreflective material within the vitreous reveals a detached posterior hyaloid face and retinal operculum, respectively. The ILM-RPE (G) overlay reveals the area of small retinal defect.

She subsequently underwent pars plana vitrectomy. Visual acuity returned to 20/30. Dilated fundus exam (H) reveals trace RPE changes. Horizontal OCT scan (I) demonstrates a hyporeflective space at the level of the RPE. The ILM-RPE map (J) demonstrates the retinal contour.

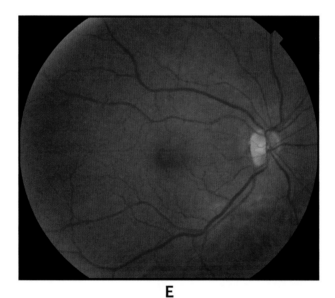

E

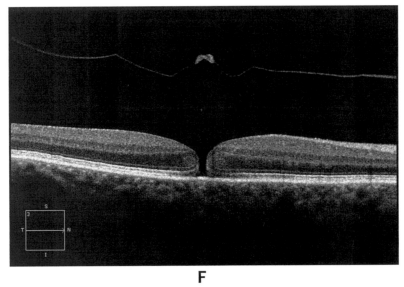

F

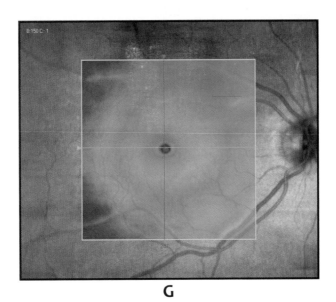

G

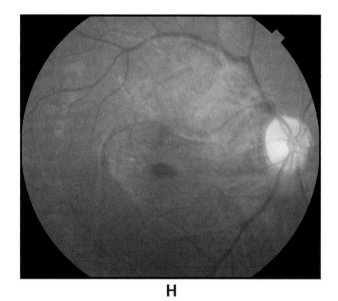

H

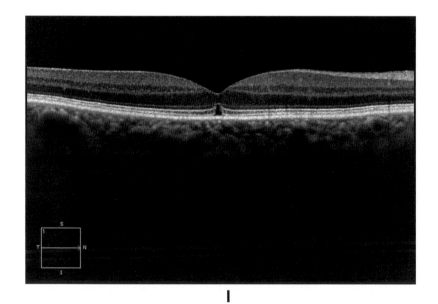

I

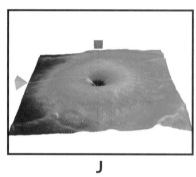

J

Case 3-7A. Full-Thickness Macular Hole

Clinical Summary

An 83-year-old female complains of blurry central vision for several weeks. Her visual acuity in the left eye measures 20/200. Dilated fundus examination reveals a 30-μm red spot in the fovea, suggestive of a full-thickness macular hole (A). There is no evidence of posterior vitreous detachment on examination. She undergoes 23-gauge pars plana vitrectomy, indocyanine green staining of the ILM, and membrane peel. Four weeks after surgery, her visual acuity is 20/200. Dilated fundus examination shows retinal pigment mottling in the fovea, but no evidence of a macular hole (B).

Optical Coherence Tomography

Initial horizontal OCT scan (C) reveals a full-thickness macular hole with a subretinal fluid cuff. Posterior hyaloid face is not visible. The edges are thickened with cavities of reduced reflectivity, suggestive of edema. Parafoveal thickness reaches 599 μm (D). The ILM-RPE map (E) demonstrates the surface contour, while the ILM map (F) reveals the ILM contour. Postoperative horizontal OCT scan (G) demonstrates the absence of a macular hole, foveal thinning, irregular contour, and interruption of the nerve fiber layer along the nasal retina. Postoperative central retinal thickness is 145 μm (H). The ILM-RPE map reveals the overall retinal contour, with absence of macular hole, and irregular retinal surface (I).

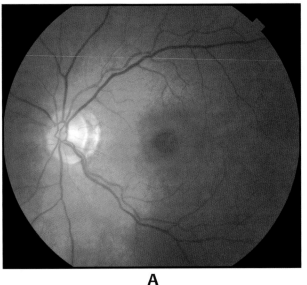

A

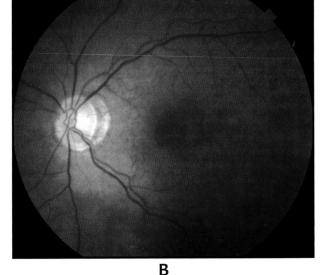

B

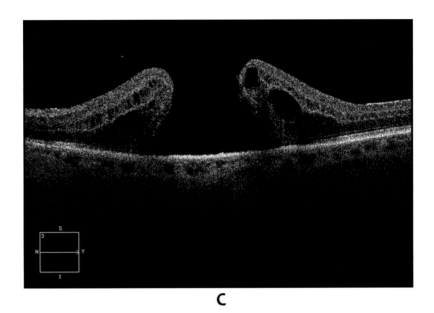

C

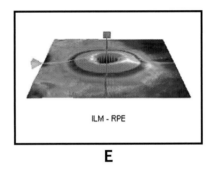

ILM-RPE Thickness (µm)

D

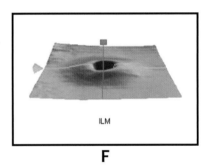

ILM - RPE

E

ILM

F

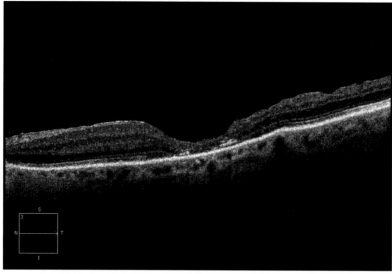

G

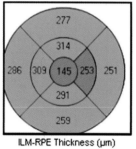

ILM-RPE Thickness (µm)

H

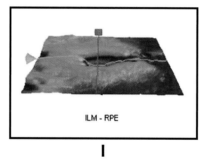

ILM - RPE

I

Case 3-7B. Full-Thickness Macular Hole

Clinical Summary

A 74-year-old female presents with poor vision in the left eye, which has been stable for more than 6 years. Visual acuity is 20/100. Dilated fundus exam of the left eye (A) reveals a central macular hole with a small cuff of subretinal fluid.

Optical Coherence Tomography

Horizontal OCT scan (B) reveals a full-thickness defect in the retina. Intraretinal spaces suggest cystoid macular edema. The ILM-RPE map (C) reveals the area of thickening.

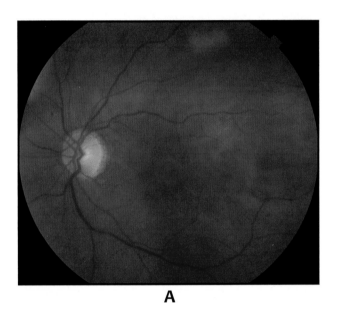

A

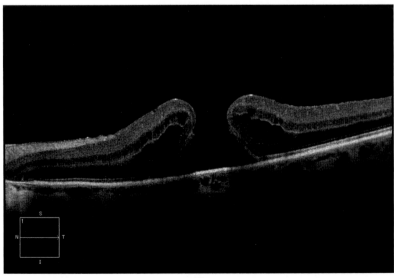

B

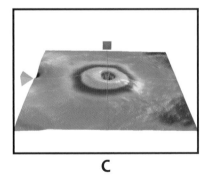

C

Case 3-8A. Full-Thickness Macular Hole—Traumatic

Clinical Summary

A 32-year-old male presents with sudden vision loss in the right eye 6 months after blunt trauma to the right eye. Dilated fundus exam reveals a 500-µm full-thickness macular hole with an associated small cuff of subretinal fluid and mottling of the pigment epithelium. Intraretinal pigment is present in a papillomacular bundle (A).

Optical Coherence Tomography

Horizontal OCT scan (B) shows a full-thickness retinal defect. Hyporeflective spaces within the retina at the temporal aspect of the defect suggest mild edema. A hyperreflective particle on the pigment epithelium may be a macrophage. Retinal thinning is noted along the nasal aspect of the defect. A hyperreflective line in the vitreous is suggestive of a detached posterior hyaloid. The ILM-RPE overlay (C) better demonstrates this tissue defect and retinal thinning nasal to the fovea.

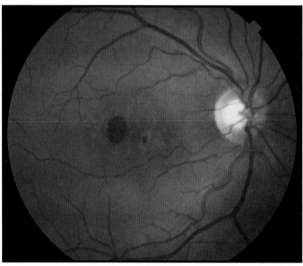

A

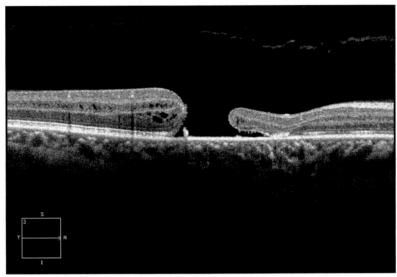

B

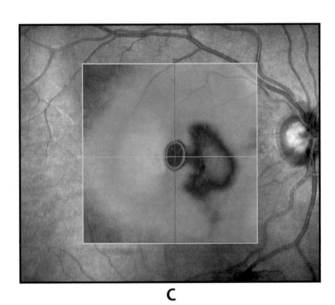

C

Case 3-8B. Full-Thickness Macular Hole—Traumatic

Clinical Summary

A 47-year-old male presents after a history of remote trauma with sustained loss of vision in the left eye for years. He had undergone pars plana vitrectomy without improvement in vision 3 years ago. Visual acuity in the left eye is 20/400. Dilated fundus exam (A) reveals a full-thickness macular hole with retinal pigment mottling surrounding the hole.

Optical Coherence Tomography

Horizontal OCT scan (B) demonstrates the retinal defect. Hyporeflective spaces within the deep retinal layers suggest chronic fluid accumulation. Loss of photoreceptor layer is noted at both edges of the macular hole. The ILM-RPE map (C) illustrates the retinal defect and contour. Central foveal thickness is 120 μm (D).

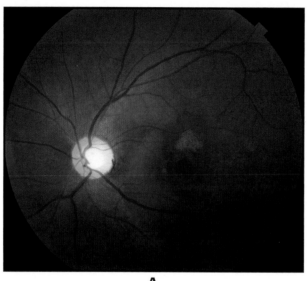

A

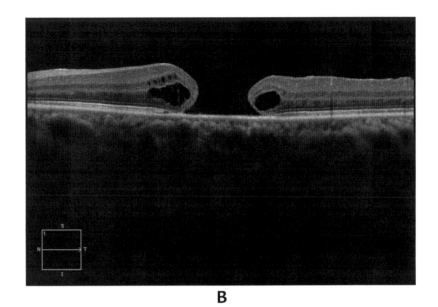

B

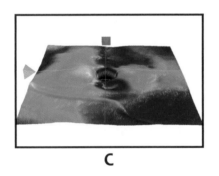

C

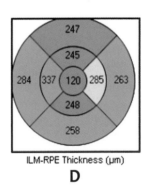

ILM-RPE Thickness (μm)

D

Case 3-9. Macular Holes Stage 1 Bilateral

Clinical Summary

A 69-year-old female presents for her annual diabetic eye exam with no complaints. Visual acuity in the right eye is 20/40 and the left eye is 20/50. Dilated fundus exam of the right eye (A) reveals a few dot-blot hemorrhages and a yellow cyst in the fovea. Dilated fundus exam of the left eye (B) demonstrates hard exudates superior to the fovea and a faint yellow cyst in the left eye.

Optical Coherence Tomography

Horizontal OCT scans of the right eye (C) and left eye (D) reveal a hyperreflective line in the vitreous with focal attachment to the fovea, suggestive of focal traction of the posterior hyaloid face at the fovea. Hyporeflective spaces within the retina reveal bilateral Stage 1 macular holes due to traction. The ILM-RPE overlays of the right eye (E) and left eye (F) demonstrate focal elevation within the fovea. Central foveal thickness of the right eye is 291 μm (G) and that of the left eye is 255 μm (H).

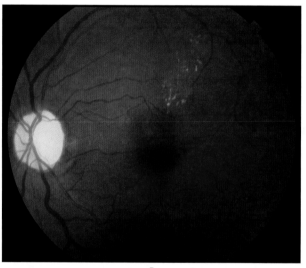

A

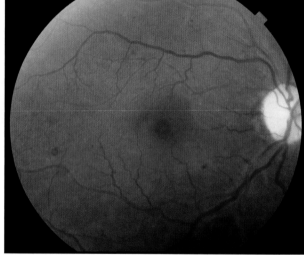

B

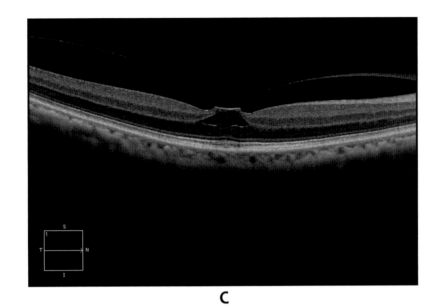

C

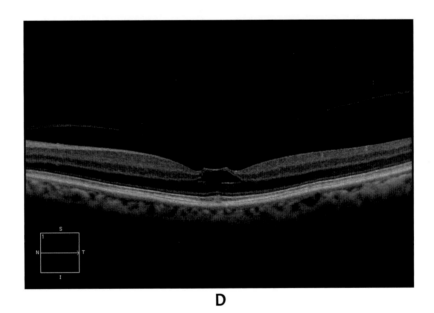

D

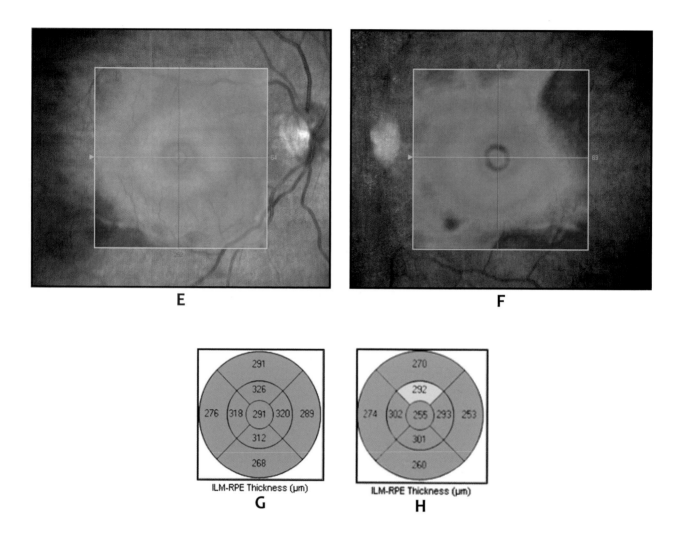

E

F

ILM-RPE Thickness (µm)

G

ILM-RPE Thickness (µm)

H

Case 3-10. Macular Hole Formation and Surgical Management

Clinical Summary

A 64-year-old male reports decreased central vision in his left eye for 2 weeks. His visual acuity is 20/50 in this eye, and dilated fundus exam shows a yellow spot in the fovea. There is no evidence of posterior vitreous detachment on clinical exam. Over the next 3 weeks, he notices increasing central distortion and decreasing vision. His visual acuity declines to 20/70, and dilated fundus exam now shows a small full-thickness macular hole. He undergoes pars plana vitrectomy, membrane peel, and C3F8 injection for management of this macular hole. Five weeks after surgery, his visual acuity is 20/70 with mild cataract formation. Dilated fundus exam shows mottling in the fovea but no evidence of macular hole.

Optical Coherence Tomography

Initial OCT examination (A) shows loss of the normal foveal contour with retinal thinning and a small nonreflective space under the fovea consistent with a foveal detachment. There was no evidence of a full-thickness retinal defect on multiple OCT scans through this area. The posterior hyaloid can be seen shallowly detached from the perifoveal retina but appears to be persistently attached in the foveal region. This configuration corresponds to a Stage 1 macular hole with persistent vitreomacular traction. Three weeks later, OCT examination (B) now confirms the full-thickness defect in the retina with an operculum attached to one edge. The posterior hyaloid can again be seen as a faint membrane above the perifoveal retina that continues to be attached to this operculum. This configuration is consistent with a Stage 2 macular hole and highlights the role of vitreomacular traction in hole development. Postoperative OCT examination (C) confirms complete closure of the macular hole with resolution of the previously identified vitreomacular traction. The retina is still mildly thickened and has not yet regained the normal foveal contour.

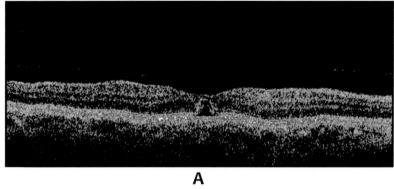

A

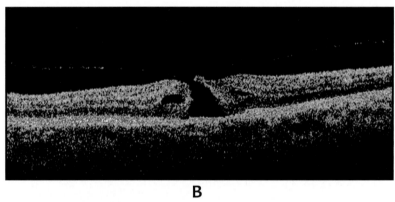

B

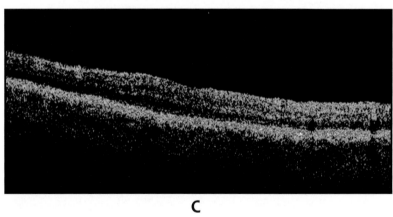

C

Case 3-11. *Myopic Degeneration With a Full-Thickness Macular Hole*

Clinical Summary

A 60-year-old female with a history of myopic degeneration has poor visual acuity in the right eye after developing choroidal neovascularization 2 years earlier. She now complains of worsening visual acuity in her left eye over the past 2 months. Her current visual acuity in the left eye is 20/200. Dilated fundus exam (A) shows a tilted optic nerve with peripapillary atrophy. There is extensive pigmentary mottling in the macular region that limits visualization of the macular hole on clinical exam.

Optical Coherence Tomography

A horizontal OCT image (B) taken through the macula confirms the presence of a full-thickness macular hole. The posterior hyaloid face is not identified on the OCT cuts, and there is no evidence of persistent vitreous traction on the retina. The macular hole and adjacent retina appear similar on OCT to cases of idiopathic macular hole formation. The myopic pigmentary atrophy, however, allows greater penetration and reflectivity of the signal, resulting in a thicker and brighter RPE/choroidal band. Choroidal vessels can be seen as nonreflective spaces within this highly reflective band.

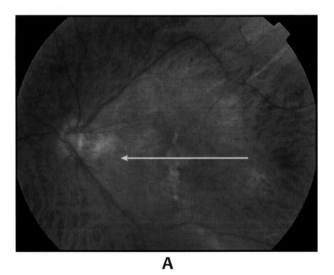

A

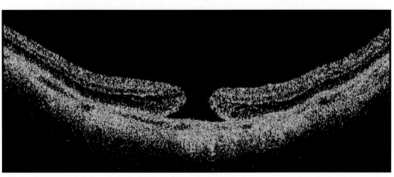

B

Case 3-12A. Lamellar Hole

Clinical Summary

A 69-year-old male presents with complaints of blurry central vision in the left eye. Visual acuity measures 20/20 in the right eye and 20/30 in the left eye. A central scotoma is present in the left visual field examination. Dilated fundus exam of the left eye reveals a mild ERM with a red, circular area in the central macula, suggestive of a macular hole (A).

Optical Coherence Tomography

Horizontal OCT scan (B) shows a hyperreflective linear density at the retinal surface, suggestive of an ERM. A central, irregular foveal retinal defect extends to just above the photoreceptor layer. A second horizontal OCT scan (C), inferior than the previous, reveals a defect wider than previously shown. Central foveal thickness is 290 µm (D). The ILM-RPE overlay reveals a central, irregular decrease in retinal thickness (E).

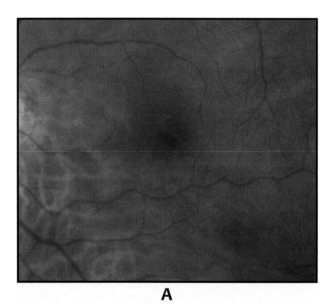

A

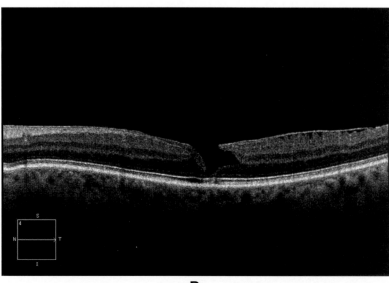

B

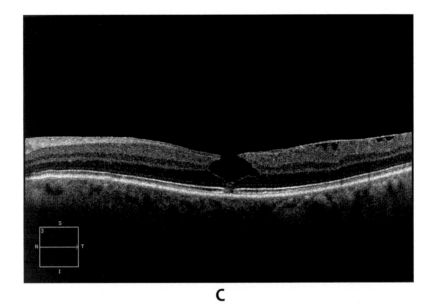

C

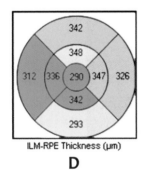

ILM-RPE Thickness (µm)

D

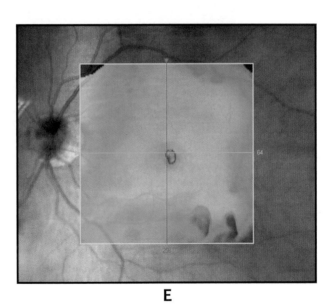

E

Case 3-12B. Lamellar Hole

Clinical Summary

A 60-year-old male presents with complaints of a "black area in my central vision" in the right eye. Visual acuity is 20/50. Dilated fundus exam of the right eye (A) reveals peripheral drusen and a central cyst in the fovea.

Optical Coherence Tomography

Horizontal OCT scan (B) reveals missing retinal tissue in the central fovea and nasal to the fovea, with focal disruption of the photoreceptor layer. Central foveal thickness is 323 µm (C). The ILM-RPE map reveals the general retinal contour (D).

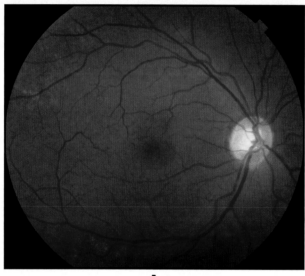

A

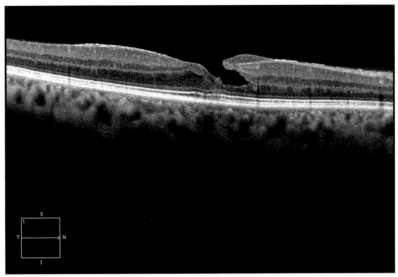

B

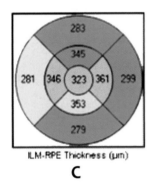

ILM-RPE Thickness (μm)

C

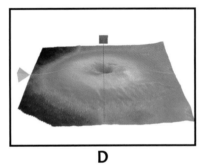

D

Chapter 4

Retinal Vascular Diseases

Heeral R. Shah, MD; Vanessa Cruz-Villegas, MD;
Carmen A. Puliafito, MD, MBA; James G. Fujimoto, PhD; and Jay S. Duker, MD

- Branch Retinal Artery Occlusion
- Central Retinal Artery Occlusion
- Branch Retinal Vein Occlusion
- Central Retinal Vein Occlusion
- Bilateral Idiopathic Juxtafoveal Retinal Telangiectasis
- Retinal Arterial Macroaneurysm

Retinal vascular diseases are common etiologies for central visual loss. Optical coherence tomography (OCT) complements the information obtained from clinical examination and angiographic studies on these conditions. Furthermore, OCT provides objective information in a reproducible way such that monitoring the natural course of evolution of these conditions and assessing response to therapeutic interventions are feasible.

Branch Retinal Artery Occlusion

Branch retinal artery occlusion (BRAO) is usually characterized by sudden visual field loss or vision decrease. The mechanism of occlusion usually involves embolization or thrombosis of the affected vessel. Superficial retinal whitening occurs in the distribution of the occluded arteriole. Fluorescein angiography confirms a delay or lack of perfusion of the involved branch retinal artery. Histopathologic

studies of acute retinal artery occlusions reveal intracellular edema and ischemia of the inner retinal layers. The findings of acute BRAO on OCT correlate with the aforementioned histopathologic reports. The area affected by the obstructed vessel shows increased retinal thickness without cystic spaces of low reflectivity. This finding probably correlates with the fact that the edema that occurs in retinal artery occlusions is in the intracellular instead of the extracellular space. Also, the inner retinal layers tend to be more highly reflective in OCT, probably due to ischemia or coagulative necrosis of these layers. This high reflectivity of the inner retinal layers causes shadowing of the optical signal of the outer retinal layers and retinal pigment epithelium (RPE)/choriocapillaris complex beneath.

Central Retinal Artery Occlusion

Central retinal artery occlusion (CRAO) shares the same thromboembolic etiologic mechanism with BRAO. Patients with CRAO experience sudden severe visual loss unless sparing of the fovea occurs due to the presence of a patent cilioretinal artery, which is present in 15% of the population. The clinical picture of an acute CRAO is characterized by retinal whitening with a central cherry-red spot in the foveola. On intravenous fluorescein angiography, delayed filling

Schuman JS, Puliafito CA, Fujimoto JG, Duker JS, eds.
Optical Coherence Tomography of Ocular Diseases,
Third Edition (pp 111-144).
© 2013 SLACK Incorporated.

of the central retinal artery with boxcarring of the blood column is observed. This lack of adequate perfusion results in ischemia of the inner retinal layers as reported in histopathologic studies.[1,2] OCT makes an understanding of the pathophysiology of this condition possible. The inner retinal layers typically show enhanced reflectivity, which may represent ischemic cellular damage and accumulation of byproducts. The increased thickness of the inner retina typically seen in acute artery occlusions corresponds to the intracellular edema. Histopathologic studies report the presence of edema in the intracellular instead of the extracellular compartment in acute occlusions.[1,2] This accounts for the usual lack of low reflective intraretinal fluid spaces in OCT with artery occlusions. Blocking of the optical reflections from the outer retinal layers and RPE/choriocapillaris complex occurs secondarily to the presence of a thickened, highly reflective inner retina. OCT images of chronic CRAO are characterized by thinning and atrophy of the inner retinal layers as described in histopathologic reports. A patient with a chronic CRAO usually presents with a featureless retinal appearance, but by performing an OCT scan, the diagnosis may be established.

Branch Retinal Vein Occlusion

Branch retinal vein occlusion (BRVO) may produce sudden onset or slow, progressive decreased vision and metamorphopsia. Clinical signs include intraretinal hemorrhages, dilated tortuous retinal veins, cotton-wool spots, and retinal thickening in the sector drained by the obstructed vein. Macular edema is often responsible for central visual loss. OCT is very valuable in diagnosing, monitoring, and managing macular edema secondary to retinal vein occlusions.[3,4] By furnishing objective qualitative and quantitative information in a noninvasive way, detecting and monitoring the effect of therapeutic interventions such as focal laser photocoagulation, intravitreal triamcinolone acetonide injection, adventitial sheathotomy, and pars plana vitrectomy are possible.[5,6] Macular edema due to BRVO is represented by an increase in the retinal thickness and areas of intraretinal-reduced reflectivity on OCT. Usually, this fluid accumulation has a cystic appearance. It is not unusual to observe subretinal fluid accumulation and neurosensory detachment in these cases.[7] BRVO OCT findings may also include epiretinal membranes, pseudoholes, lamellar holes, and subhyaloid or preretinal hemorrhages. Subhyaloid hemorrhages are visualized as high reflective areas

underneath a reflective band (posterior hyaloid). See Chapter 3 for information on epiretinal membranes, pseudoholes, and lamellar holes.

The utility of OCT findings may be greater with both new and old treatment options for macular edema associated with BRVO. Recent data from a Phase III trial suggest that intravitreal ranibizumab results in a gain in visual acuity and decrease in central foveal thickness at 6-month follow-up.[8] The SCORE study confirms that grid laser photocoagulation remains the standard of care compared with 1- and 4-mg doses of intravitreal triamcinolone.[9] Regardless of the treatment, OCT findings, including central foveal thickness, provide significant accuracy for evaluation and monitoring after treatment.

Central Retinal Vein Occlusion

Central retinal vein occlusion (CRVO) is also a common retinal vascular condition usually affecting individuals older than 50 years. Patients typically experience visual loss and present with dilated tortuous retinal veins and scattered intraretinal hemorrhages in all 4 quadrants. Cotton-wool spots, optic disc swelling, and macular edema may be appreciated. Intravenous fluorescein angiography may show areas of blocked fluorescence from the intraretinal blood, staining of the vessel walls, a delayed arteriovenous phase, nonperfused areas, and perifoveal leakage. However, perifoveal leakage sometimes may not be visualized on intravenous fluorescein angiography despite the presence of macular edema due to the presence of a marked hemorrhagic component or because of the lack of intact perifoveal vessels. OCT detects macular edema in spite of these circumstances. Recent studies have shown the efficacy of intravitreal triamcinolone injection in macular edema secondary to CRVO, both individually and compared to observation.[10-12] Furthermore, intravitreal ranibizumab has been shown to provide rapid improvement in 6-month visual acuity and macular edema following a CRVO.[13] OCT plays a pivotal role in quantitatively monitoring changes in retinal thickness after this treatment modality.

Bilateral Idiopathic Juxtafoveal Retinal Telangiectasis

Idiopathic juxtafoveal retinal telangiectasis is a bilateral retinal vascular disorder consisting of an incompetent and ectatic capillary bed in the juxtafoveal temporal region. Central vision may become affected due to exudation. Gass described a classification of 3 subgroups.[14,15] Group IA (unilateral congenital parafoveolar telangiectasis) is characterized by telangiectatic capillaries temporal to the fovea often associated with a circinate ring of exudation. Group IB (unilateral idiopathic focal juxtafoveolar telangiectasis) consists of a small focal area of incompetent capillaries next to the foveal avascular zone. Exudative alterations may be present. Group IIA (bilateral idiopathic acquired parafoveolar telangiectasis) is characterized by bilateral regions of retinal thickening temporal to the fovea. Right-angled venules, retinal pigment epithelial hyperplastic plaques, subretinal neovascularization, and crystalline deposits may be observed. Gass described retinal telangiectasis in 2 siblings.[14,15] He described this group as IIB, or juvenile occult familial idiopathic juxtafoveolar retinal telangiectasis. Patients with Group IIIA (occlusive idiopathic juxtafoveolar retinal telangiectasis) may experience visual loss due to obliteration of perifoveal capillaries. Patients with Group IIIB (occlusive idiopathic juxtafoveolar retinal telangiectasis associated with central nervous system vasculopathy) share the same findings from Group IIIA plus central nervous system involvement.[14,15] OCT depicts clearly the involvement of the intraretinal and subretinal spaces in this condition. This vascular disorder may show low reflective intraretinal areas of macular edema and highly reflective lipid exudates in OCT. Plaques of retinal pigment hyperplasia appear as intraretinal hyperreflective spots associated with shadowing of the reflections from the tissues below.[16] For details about OCT findings of subretinal neovascularization associated with juxtafoveal telangiectasis, refer to Chapter 8.

Retinal Arterial Macroaneurysm

Retinal arterial macroaneurysms are vascular dilations that may present in association with macular edema, retinal lipid exudation, or hemorrhage. Visual loss may result if the macula becomes involved. Hemorrhage may occur in different levels: vitreous, subhyaloid or preretinal, intraretinal, or subretinal. OCT depicts clearly the hemorrhagic component of ruptured retinal arterial macroaneurysms. Subhyaloid hemorrhages are represented as regions of high backscattering below the reflective posterior hyaloid band. Hemorrhagic lesions

beneath the internal limiting membrane (ILM) also can be appreciated by OCT. The ILM tends to be more reflective than the posterior hyaloid. Subretinal hemorrhages appear as dense highly reflective bands below the neurosensory retina. Shadowing of the optical reflections from the tissues under those hemorrhagic lesions is usually observed. In the case of subhyaloid or preretinal blood, blocking of the neurosensory retina and RPE/choriocapillaris reflections is observed. Subretinal blood blocks the reflections from the RPE/choriocapillaris only. Other morphological findings associated with retinal arterial macroaneurysm seen in OCT are hard lipid exudates, which appear as intraretinal dots or areas of increased reflectivity, and low reflective intraretinal fluid accumulation and edema. The natural course of this condition can be followed with OCT as well as the response to therapeutic interventions.

References

1. Dahrling BE II. The histopathology of early central retinal artery occlusion. *Arch Ophthalmol*. 1965;73:506-510.
2. Kroll AJ. Experimental central retinal artery occlusion. *Arch Ophthalmol*. 1968;79:453-469.
3. Lerche RC, Schaudig U, Scholz F, Walter A, Richard G. Structural changes of the retina in retinal vein occlusion—imaging and quantification with optical coherence tomography. *Ophthalmic Surg Lasers*. 2001;32(4):272-280.
4. Imasawa M, Iijima H, Morimoto T. Perimetric sensitivity and retinal thickness in eyes with macular edema resulting from branch retinal vein occlusion. *Am J Ophthalmol*. 2002;133:428-429.
5. Saika S, Tanaka T, Miyamoto T, Ohnishi Y. Surgical posterior vitreous detachment combined with gas/air tamponade for treating macular edema associated with branch retinal vein occlusion: retinal tomography and visual outcome. *Graefes Arch Clin Exp Ophthalmol*. 2001;239(10):729-732.
6. Fujii GY, De Juan E Jr, Humayun MS. Improvements after sheathotomy for branch retinal vein occlusion documented by optical coherence tomography and scanning laser ophthalmoscope. *Ophthalmic Surg Lasers Imaging*. 2003;34(1):49-52.
7. Spaide RF, Lee JK, Klancnik JM Jr, Gross NE. Optical coherence tomography of branch retinal vein occlusion. *Retina*. 2003;23(3):343-347.
8. Campochiaro PA, Heier JS, Feiner L, et al; BRAVO Investigators. Ranibizumab for macular edema following branch retinal vein occlusion: six-month primary end point results of a phase III study. *Ophthalmology*. 2010;117(6):1102-1112.e1.
9. Scott IU, Ip MS, VanVeldhuisen PC, et al; SCORE Study Research Group. A randomized trial comparing the efficacy and safety of intravitreal triamcinolone with standard care to treat vision loss associated with macular edema secondary to branch retinal vein occlusion: the Standard Care vs Corticosteroid for Retinal Vein Occlusion (SCORE) study report 6. *Arch Ophthalmol*. 2009;127(9):1115-1128.

10. Jonas JB, Kreissig I, Degenring RF. Intravitreal triamcinolone acetonide as treatment of macular edema in central retinal vein occlusion. *Graefes Arch Clin Exp Ophthalmol.* 2002;240(9):782-783.

11. Greenberg PB, Martidis A, Rogers AH, Duker JS, Reichel E. Intravitreal triamcinolone acetonide for macular edema due to central retinal vein occlusion. *Br J Ophthalmol.* 2002;86(2):247-248.

12. Ip MS, Scott IU, VanVeldhuisen PC, et al; SCORE Study Research Group. A randomized trial comparing the efficacy and safety of intravitreal triamcinolone with observation to treat vision loss associated with macular edema secondary to central vein occlusion: the Standard Care vs Corticosteroid for Retinal Vein Occlusion (SCORE) study report 5. *Arch Ophthalmol.* 2009;127(9):1101-1114.

13. Brown DM, Campochiaro PA, Singh RP, et al; CRUISE Investigators. Ranibizumab for macular edema following central retinal vein occlusion: six-month primary end point results of a phase III study. *Ophthalmology.* 2010;117(6):1124-1133.e1.

14. Gass JDM, Blodi BA. Idiopathic juxtafoveolar retinal telangiectasis; update of classification and follow-up study. *Ophthalmology.* 1993;100:1536-1546.

15. Gass JDM. *Stereoscopic Atlas of Macular Diseases.* 4th ed. St. Louis, MO: CV Mosby; 1997:374-376.

16. Trabucchi G, Brancato R, Pierro L, Introini U, Sannace C. Idiopathic juxtafoveolar retinal telangiectasis and pigment epithelial hyperplasia: an optical coherence tomographic study. *Arch Ophthalmol.* 1999;117(3):405-406.

Index to Cases

Case 4-1A. Acute Branch Retinal Artery Occlusion

Clinical Summary

A 56-year-old female complains of blurry vision in the inferior visual field of the right eye for 3 hours. She had undergone an aortic valve replacement 3 months prior to presentation. Visual acuity measures 20/60 in the right eye, with loss of inferior field. Dilated fundus examination reveals an intra-arterial embolus along the superotemporal arcade with smaller embolus distally, with associated retinal whitening (A).

Optical Coherence Tomography

Horizontal OCT scan (B) through the corresponding area (C) shows intraretinal thickening with hyperreflectivity of inner retinal layers (arrows). Additionally, focal areas of shadowing correspond to retinal arteries and veins. The superior macula is thickened to 302 µm (D). The patient's Humphrey visual field defect correlates to the area of ischemic retina (E).

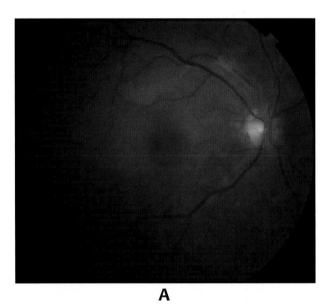

A

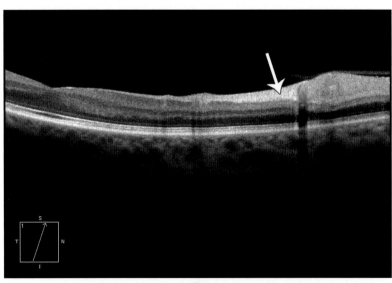

B

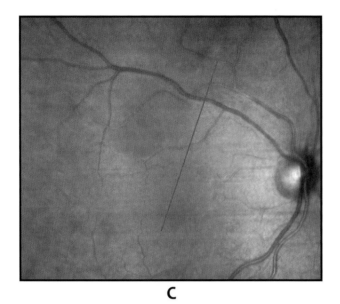

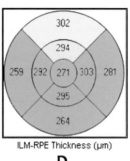

C

ILM-RPE Thickness (μm)

D

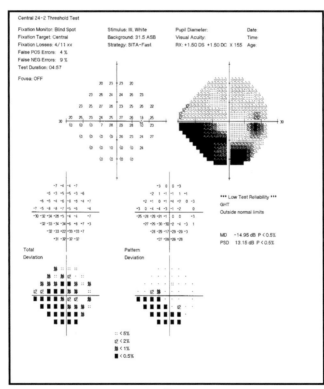

E

Case 4-1B. Acute Branch Retinal Artery Occlusion

Clinical Summary

A 51-year-old male experiences loss of the superior visual field in his left eye. The visual acuity in this eye is 20/25. Dilated fundus examination shows retinal whitening in the distribution of an inferotemporal branch retinal artery (A). Fluorescein angiography (B) reveals delayed filling of the involved branch retinal artery.

Optical Coherence Tomography

OCT (C) shows increased reflectivity and thickness of the inner retinal layers compatible with the acute ischemic tissue insult. Shadowing of the outer retinal layers and RPE/choriocapillaris optical signals is appreciated.

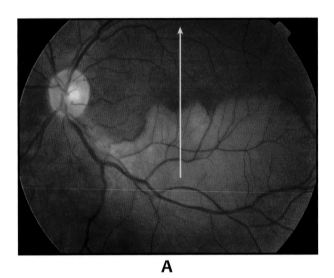

A

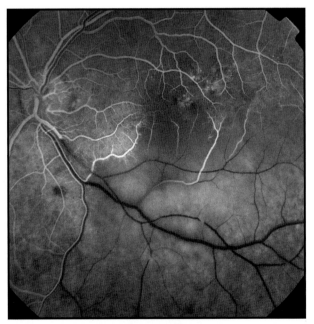

B—early

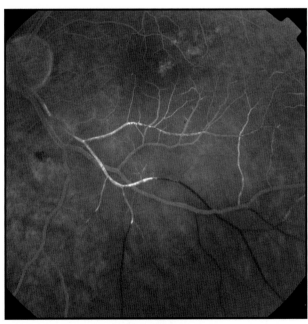

B—late

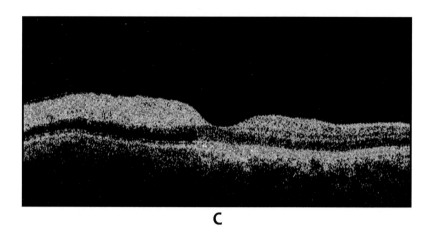

C

Case 4-2. Chronic Central Retinal Artery Occlusion

Clinical Summary

A 66-year-old male presents with a history of sudden loss of vision in the left eye 2 months ago. He had undergone phacoemulsification and intraocular lens implantation 2 weeks previously. Medical history is significant for coronary artery disease, cholesterolemia, and hypertension. Visual acuity measures hand movements in the left eye. Dilated fundus exam reveals diffusely attenuated arteries, tortuous veins, retinal thickening within the macula, and the presence of a cherry-red spot (A).

Optical Coherence Tomography

Horizontal OCT scan (B) shows diffuse thinning of the inner retinal layers and a relatively intact photoreceptor layer. Central retinal thickness is 197 μm (C). The ILM-RPE overlay illustrates areas of retinal thinning (D).

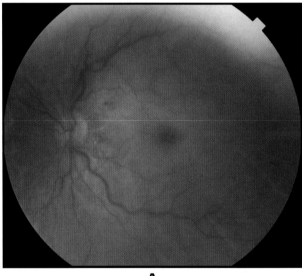

A

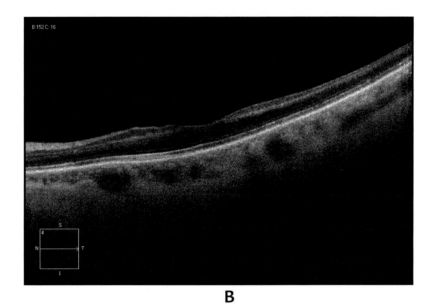

B

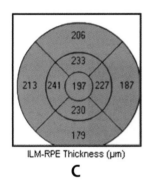

ILM-RPE Thickness (µm)

C

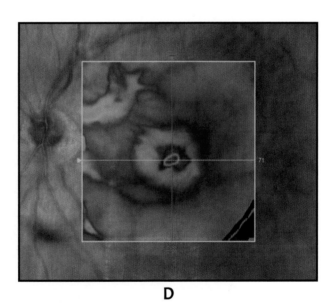

D

Case 4-3A. Branch Retinal Vein Occlusion

Clinical Summary

A 51-year-old male presents with blurry vision in the left eye. Visual acuity measures 20/400 in the affected eye. Dilated fundus examination (A) reveals intraretinal hemorrhage and cotton-wool spots along the superior arcade with macular edema.

Optical Coherence Tomography

Horizontal OCT scan (B) demonstrates numerous hyporeflective spaces within the outer plexiform layer and larger hyporeflective cavities within the outer retina, indicating fluid accumulation in the superonasal macula. Intraretinal thickening leads to an elevation of neurosensory retina and a loss of foveal contour.

Treatment With Intravitreal Bevacizumab

The patient was treated with intravitreal bevacizumab on presentation. He returned 6 weeks later with stable visual acuity and mild reduction in intraretinal hemorrhage (C). Horizontal OCT scan (D) shows fewer hyporeflective cystic spaces. Central foveal thickness is 402 μm (E).

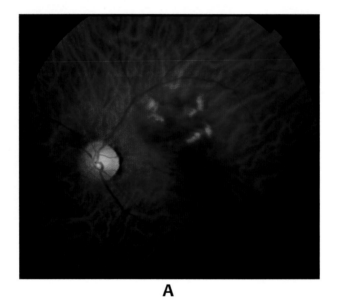

A

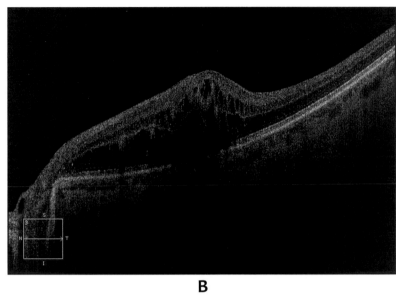

B

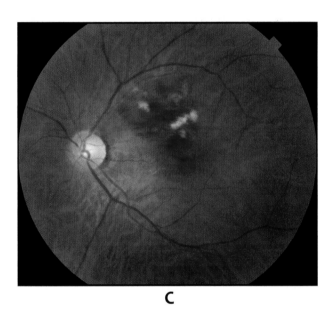

C

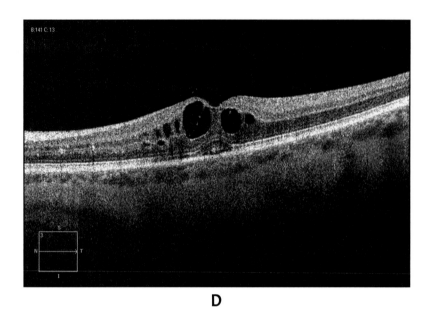

D

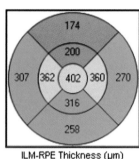

ILM-RPE Thickness (µm)

E

Case 4-3B. Branch Retinal Vein Occlusion

Clinical Summary

A 48-year-old male with a history of a branch retinal vein occlusion in the left eye is examined. His visual acuity is 20/20 in this eye. Dilated fundus examination shows a sclerotic superonasal branch retinal vein associated with telangiectatic vessels and old dehemoglobinized subhyaloid blood superior to the optic nerve (A). Fluorescein angiography (B) shows a delayed filling of the involved vein and minimal leakage from the telangiectatic vessels.

Optical Coherence Tomography

OCT scan (C) acquired through the subhyaloid blood shows an area of high reflectivity, which shadows the optical signals from the retinal, RPE, and choriocapillaris layers underneath. Superiorly (right side of the scan), a reflective band is appreciated consistent with the posterior hyaloid. The subhyaloid space is visualized as a low reflective area beneath that reflective band.

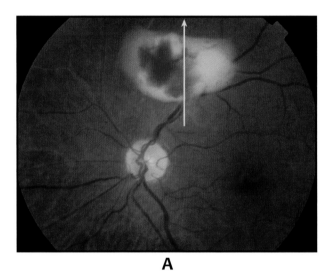

A

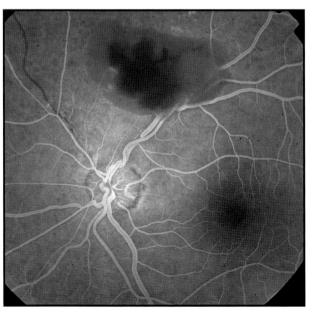

B—early

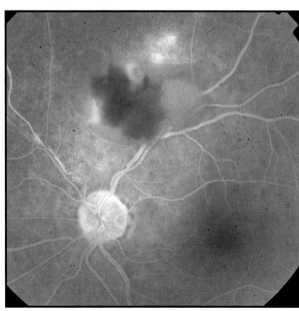

B—late

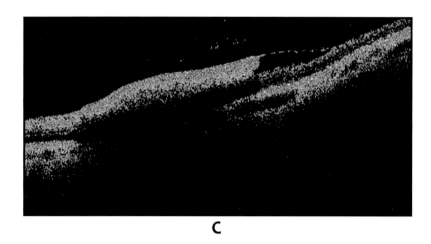

C

Case 4-4A. Central Retinal Vein Occlusion

Clinical Summary

A 68-year-old female presents with a sudden decline in visual acuity of the left eye. Visual acuity of the right eye measures 20/25 and the left eye is 20/200. Past medical history is significant for diabetes mellitus type 2, hypercholesterolemia, and hypertension. Ocular history includes primary open-angle glaucoma. IOP is 20 mm Hg right eye and 18 mm Hg left eye. Dilated fundus examination of the left eye shows diffuse intraretinal hemorrhage in all quadrants and dilated tortuous veins (A). Late-phase fluorescein angiography reveals dilated tortuous veins and blocking of choroidal flush and vessels by intraretinal blood. Perifoveal leakage is difficult to assess due to the diffuse retinal hemorrhage (B).

Optical Coherence Tomography

Horizontal OCT scan (C) shows diffuse hyporeflective spaces within the outer plexiform layer and outer retinal layers, consistent with macular edema. A hyperreflective linear density in the vitreous suggests a detached posterior hyaloid face. Central foveal thickness measures 719 μm (D). The ILM-RPE map reveals the general retinal contour (E).

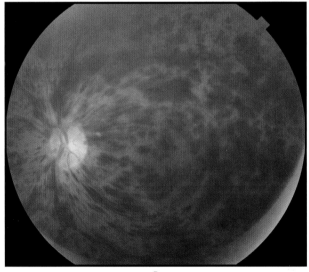

A

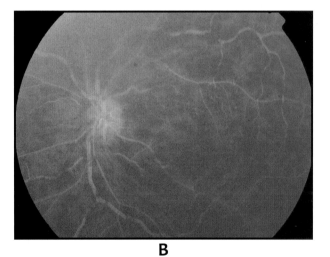

B

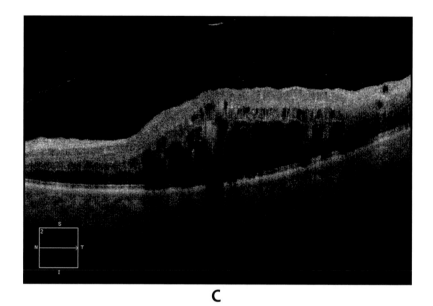

C

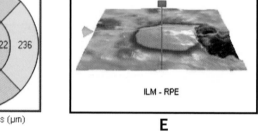

ILM-RPE Thickness (µm)

D

ILM - RPE

E

Case 4-4B. Central Retinal Vein Occlusion

Clinical Summary

A 70-year-old male presents for a decline in vision in the left eye over 1 month. Visual acuity is 20/200 in the left eye. Dilated fundus exam (A) reveals dilated tortuous veins, diffuse intraretinal hemorrhage in all quadrants, and macular edema.

Optical Coherence Tomography

Horizontal OCT scan (B) of the left eye reveals large intraretinal hyporeflective spaces, suggestive of diffuse macular edema. Vertical linear structures within the retina are suggestive of Müller cells. The ILM-RPE map (C) demonstrates the area of edema. Central foveal thickness is 730 μm (D).

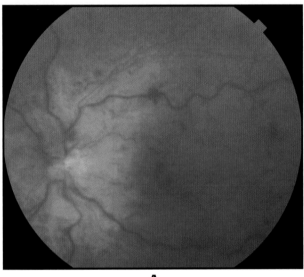

A

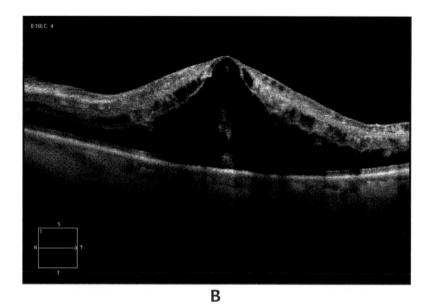

B

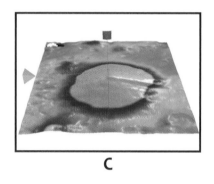

C

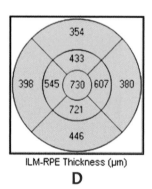

ILM-RPE Thickness (µm)

D

Case 4-5. Hemiretinal Vein Occlusion

Clinical Summary

A 58-year-old female presents with complaints of decline in vision in the left eye over 1 month. Visual acuity in the right eye is 20/20 and the left eye is 20/200. Dilated fundus exam of the left eye (A) reveals diffuse intraretinal hemorrhages and dilated tortuous veins in the inferior hemifield with macular edema.

Optical Coherence Tomography

Horizontal OCT scan (B) of the left eye demonstrates a large hyporeflective space within the retina, suggestive of macular edema. The ILM-RPE overlay (C) partially reveals the area of thickening. Due to the degree of edema inferior to the fovea, the retina is not detected. Central foveal thickness is 518 μm (D).

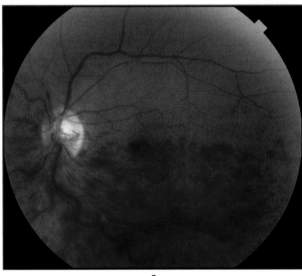

A

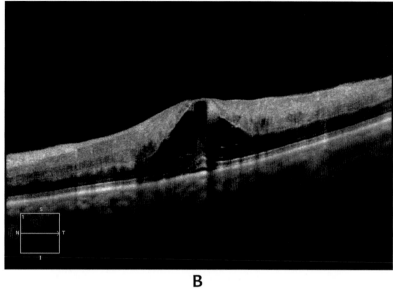

B

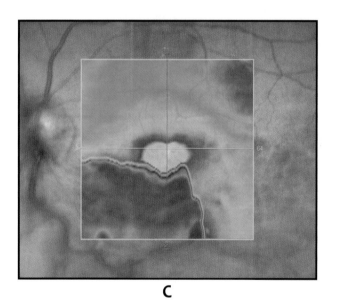

C

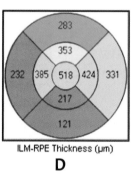

ILM-RPE Thickness (µm)

D

Case 4-6A. Bilateral Idiopathic Juxtafoveal Retinal Telangiectasis

Clinical Summary

A 53-year-old male presents with complaints of "crescent halos" in both eyes. Visual acuity measures 20/20 in the right eye and 20/25 in the left eye. Dilated fundus examination of both eyes reveal faint bilateral telangiectatic vessels with cystic changes (A, B).

Optical Coherence Tomography

Horizontal OCT scan of the right eye (C) shows loss of foveal inner retinal tissue and foveal contour. A linear density along the surface may represent an intact posterior hyaloid face. Central foveal thickness is reduced to 237 μm (D). Horizontal OCT scan of the left eye (E) shows loss of inner foveal tissue, again with a visible intact posterior hyaloid face. The ILM-RPE map (F) reveals the subtle surface contour abnormality. Central foveal thickness is reduced to 247 μm (G).

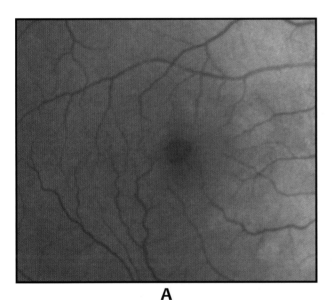

A

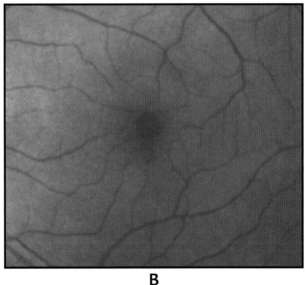

B

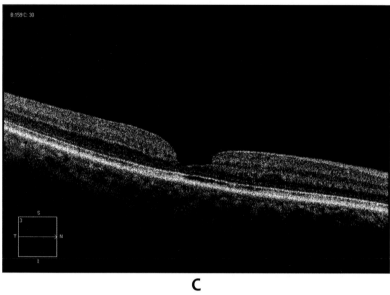

C

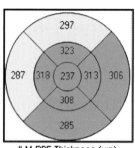

ILM-RPE Thickness (µm)

D

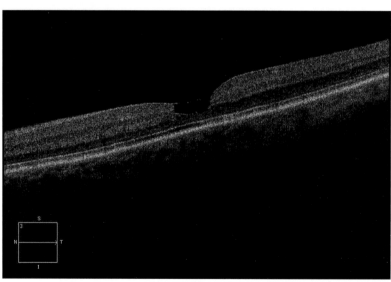

E

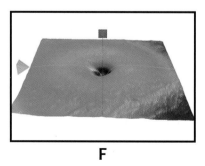

F

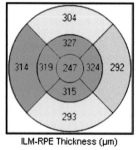

ILM-RPE Thickness (µm)

G

Case 4-6B. Bilateral Idiopathic Juxtafoveal Retinal Telangiectasis

Clinical Summary

A 64-year-old male reports central distortion in his right eye over the past year. His visual acuity in this eye is 20/50. On examination, there is evidence of a grayish discoloration and retinal thickening in the temporal portion of the fovea (A). Fluorescein angiography (B) shows telangiectatic vessels and late leakage of dye.

Optical Coherence Tomography

A vertical OCT scan (C) obtained through fixation reveals a small central area of low intraretinal reflectivity in a slit configuration consistent with fluid accumulation. No other pockets or spaces of low reflectivity are identified. In spite of that area of fluid accumulation, the central retinal thickness measures 193 μm (D).

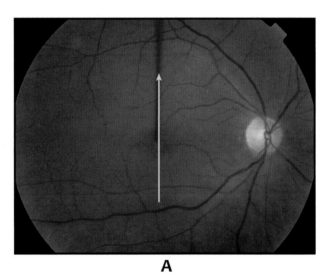

A

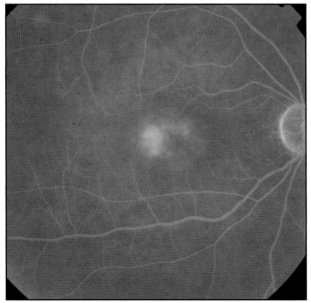

B—early

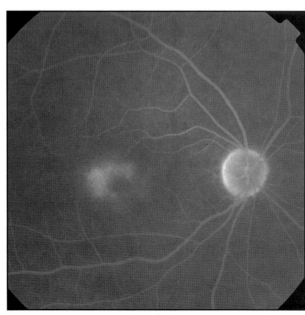

B—late

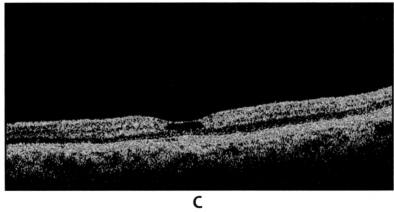

C

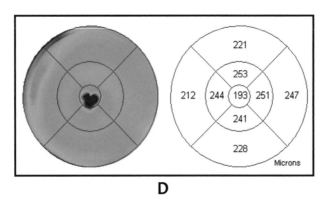

D

Case 4-6B. Bilateral Idiopathic Juxtafoveal Retinal Telangiectasis (continued)

Clinical Summary

Examination of the patient's left eye reveals subretinal fibrosis, right-angle venules, intraretinal pigment migration, and lipid exudates temporal to the fovea (E). The visual acuity in this eye measures 20/200. Fluorescein angiography (F) shows staining.

Optical Coherence Tomography

OCT (G) reveals a region of increased optical reflectivity in the macular area at the level of RPE/choriocapillaris complex consistent with subretinal fibrosis. Central retinal thickness measures 195 μm (H).

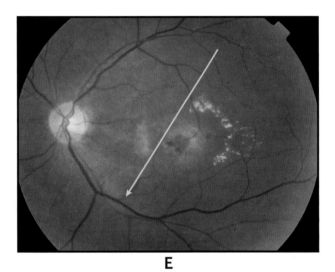

E

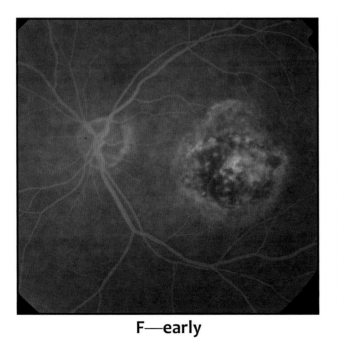

F—early

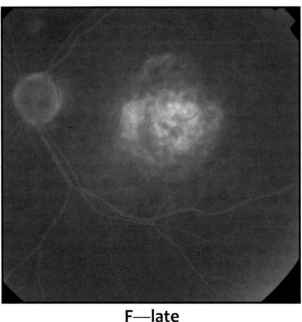

F—late

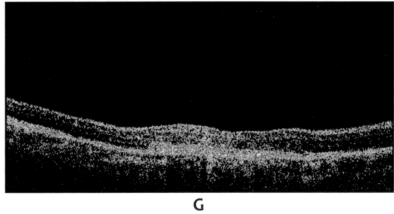

G

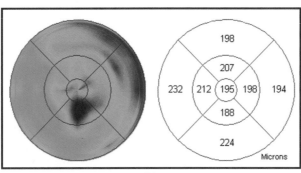

H

Case 4-7. Unilateral Idiopathic Juxtafoveal Retinal Telangiectasis

Clinical Summary

A 75-year-old male is referred for macular changes. He denies any ocular complaints. Visual acuity measures 20/20 in the right eye and 20/25 in the left eye. Dilated fundus exam of the right eye shows a vitelliform-like lesion in the center of the fovea, with telangiectases superior and inferior to this lesion (A). Fundus exam of the left eye is normal (B). Fluorescein angiography of the right eye reveals widened foveal intracapillary spaces and telangiectases at the margin (C).

Optical Coherence Tomography

Horizontal OCT scan (D) of the right eye through a telangiectatic vessel reveals a hyperreflective, subfoveal lesion at the level of the RPE, with no intraretinal or subretinal fluid.

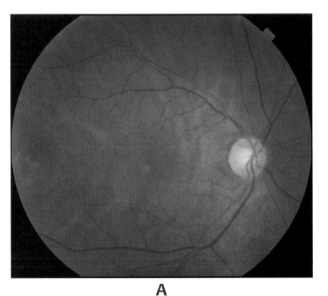

A

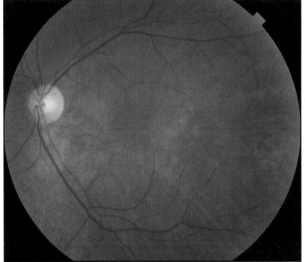

B

C

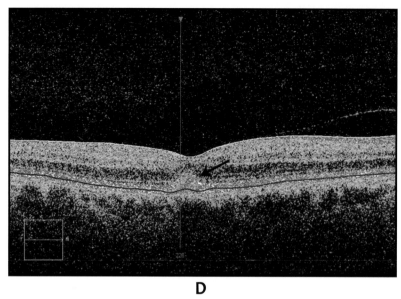

D

Case 4-8. Retinal Arterial Macroaneurysm

Clinical Summary

A 72-year-old male had a 3-day history of vision loss in his left eye. His vision measures 1/200 in this eye. On examination, intraretinal and subretinal hemorrhages are evident in the macular region extending toward the inferior arcade. An arterial macroaneurysm is visualized along the course of an arteriole inferotemporally (A). Fluorescein angiography (B) shows early filling of the macroaneurysm with late staining. Blocked fluorescence of the choroidal vasculature from the intraretinal and subretinal blood is appreciated.

Optical Coherence Tomography

An OCT scan (C) obtained through fixation shows marked elevation of the macula with cystic spaces of low reflectivity at the level of the outer plexiform layer corresponding to fluid accumulation. High backscattering is appreciated in the subretinal space as well as intraretinally, which shadows the optical reflections from the choriocapillaris and choroid layers underneath. A horizontal OCT scan (D) depicts that much of the hemorrhagic component lay in the sub-RPE space.

Six weeks later, vision measures 8/200. On examination, dehemoglobinized blood is still present (E). An OCT scan (F) obtained at that time reveals resolution of the intraretinal fluid accumulation. The blood looks more organized in the sub-RPE space. The macroaneurysm is visualized in one of the images (G) as a round focal area of enhanced reflectivity that blocks the optical signals from the tissues below.

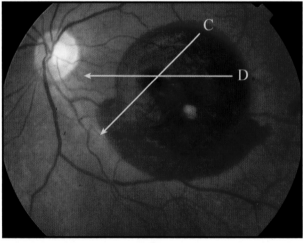

A

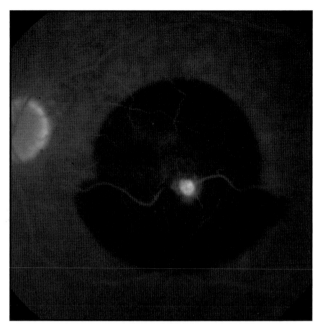
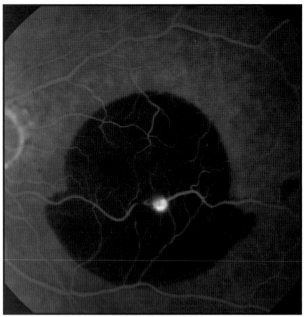
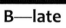

B—early

B—late

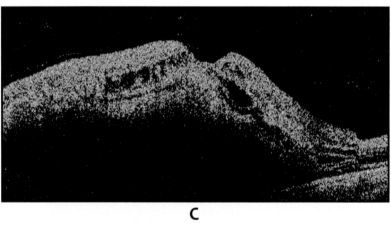

C

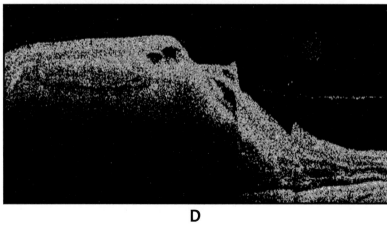

D

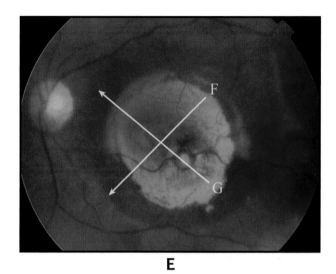

E

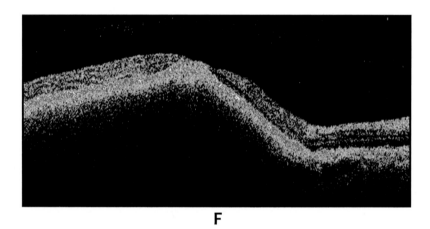

F

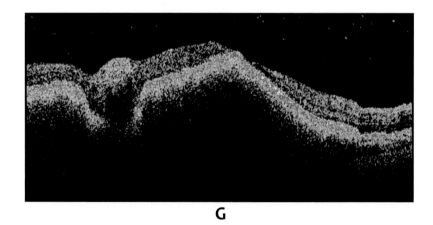

G

Chapter 5

Diabetic Retinopathy

Heeral R. Shah, MD; Vanessa Cruz-Villegas, MD;
Harry W. Flynn Jr, MD; and Jay S. Duker, MD

- Nonproliferative Diabetic Retinopathy
- Diabetic Macular Edema
- Proliferative Diabetic Retinopathy

Diabetic retinopathy is the leading cause of new blindness in individuals under 65 years of age in the United States. Diabetic retinopathy can be classified into nonproliferative diabetic retinopathy (NPDR) and proliferative diabetic retinopathy (PDR). The clinical features of NPDR include microaneurysms, intraretinal hemorrhages, hard exudates, nerve fiber layer infarcts or cotton-wool exudates, and intraretinal microvascular abnormalities. The clinical picture of PDR includes the features from NPDR in addition to proliferating new vessels on the optic nerve head, retina, or iris, which often result in vitreous hemorrhage or tractional retinal detachment.

Diabetic macular edema is a principal cause of visual loss in diabetic patients.[1,2] It can occur at any stage of diabetic retinopathy. The role of optical coherence tomography (OCT) in the assessment and management of diabetic retinopathy has become significant in understanding the vitreoretinal relationships and the internal architecture of the retina. The macular thickness can be accurately measured due to the characteristic and well-defined optical reflectivity of the anterior and posterior margins or boundaries of the neurosensory retina.[3] Studies have shown that OCT may be more sensitive in evaluating diabetic macular edema than slit-lamp examination.[3,4] In addition, central macular thickness correlates with visual acuity even better than fluorescein leakage.[3,5] OCT also allows quantification of macular thickness in a reproducible manner.[6,7] With this capability, the acquisition of reliable documentation of the progression of retinal thickness is possible. The response of macular edema to focal grid laser treatment as well as new treatments, such as intravitreal triamcinolone acetonide injections or intravitreal steroid devices, can be documented accurately by OCT imaging.[8-10]

OCT images of macular edema depict the presence of low intraretinal reflectivity, which corresponds to intraretinal fluid accumulation. This reduced reflectivity or backscattering tends to be more apparent in the outer retinal layers. Cystic spaces of decreased intraretinal reflectivity are evident on OCT, consistent with a cystoid macular edema configuration shown by fluorescein angiography. In addition to increased retinal thickness and cystoid macular edema, diabetic eyes can show neurosensory retinal detachments with subretinal fluid accumulation.[11] Other morphological features of diabetic retinopathy that can be appreciated by OCT are intraretinal hard lipid exudates and intraretinal hemorrhages. Hard exudates are represented as highly reflective intraretinal areas. Shadowing of the optical reflection from the retinal tissue and choroid beneath the exudate is sometimes observed. Hemorrhages also appear as areas of high backscattering with shadowing of the reflection of deeper tissue layers.

Schuman JS, Puliafito CA, Fujimoto JG, Duker JS, eds.
Optical Coherence Tomography of Ocular Diseases,
Third Edition (pp 145-170).
© 2013 SLACK Incorporated.

OCT also helps to distinguish those patients with diabetic macular edema, which has a component of vitreous traction or retinoschisis. Vitreoretinal adhesions are detected more precisely by OCT than with slit-lamp examination.[12] A taut posterior hyaloid or vitreoretinal adhesion is seen as a reflective membrane with persistent focal attachment to the fovea. Moreover, a shallow traction macular detachment or retinoschisis may be present but only visualized by OCT.[13] Studies have shown a benefit from pars plana vitrectomy in those patients with diabetic macular edema and vitreomacular traction.[14-17] Diabetic patients with macular retinoschisis generally have a poor visual prognosis. Thus, OCT is effective in determining the necessity of, as well as the response to, surgical management.[17-19]

PDR could be visualized in OCT as highly reflective preretinal bands anterior to the retinal surface consistent with preretinal fibrovascular or fibroglial proliferation. Diffuse retinal thickening, distortion, and irregularity of the retinal contour can also occur as a result of the contraction of these preretinal membranes. An associated retinal traction detachment may be observed. OCT is valuable in determining the extent of the tractional component as well as the presence of foveal involvement. Again, OCT assists in the decision-making process of surgical intervention.

References

1. Moss SE, Klein R, Klein BE. Ten-year incidence of visual loss in a diabetic population. *Ophthalmology*. 1994;101(6):1061-1070.
2. Moss SE, Klein R, Klein BE. The 14-year incidence of visual loss in a diabetic population. *Ophthalmology*. 1998;105(6):998-1003.
3. Hee MR, Puliafito CA, Wong C, et al. Quantitative assessment of macular edema with optical coherence tomography. *Arch Ophthalmol*. 1995;113(8):1019-1029.
4. Yang CS, Cheng CY, Lee FL, Hsu WM, Liu JH. Quantitative assessment of retinal thickness in diabetic patients with and without clinically significant macular edema using optical coherence tomography. *Acta Ophthalmol Scand*. 2001;79(3):266-270.
5. Hee MR, Puliafito CA, Duker JS, et al. Topography of diabetic macular edema with optical coherence tomography. *Ophthalmology*. 1998;105(2):360-370.
6. Massin P, Vicaut E, Haouchine B, Erginay A, Paques M, Gaudric A. Reproducibility of retinal mapping using optical coherence tomography. *Arch Ophthalmol*. 2001;119(8):1135-1142.
7. Goebel W, Kretzchmar-Gross T. Retinal thickness in diabetic retinopathy: a study using optical coherence tomography (OCT). *Retina*. 2002;22(6):759-767.
8. Rivellese M, George A, Sulkes D, Reichel E, Puliafito CA. Optical coherence tomography after laser photocoagulation for clinically significant macular edema. *Ophthalmic Surg Lasers*. 2000;31(3):192-197.
9. Lattanzio R, Brancato R, Pierro L, et al. Macular thickness measured by optical coherence tomography (OCT) in diabetic patients. *Eur J Ophthalmol*. 2002;12(6):482-487.
10. Martidis A, Duker JS, Greenberg PB, et al. Intravitreal triamcinolone for refractory diabetic macular edema. *Ophthalmology*. 2002;109(5):920-926.
11. Otani T, Kishi S, Maruyama Y. Patterns of diabetic macular edema with optical coherence tomography. *Am J Ophthalmol*. 1999;127(6):688-693.
12. Gallemore RP, Jumper JM, McCuen BW II, Jaffe GJ, Postel EA, Toth CA. Diagnosis of vitreoretinal adhesions in macular disease with optical coherence tomography. *Retina*. 2000;20(2):115-120.
13. Kaiser PK, Rieman CD, Sears JE, Lewis H. Macular traction detachment and diabetic macular edema associated with posterior hyaloidal traction. *Am J Ophthalmol*. 2001;131(1):44-49.
14. Lewis H, Abrams GW, Blumenkranz MS, Campo RV. Vitrectomy for diabetic macular traction and edema associated with posterior hyaloidal traction. *Ophthalmology*. 1992;99(5):753-759.
15. Harbour JW, Smiddy WE, Flynn HW Jr, Rubsamen PE. Vitrectomy for diabetic macular edema associated with a thickened and taut posterior hyaloid membrane. *Am J Ophthalmol*. 1996;121(4):405-413.
16. Pendergast SD, Hassan TS, Williams GA, et al. Vitrectomy for diffuse diabetic macular edema associated with a taut premacular posterior hyaloid. *Am J Ophthalmol*. 2000;130(2):178-186.
17. Massin P, Duguid G, Erginay A, Haouchine B, Gaudric A. Optical coherence tomography for evaluating diabetic macular edema before and after vitrectomy. *Am J Ophthalmol*. 2003;135(2):169-177.
18. Otani T, Kishi S. Tomographic assessment of vitreous surgery for diabetic macular edema. *Am J Ophthalmol*. 2000;129(4):487-494.
19. Giovannini A, Amato G, Mariotti C, Scassellati-Sforzolini B. Optical coherence tomography findings in diabetic macular edema before and after vitrectomy. *Ophthalmic Surg Lasers*. 2000;31(3):187-191.

Index to Cases

Case 5-1. Nonproliferative Diabetic Retinopathy

Clinical Summary

An 86-year-old female with poorly controlled diabetes mellitus type 2 presents with a decline in visual acuity in the left eye over 6 months. She has a prior history of focal laser treatment in both eyes for clinically significant macular edema. Dilated fundus exam of the right eye reveals a prominent epiretinal membrane, old laser scars, and scattered microaneurysms (A). Examination of the left eye reveals macular edema with intraretinal hemorrhage and exudates, consistent with diabetic retinopathy. Also noted is a prominent epiretinal membrane, leading to stretching and tortuosity of vessels (B).

Optical Coherence Tomography

Horizontal OCT scan (C) of the right eye shows a hyperreflective linear density on the surface of the retina, consistent with an epiretinal membrane. A few small hyporeflective intraretinal spaces reveal macular edema. Associated retinal thickening with loss of foveal contour is noted. The ILM-RPE overlay (D) reveals an increase in macular thickness with retinal striae. Central foveal thickness is 360 μm (E). Horizontal OCT scan (F) of the left eye shows a fragmented hyperreflective linear density on the retinal surface, consistent with an epiretinal membrane. Large, hyporeflective cavities indicate macular edema with intraretinal thickening. A central break in the epiretinal membrane is associated with prolapse of intraretinal material into the vitreous cavity. Arrows in the scan indicate intraretinal hard exudates. The ILM-RPE overlay (G) shows a diffuse increase in macular thickness. Central foveal thickness is 678 μm (H).

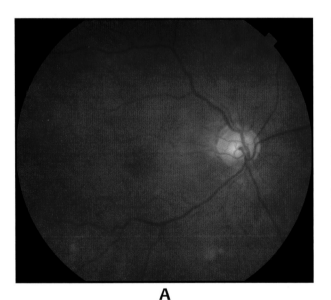

A

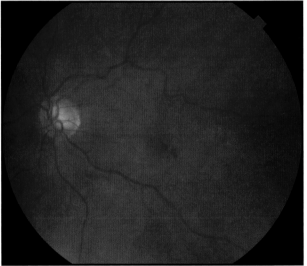

B

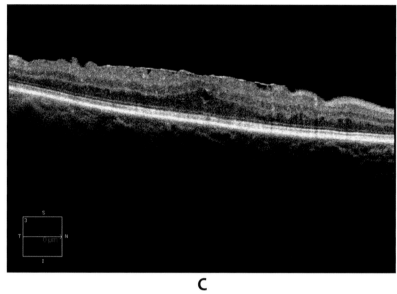

C

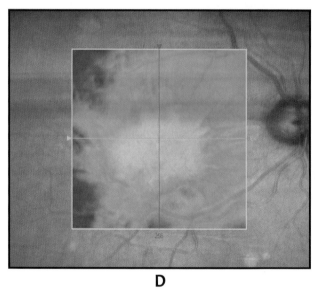

D

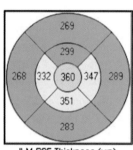

ILM-RPE Thickness (μm)

E

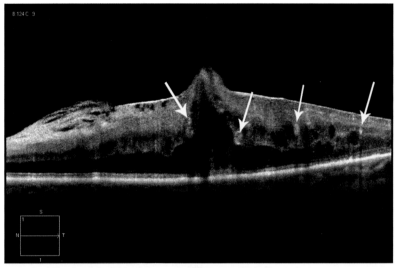

F

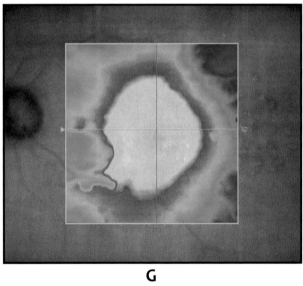

G

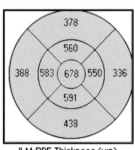

ILM-RPE Thickness (µm)

H

Case 5-2. Nonproliferative Diabetic Retinopathy With Epiretinal Membrane Formation and Macular Edema

Clinical Summary

A 67-year-old male with a history of nonproliferative diabetic retinopathy underwent focal/grid laser photocoagulation approximately 10 months earlier for clinically significant macular edema in his left eye. His visual acuity in this eye is 20/50. Dilated fundus examination of this eye shows laser scars, microaneurysms, hard lipid exudates, and retinal thickening temporal to the fovea consistent with clinically significant macular edema. An epiretinal membrane is also observed (A). Fluorescein angiography (B) demonstrates laser scars, dots of hyperfluorescence corresponding to microaneurysms, and perifoveal late leakage.

Optical Coherence Tomography

OCT (C) illustrates loss of the normal foveal contour and retinal thickening. Areas of reduced optical backscattering correspond to intraretinal fluid accumulation. Hard retinal exudates are visible as highly reflective intraretinal dots (left side of the scan). A highly reflective band corresponding to the epiretinal membrane is seen in the retinal surface. This membrane is slightly separated from the retina superotemporally (left side of the scan) and more adherent inferonasally (right side of the scan). Central macular thickness measures 519 µm (D). Focal/grid laser photocoagulation is performed.

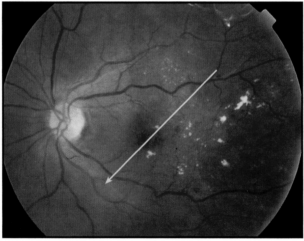

A

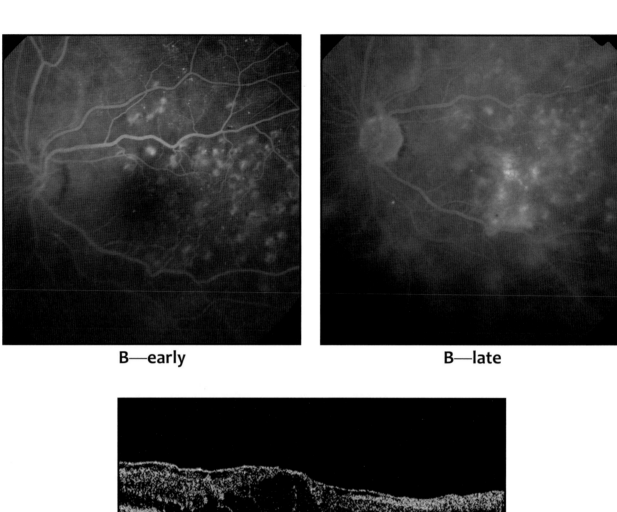

B—early   B—late

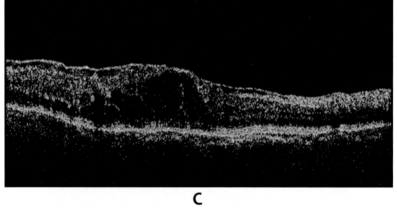

C

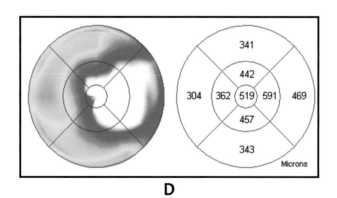

D

Case 5-3A. Diabetic Macular Edema

Clinical Summary

A 64-year-old male is referred for a decline in vision in both eyes, with a history of poorly controlled diabetes. Visual acuity measures 20/100 in the right eye and 20/40 in the left eye. Dilated fundus exam of the right eye shows diffuse dot-blot hemorrhages in the temporal macula and hard exudates temporal to and within the fovea (A). Dilated fundus exam of the left eye reveals diffuse intraretinal hemorrhages and microaneurysms. Hard exudates surround the fovea, with the maximal density temporally (B).

Optical Coherence Tomography

Horizontal OCT scan (C) of the right eye shows thickening of the retina, hyporeflective spaces within and beneath the retina, indicative of fluid accumulation. Hyperreflective particles within the retina may represent lipid particles. The ILM-RPE overlay of the right eye demonstrates areas of thickening (D). Central foveal thickness is 267 µm (E). Horizontal OCT scan (F) of the left eye reveals a normal foveal contour. Again, hyperreflective particles (arrows) within the retina likely represent lipid. The ILM-RPE overlay reveals thickening areas of the macula, sparing the fovea (G). Central foveal thickness is 215 µm (H).

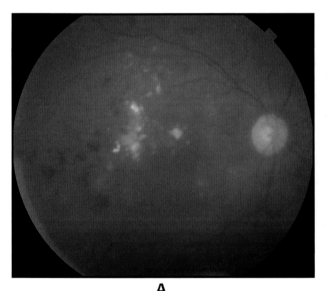

A

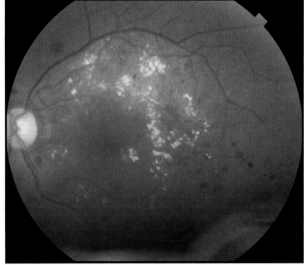

B

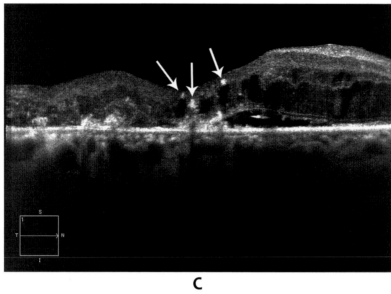

C

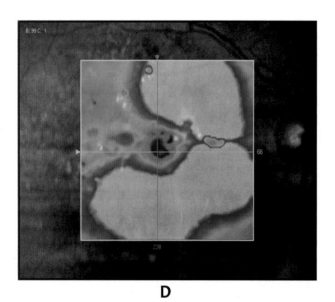

D

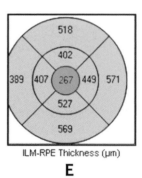

ILM-RPE Thickness (µm)

E

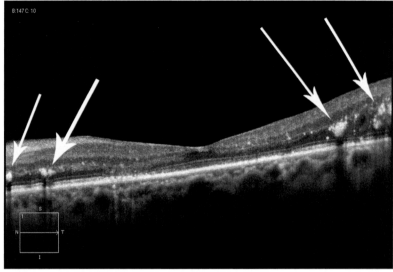

F

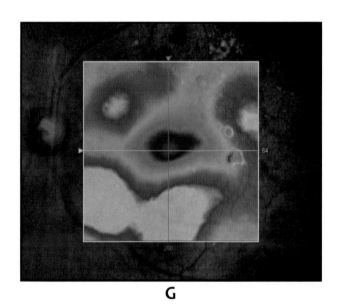

G

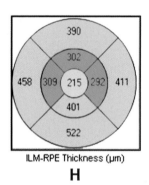

ILM-RPE Thickness (µm)

H

Case 5-3B. Diabetic Macular Edema

Clinical Summary

A 57-year-old female presents for a regular diabetic eye exam. She has no complaints. There was a history of focal laser performed for diabetic macular edema in the right eye. Visual acuity in each eye is 20/25. Dilated fundus exam of the right eye (A) reveals few dot-blot hemorrhages, laser scars inferior to the fovea, and trace thickening within the fovea. Dilated fundus exam of the left eye (B) reveals few hard exudates in the temporal macula and trace thickening within the fovea.

Optical Coherence Tomography

Horizontal OCT scan (C) of the right eye reveals 3 to 4 hyporeflective spaces within the retina, suggestive of cystoid macular edema. The ILM-RPE map (D) illustrates the area of edema. Central foveal thickness is 368 µm (E). Horizontal OCT scan (F) of the left eye reveals 2 hyporeflective intraretinal spaces suggestive of cystoid macular edema. A hyperreflective line along the surface indicates an epiretinal membrane. Again, the ILM-RPE overlay (G) demonstrates the area of edema. Central foveal thickness is 331 µm (H).

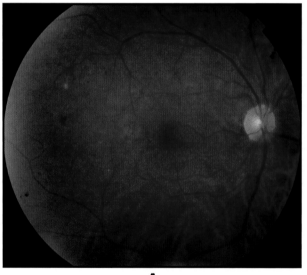

A

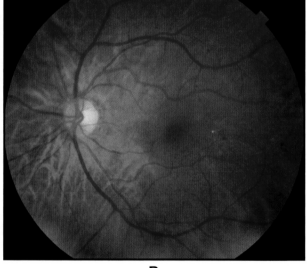

B

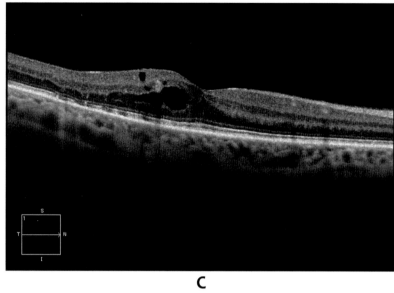

C

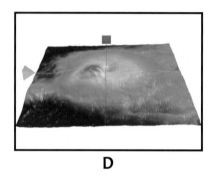

D

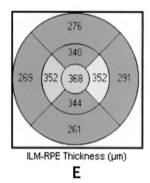

ILM-RPE Thickness (µm)

E

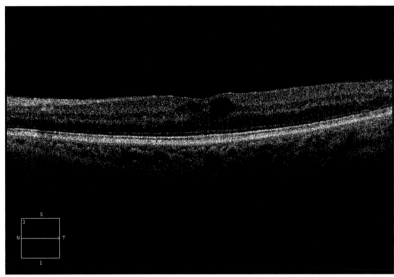

F

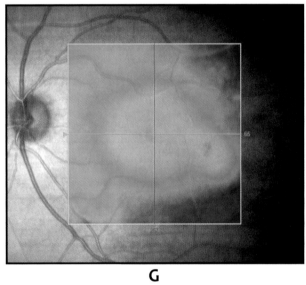

G

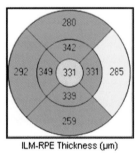

ILM-RPE Thickness (μm)

H

Case 5-4. Proliferative Diabetic Retinopathy

Clinical Summary

A 63-year-old male is referred for bleeding in the left eye. He had undergone a pars plana vitrectomy in the left eye 5 months prior. He complains of poor vision in the left eye without recent change. Visual acuity measures 20/25 in the right eye and 20/800 in the left eye. Dilated fundus examination of the left eye reveals complete panretinal photocoagulation scars, a combined rhegmatogenous and tractional detachment with an eccentric macular hole, and a preretinal membrane inferiorly (A). The patient underwent pars plana vitrectomy for repair of the detachment. Visual acuity at the 2-month follow-up improved to 20/200. Fundus exam reveals a flat retina and laser around the macular hole (B).

Optical Coherence Tomography

Initial horizontal OCT scan (C) shows a large hyporeflective cavity beneath the neurosensory retina, causing bullous elevation of the neurosensory retina, suggestive of a retinal detachment. Hyporeflective spaces within the retina are probably due to fluid accumulation. Isoreflective linear densities within the retina likely suggest Müller's cells. Central foveal thickness is 772 μm (D). The ILM-RPE overlay reveals the area of the macula not captured due to elevation of the retina (E). Horizontal OCT scan (F) 2 months following surgical repair shows an absence of subretinal fluid, mild thickening of the retina with few hyporeflective spaces, and a mildly abnormal foveal contour. Central foveal thickness is 366 μm (G). The ILM-RPE overlay reveals the improved macular contour (H).

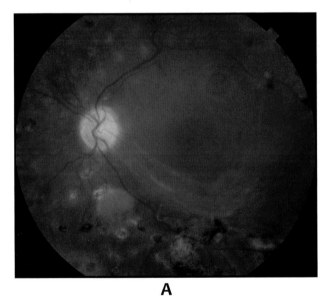

A

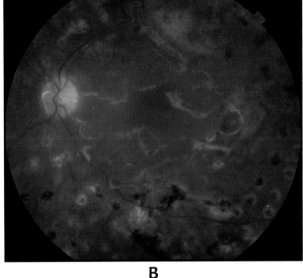

B

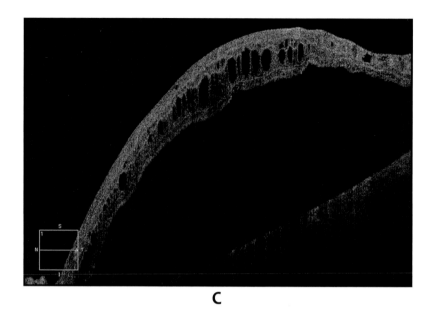

C

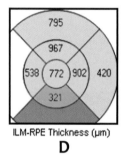

ILM-RPE Thickness (μm)

D

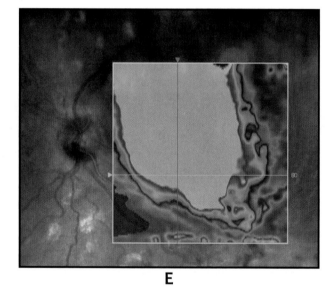

E

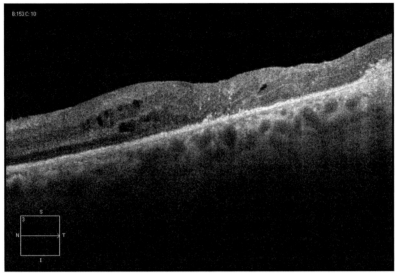

F

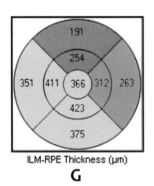

ILM-RPE Thickness (µm)

G

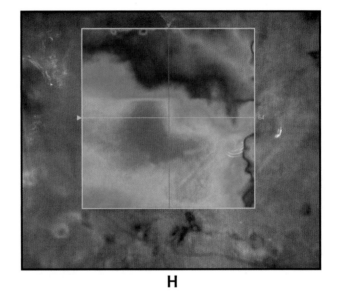

H

Case 5-5. Proliferative Diabetic Retinopathy With Macular Edema

Clinical Summary

A 62-year-old male presents for a diabetic eye exam. He has a history of proliferative diabetic retinopathy and laser for this in the past. Visual acuity is 20/400 in the right eye and 20/60 in the left eye. Dilated fundus exam of the right eye (A) reveals peripheral laser scars, scattered intraretinal hemorrhages, macular edema, and sclerotic vessels temporal to the fovea. Fundus exam of the left eye (B) reveals intraretinal hemorrhages, hard exudates inferior and temporal to the fovea, and intraretinal microvascular abnormalities along the superior arcade.

Optical Coherence Tomography

Horizontal OCT scan (C) of the right eye reveals large intraretinal hyporeflective spaces, suggestive of macular edema. Nasally, a small hyperreflective line at the retinal surface demonstrates an epiretinal membrane. Diffuse loss of foveal contour is noted. The ILM-RPE overlay (D) illustrates the retinal contour. Central foveal thickness is 372 µm (E). Horizontal OCT scan (F) of the left eye reveals a few large hyporeflective spaces within the retina, again suggestive of macular edema. An epiretinal membrane is evident. Several hyperreflective particles within the retina likely represent intraretinal lipid. The ILM-RPE overlay (G) illustrates the retinal contour. Central retinal thickness is 353 µm (H).

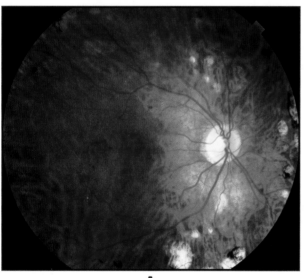

A

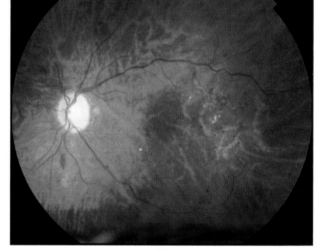

B

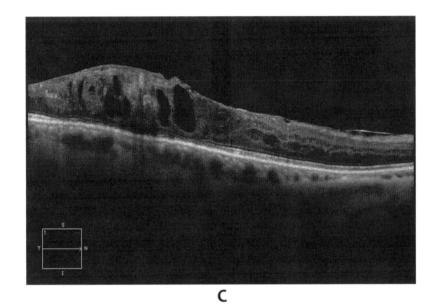

C

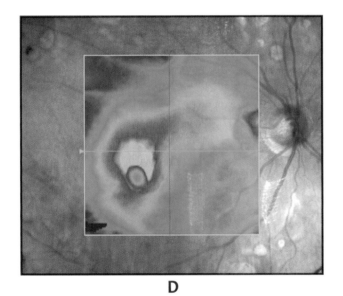

D

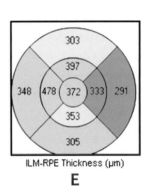

ILM-RPE Thickness (µm)

E

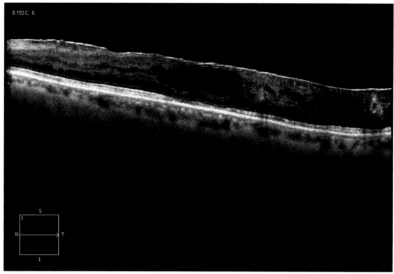

F

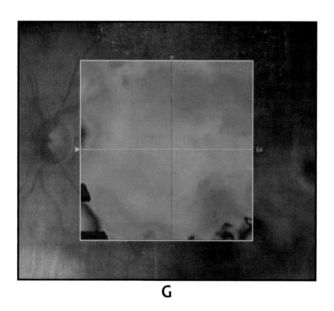

G

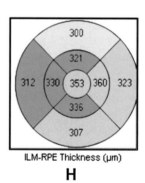

ILM-RPE Thickness (µm)

H

Case 5-6. Proliferative Diabetic Retinopathy and Taut Posterior Hyaloid

Clinical Summary

A 59-year-old female with proliferative diabetic retinopathy had received panretinal laser photocoagulation 12 months earlier. Her visual acuity in the right eye is 20/200. Dilated fundus examination reveals panretinal laser scars, retinal thickening in the macular region, and no evidence of active neovascularization (A). Fluorescein angiography (B) reveals perifoveal leakage in a petalloid fashion consistent with cystoid macular edema.

Optical Coherence Tomography

A vertical OCT scan (C) through the fovea reveals a taut posterior hyaloid represented as hyperreflective bands exerting traction on the macular region. Macular thickening and large areas of low intraretinal reflectivity, corresponding to intraretinal cysts and fluid accumulation, are also appreciated. The retinal map analysis reveals a foveal thickness of 503 μm (D). Pars plana vitrectomy is offered to the patient.

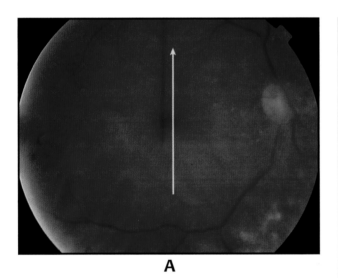

A

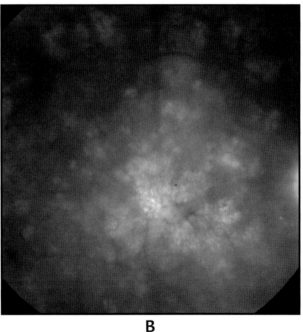

B

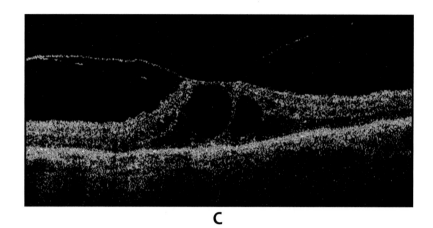

C

D

Microns

Case 5-7. Proliferative Diabetic Retinopathy With Preretinal Fibroglial Tissue

Clinical Summary

A 55-year-old female with a history of proliferative diabetic retinopathy and macular ischemia is evaluated. The left eye has a visual acuity of 20/300. Dilated fundus examination (A) reveals scattered dot-blot hemorrhages throughout the posterior pole and fibroglial tissue extending from the superotemporal arcade toward the inferior peripapillary area. Panretinal photocoagulation laser scars are noted in the periphery.

Optical Coherence Tomography

OCT images (B) illustrate loss of the normal foveal contour and a preretinal hyperreflective band adherent to the retinal surface. This preretinal membrane is separated from the retina inferonasally (right side of the scan). The retinal map analysis reveals a foveal thickness of 317 μm (C).

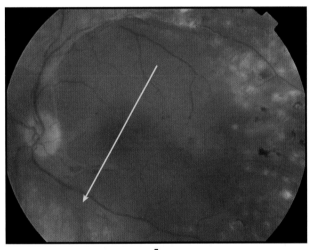

A

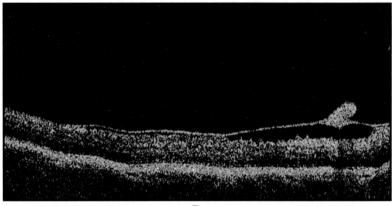

B

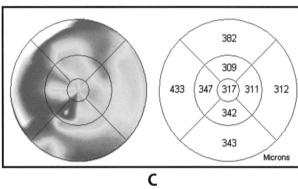

C

Case 5-8. *Proliferative Diabetic Retinopathy With Macular Schisis Formation*

Clinical Summary

A 77-year-old female with a history of proliferative diabetic retinopathy and poor vision in the right eye is examined. Her visual acuity is hand motions in this eye. Clinical examination reveals sclerotic retinal vessels and diffuse pigmentary and cystic alterations in the macular region (A). Fluorescein angiography (B) shows staining and diffuse leakage in the posterior pole.

Optical Coherence Tomography

A vertical OCT scan (C) illustrates a splitting at the level of the outer retinal layers forming a schisis. An opening of the inner retina is observed. Another OCT image (D) shows cystic low reflective intraretinal spaces. Again, the hole or opening of the inner retina is visualized reminiscent of a giant lamellar hole with a schitic configuration. Probably rupture of the macular cysts created this configuration. Central foveal thickness measures 434 µm (E).

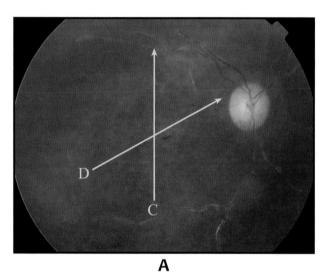

A

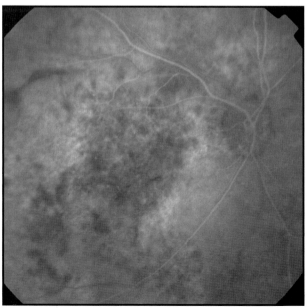

B—early

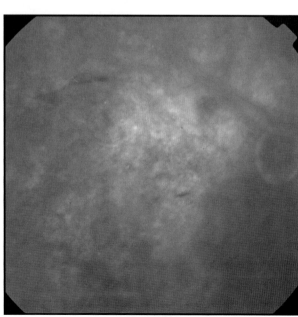

B—late

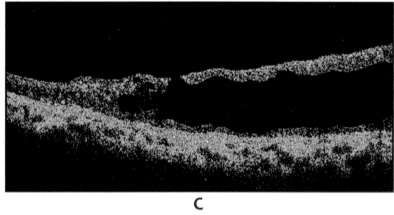

C

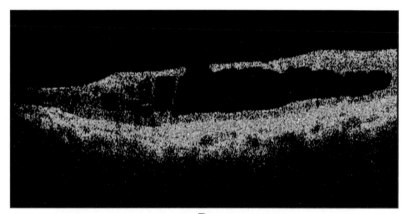

D

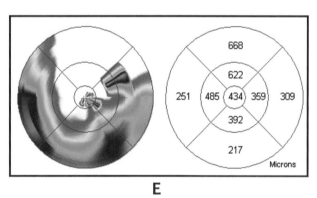

E

Chapter 6

Central Serous Chorioretinopathy

Heeral R. Shah, MD; Elias C. Mavrofrides, MD;
Carmen A. Puliafito, MD, MBA; James G. Fujimoto, PhD; and Jay S. Duker, MD

- Typical Central Serous Chorioretinopathy
- Chronic Central Serous Chorioretinopathy
- Bullous Central Serous Chorioretinopathy
- Laser Treatment for Central Serous Chorioretinopathy
- Central Serous Chorioretinopathy RTVue-100
- Photodynamic Therapy Treatment for Central Serous Chorioretinopathy

Central serous chorioretinopathy (CSCR) is characterized by serous detachment of the neurosensory retina in the macular region. This condition occurs most commonly in healthy individuals between 20 to 50 years of age, and there is a strong male predominance.[1,2] Stressful events, "type A" personality, pregnancy, and steroid use are common predisposing factors to this condition.[3-6]

Patients usually present with complaints of decreased and distorted central visual acuity. Micropsia, central scotoma, and decreased color vision are also common complaints. Most patients show evidence of a well-circumscribed neurosensory detachment in the macular region. The fovea is frequently involved, and small associated pigment epithelial detachments are commonly seen.[1,2]

Fluorescein angiography shows one or more focal leaks at the level of the retinal pigment epithelium (RPE) with subsequent pooling of dye in the subretinal space. Indocyanine green angiography typically demonstrates large hyperfluorescent patches with late leakage, suggesting abnormal choroidal hyperpermeability as an etiologic factor.[1,2,7]

Optical coherence tomography (OCT) has become an effective means for both qualitative and quantitative evaluation of patients with CSCR. Serous detachment of the neurosensory retina can be seen on the OCT image as elevation of the retinal layers above an optically clear fluid-filled cavity. When the underlying pigment epithelium remains attached, this can be seen as a highly reflective band at the base of this clear cavity.

The serous pigment epithelial detachments that frequently accompany elevation of the neurosensory retina are also readily identified on the OCT image. These appear as localized elevations of the highly reflective RPE signal over a clear cavity. The detached RPE causes attenuation of the reflected light, resulting in extensive shadowing of the underlying choroidal signal. This sign can be helpful in distinguishing retinal detachment from larger serous RPE detachments. Occasionally, the reflection from the posterior surface of detached neurosensory retina may be increased and mimic a detachment of the RPE; however, in this case, there is only minimal shadowing of the choroidal signal.[8]

In some cases, diagnosis of CSCR can be difficult due to shallow subretinal fluid. Despite significant visual complaints, there may be minimal changes identified on clinical exam. OCT is highly sensitive in establishing small elevations of the retina because of the clear difference in optical reflectivity between retinal tissue and serous fluid. Wang and associates reported on a series of 7 patients with classic

Schuman JS, Puliafito CA, Fujimoto JG, Duker JS, eds.
Optical Coherence Tomography of Ocular Diseases,
Third Edition (pp 171-196).
© 2013 SLACK Incorporated.

symptoms of CSCR in which the presence of sub-retinal fluid could not be definitely established with biomicroscopy or fluorescein angiography.[9] All of these patients showed shallow elevation of the neurosensory retina on OCT imaging, demonstrating that OCT is superior to these other techniques in identifying such detachments.

OCT imaging can be useful in defining anatomic changes of the detached neurosensory retina. Hee and associates were the first to describe thickening of the detached neurosensory retina with intraretinal cystic changes in a case of CSCR.[8] Iida and associates have subsequently demonstrated thickening of the detached retina in 23 patients during the acute phase of CSCR. Despite this thickening, most patients maintained some evidence of a foveal pit in the area of detachment. All patients showed a statistically significant decrease in foveal thickness following resolution of the neurosensory detachment.[10]

Although CSCR typically occurs in young patients, this condition can be seen in the elderly. In these cases, it may be difficult to differentiate this condition clinically from age-related macular degeneration and subretinal neovascularization.[11] In addition, occult choroidal neovascularization may have a similar angiographic appearance to CSCR when a focal leakage point is present. OCT can provide additional information to distinguish these conditions by confirming the presence of a serous neurosensory detachment versus the abnormalities in the RPE and choriocapillaris that result from neovascular membranes (see Chapter 7).

One of the most important applications of OCT in CSCR is quantitative monitoring of the clinical course over time. Most cases of CSCR will resolve spontaneously over 4 to 6 months. Therapeutic interventions such as focal laser or photodynamic therapy are considered when there is persistence of fluid, recurrence of fluid, and/or significant visual dysfunction.[1,2]

Quantitative measurements of subretinal fluid on OCT can be used to identify changes on follow-up examinations. This can be extremely useful in determining proper management. Small improvements may not be recognized by the patient and may be difficult to establish on clinical exam alone. Quantitatively establishing even small reductions in subretinal fluid may indicate the need for further observation. Conversely, documenting persistent or increased subretinal fluid after a period of observation can provide the impetus for intervention.

References

1. Gass JDM. Pathogenesis of disciform detachment of the neuroepithelium, II: idiopathic central serous chorioretinopathy. *Am J Ophthalmol*. 1976;63:587-615.
2. Ciardella AP, Guyer DR, Spitznas M, Yannuzzi LA. Central serous chorioretinopathy. In: Ryan SA, ed. *Retina*. St. Louis, MO: Mosby; 2001:1169-1170.
3. Gelber GS, Schatz H. Loss of vision due to central serous chorioretinopathy following psychological stress. *Am J Psychiatry*. 1987;144:46-50.
4. Yannuzzi LA. Type-A behavior and central serous chorioretinopathy. *Retina*. 1987;7:111-131.
5. Gass JDM. Central serous chorioretinopathy and white subretinal exudation during pregnancy. *Arch Ophthalmol*. 1991;109:677-681.
6. Gass JD, Little H. Bilateral bullous exudative retinal detachment complicating idiopathic central serous chorioretinopathy during systemic corticosteroid therapy. *Ophthalmology*. 1995;102:737-747.
7. Piccolino FC, Borgia L. Central serous chorioretinopathy and indocyanine green angiography. *Retina*. 1994;14:231-242.
8. Hee MR, Puliafito CA, Wong C, et al. Optical coherence tomography (OCT) of central serous chorioretinopathy. *Am J Ophthalmol*. 1995;120:65-74.
9. Wang M, Sander B, Lund-Anderson H, Larsen M. Detection of shallow detachments in central serous chorioretinopathy. *Acta Ophthalmol Scand*. 1999;77:402-405.
10. Iida T, Norikazu H, Sato T, Kishi S. Evaluation of central serous chorioretinopathy with optical coherence tomography. *Ophthalmology*. 2000;129:16-20.
11. Schatz H, Madeira D, Johnson RN, McDonald HR. Central serous chorioretinopathy occurring in patients 60 years of age and older. *Ophthalmology*. 1992;99:63-67.

Index to Cases

Case 6-1. Central Serous Chorioretinopathy—Typical

Clinical Summary

A 49-year-old male presents with a recent decline in visual acuity in the left eye. Visual acuity is 20/70 in the left eye. Dilated fundus exam (A) reveals RPE mottling and subretinal fluid within the fovea. Fluorescein angiography (B) shows a pinpoint area of leakage within the fovea and staining superonasal to the fovea.

Optical Coherence Tomography

Horizontal OCT scan (C) reveals 2 areas of elevation of the RPE, indicating detachment of the RPE, and a large hyporeflective cavity beneath the neurosensory retina, indicative of subretinal fluid. Central retinal thickness is 333 μm (D). The ILM-RPE map demonstrates the retinal contour (E).

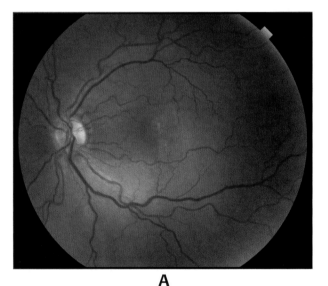

A

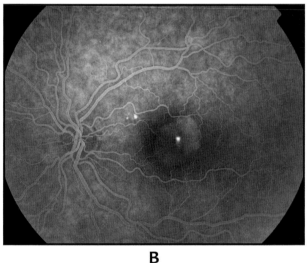

B

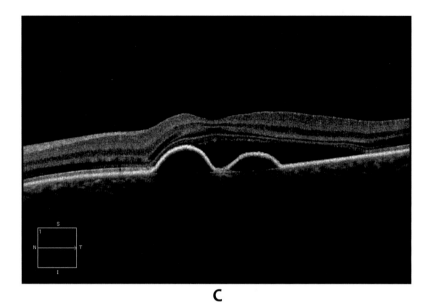

C

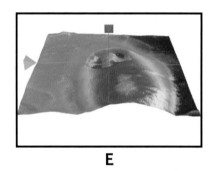

ILM-RPE Thickness (µm)

D

E

Case 6-2A. Central Serous Chorioretinopathy—Chronic

Clinical Summary

An 82-year-old male presents with fluctuating vision in both eyes over the past 4 years. Visual acuity measures 20/40 in each eye. Dilated fundus exam of the right eye shows an area of subretinal fluid superior to the fovea, retinal pigment mottling, few drusen, and choroidal folds in the temporal macula (A). Fundus examination of the left eye reveals diffuse mottling of pigment epithelium in the superior macula (B).

Optical Coherence Tomography

Horizontal OCT scan (C) of the right eye shows hyporeflective spaces nasal and temporal to the fovea, suggestive of macular edema. The posterior hyaloid face is intact at a focal point with elevation of the retina. The choroid appears thickened. Central retinal thickness is 306 µm (D). The ILM-RPE map demonstrates the retinal contour (E). Horizontal OCT scan (F) of the left eye reveals hyporeflective spaces within the outer retina, nasal to the fovea, suggestive of macular edema. Again, the choroid appears thickened. Central retinal thickness is 201 µm (G). The ILM-RPE map, again, reveals the retinal contour (H).

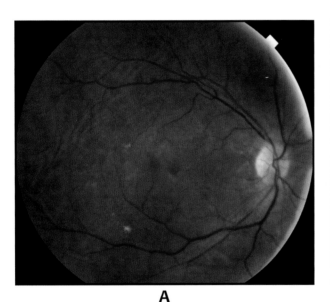

A

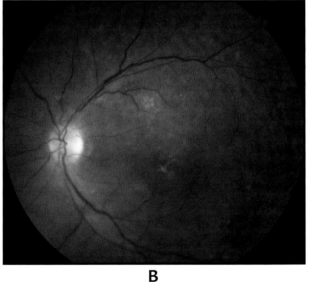

B

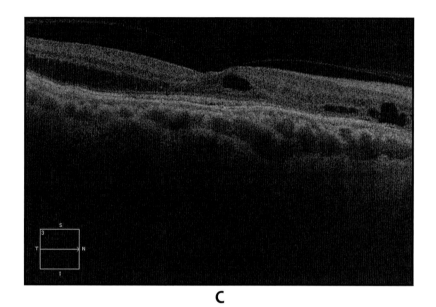

C

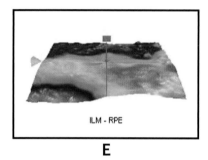

ILM-RPE Thickness (µm)

D

ILM - RPE

E

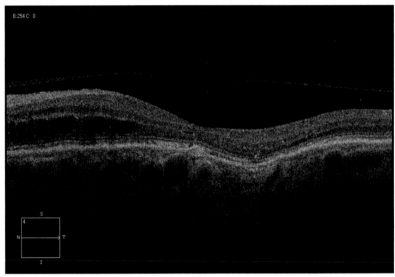

F

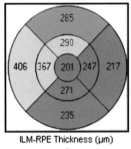

ILM-RPE Thickness (µm)

G

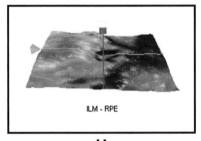

ILM - RPE

H

Case 6-2B. Central Serous Chorioretinopathy— Chronic

Clinical Summary

A 71-year-old female presents with a decline in vision in the left eye. Visual acuity in the right eye is 20/25 and in the left eye is 20/40. Dilated fundus exam of the left eye (A) reveals RPE mottling and trace subretinal fluid superior to the fovea.

Optical Coherence Tomography

Horizontal OCT scan (B) of the left eye reveals a small hyporeflective space beneath the retina. Loss of foveal contour is noted. The ILM-RPE map (C) illustrates the retinal contour. Retinal thickness in the area of fluid reaches 325 μm (D). She is treated with intravitreal bevacizumab.

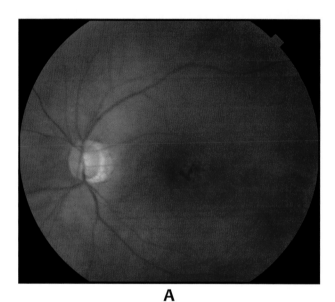

A

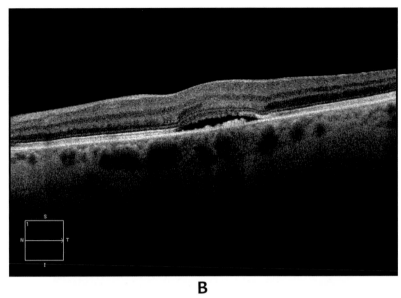

B

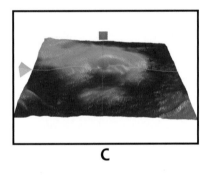

C

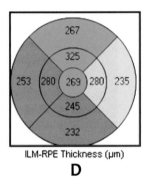

ILM-RPE Thickness (µm)

D

Case 6-2B. Central Serous Chorioretinopathy— Chronic (continued)

Follow-Up

She returns for a follow-up visit with no change in her vision. Dilated fundus exam is unchanged. Horizontal OCT scan (E) reveals persistent subretinal fluid. At the point, she is treated with reduced fluence photodynamic therapy. On follow-up visit, her visual acuity has improved to 20/25 in the left eye. Dilated fundus exam (F) reveals RPE mottling.

Horizontal OCT scan (G) demonstrates an absence of fluid, disruption of the outer retinal layers, and thickening of the RPE, while the ILM-RPE map (H) reveals the change in retinal contour. Central foveal thickness is 219 μm (I).

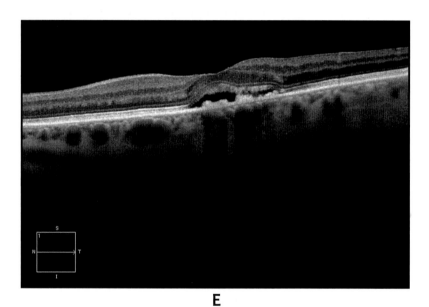

E

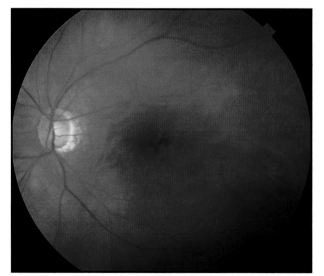

F

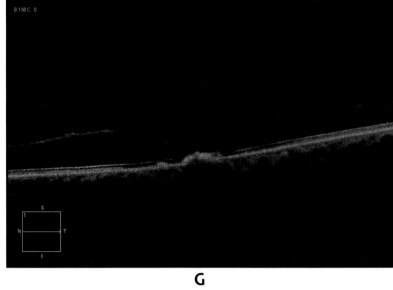

G

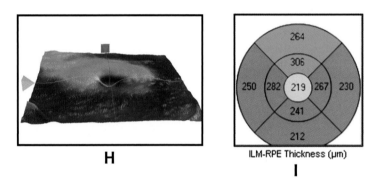

H

ILM-RPE Thickness (μm)

I

Case 6-3. Central Serous Chorioretinopathy—Bullous

Clinical Summary

A 33-year-old female presents with a decline in vision in the left eye. Visual acuity in the left eye is 20/200. Dilated fundus exam reveals a large central neurosensory detachment (A).

Optical Coherence Tomography

Obliquely oriented OCT scan (B) demonstrates a large hyporeflective cavity beneath the retina, indicating subretinal fluid. The ILM-RPE overlay (C) illustrates the area of retinal involvement. Central foveal thickness is 963 μm (D).

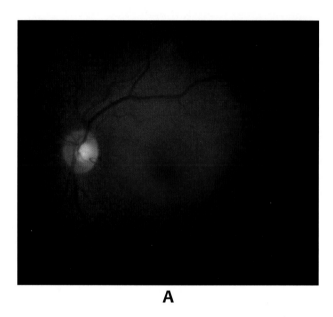

A

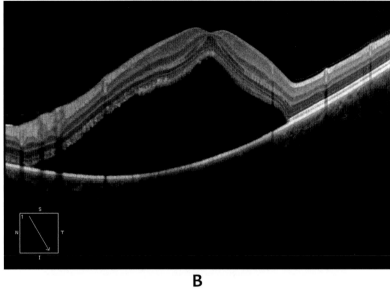

B

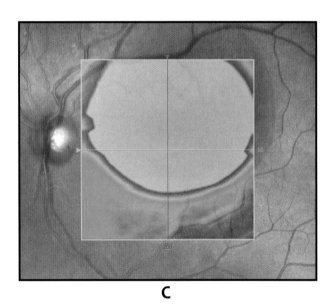

C

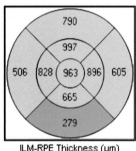

ILM-RPE Thickness (µm)

D

Case 6-4. Central Serous Chorioretinopathy Treated With Laser

Clinical Summary

A 58-year-old male presents with complaints of blurry vision in the right eye for several years. Visual acuity in the right eye is 20/60 and the left eye is 20/25. Dilated fundus exam of the right eye reveals an epiretinal membrane, RPE changes, and a small amount of subretinal fluid (A). Fluorescein angiography reveals late leakage within the papillomacular bundle of the right eye (B). This area was treated with light laser. Two months later, the patient returns with a visual acuity of 20/40 in the right eye. Fundus exam reveals RPE changes, an epiretinal membrane, and an absence of subretinal fluid (C).

Optical Coherence Tomography

Horizontal OCT scan (D) of the right eye reveals a hyperreflective linear structure along the surface of the retina, indicative of an epiretinal membrane. A shallow hyporeflective cavity present beneath the retina reveals subretinal fluid. Central foveal thickness is 364 μm (E). The ILM-RPE overlay demonstrates the retinal contour (F). Post-laser treatment, horizontal OCT scan (G) reveals an epiretinal membrane with slight irregularity of the retinal surface, trace elevation of the RPE, and no subretinal fluid. Central foveal thickness is 264 μm (H). The ILM-RPE overlay again demonstrates change in retinal contour since laser treatment (I).

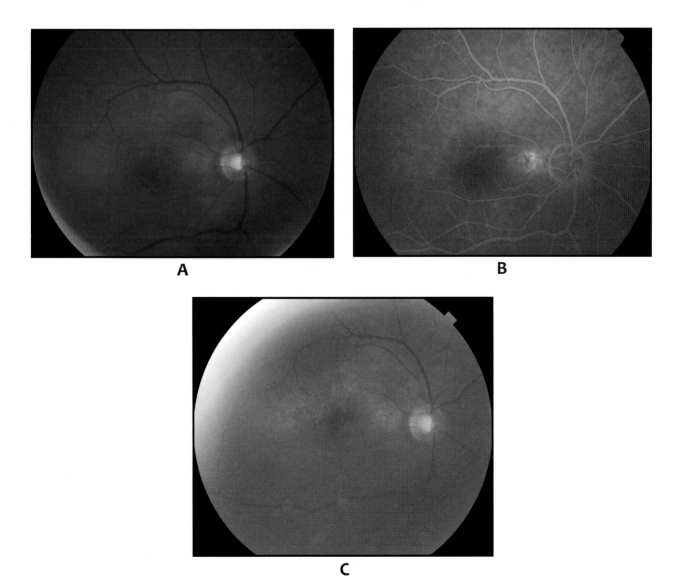

A

B

C

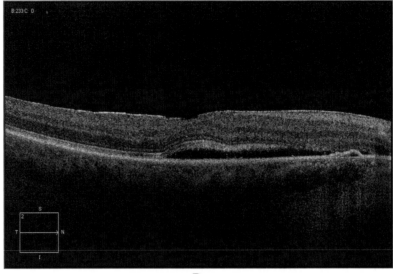

D

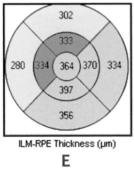

ILM-RPE Thickness (µm)

E

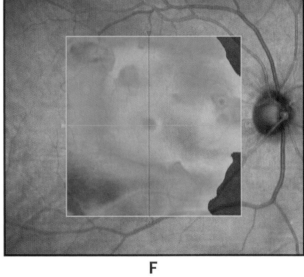

F

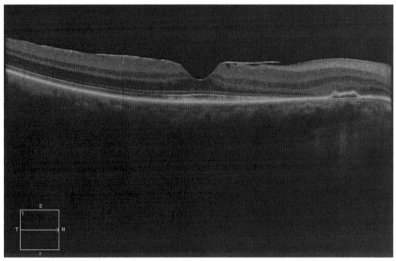

G

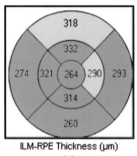

ILM-RPE Thickness (µm)

H

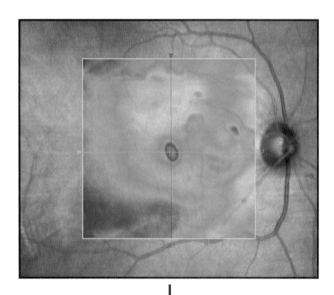

I

Case 6-5A. Central Serous Chorioretinopathy RTVue-100

Clinical Summary

A 52-year-old male presents for a decline in vision and increased distortion in the left eye. Visual acuity in the left eye is 20/25. Dilated fundus exam (A) reveals a central pigment epithelial detachment and subretinal retinal fluid in the macula.

Optical Coherence Tomography

Vertical OCT scan (B) demonstrates a diffuse hyporeflective space beneath the neurosensory retina and a focal space elevating the RPE, indicating both subretinal fluid and a detachment of the RPE. The 3D map (C) along the inferior macula reveals the retinal contour in that area.

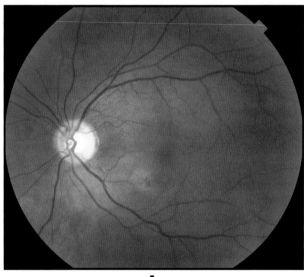

A

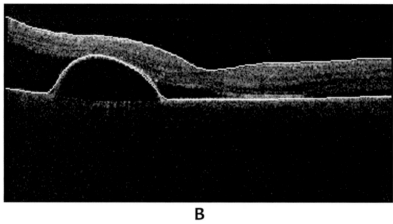

B

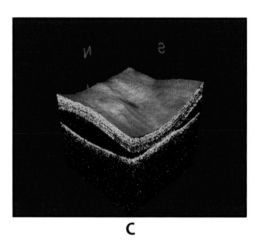

C

Case 6-5B. Central Serous Chorioretinopathy RTVue-100

Clinical Summary

A 56-year-old male presents with a recent decline in vision in the right eye. He had undergone laser treatment to the right eye 15 years ago for central serous chorioretinopathy. Visual acuity in the right eye is 20/25 and the left eye is 20/20. Dilated fundus exam of the right eye reveals trace RPE changes and subretinal fluid.

Optical Coherence Tomography

Horizontal OCT scan of the right eye (A) reveals a hyporeflective space beneath the neurosensory retina, indicating subretinal fluid. RPE-ILM overlay (B) and 3D thickness map (C) reveal the retinal contour. Central foveal thickness is 407 μm (D).

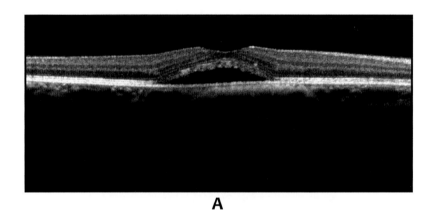

A

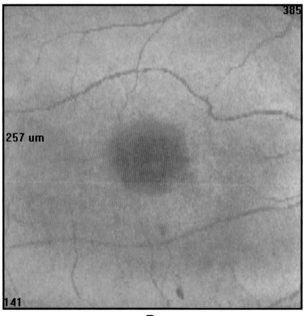

385

257 um

141

B

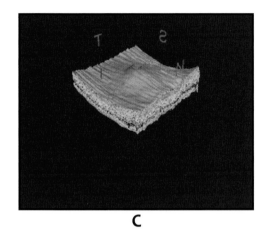

C

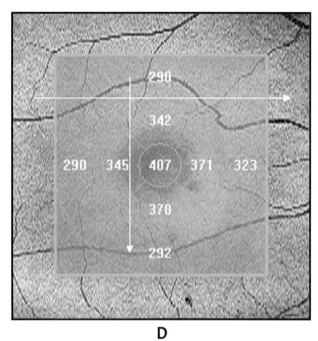

D

Case 6-6. Central Serous Chorioretinopathy Treated With Photodynamic Therapy

Clinical Summary

A 43-year-old male is referred for evaluation of chronic central serous chorioretinopathy in the left eye. His visual acuity has remained 20/70 for the past 6 months due to persistent neurosensory detachment involving the fovea (A). Fluorescein angiography (B) shows an area of leakage just superior to the fovea. Indocyanine green angiography (C) demonstrates a placoid area of hyperfluorescence under the fovea.

Optical Coherence Tomography

OCT imaging (D) acquired through the fovea confirms detachment of the neurosensory retina. The high-intensity signal beneath the fluid cavity corresponds to the RPE, indicating neurosensory detachment without RPE detachment.

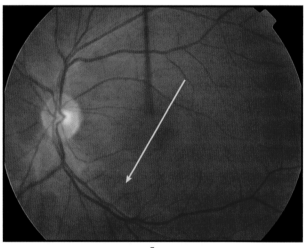

A

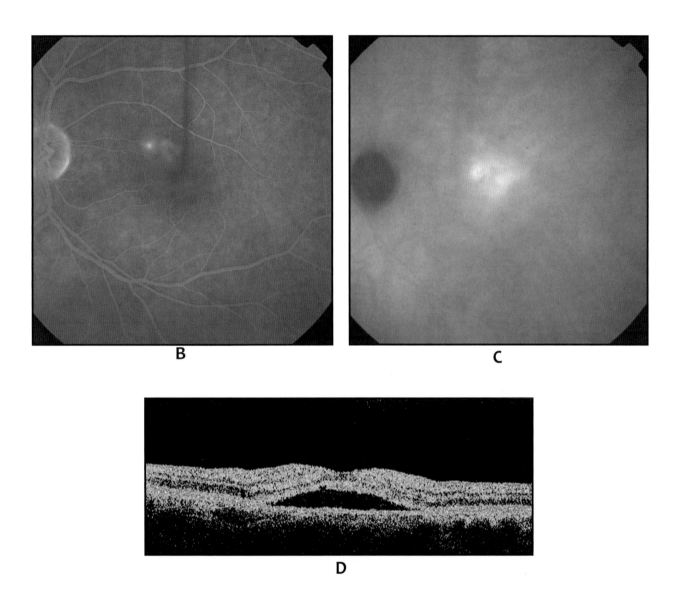

Case 6-6. Central Serous Chorioretinopathy
Treated With Photodynamic Therapy (continued)

Continuation of Clinical Summary

Because this condition is chronic and creating significant visual dysfunction, intervention is indicated. There are concerns about proceeding with focal laser to the leakage site because of the proximity to the fovea. The patient, therefore, undergoes photodynamic therapy to the area of hyperfluorescence identified on indocyanine green angiography. The patient notices normalization of his vision within 3 weeks of the treatment. At the return visit 2 months after treatment, his vision is 20/20. Dilated fundus exam (E) shows mild pigmentary mottling but no subretinal fluid. Fluorescein angiography (F) shows mottled fluorescence but no evidence of leakage.

Follow-Up
Optical Coherence Tomography

The post-treatment OCT tomogram (G) taken through the fovea shows resolution of the neurosensory detachment with normalization of the foveal contour. There is mild irregularity of the RPE signal consistent with the pigmentary changes on exam.

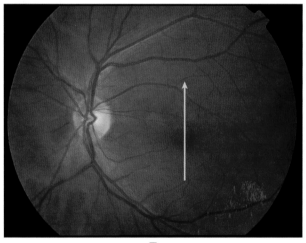

E

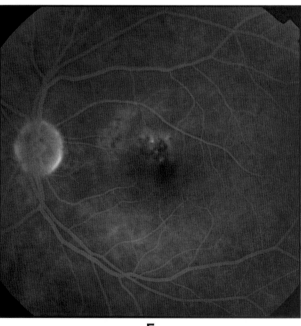

F

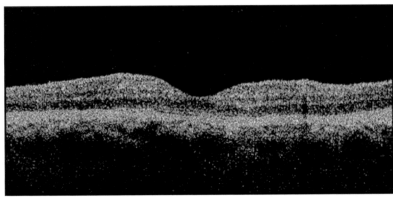

G

Chapter 7

Age-Related Macular Degeneration

Heeral R. Shah, MD; Elias C. Mavrofrides, MD;
Natalia Villate, MD; Philip J. Rosenfeld, MD, PhD;
Carmen A. Puliafito, MD, MBA; and Jay S. Duker, MD

- Drusen
- Adult Vitelliform Dystrophy
- Geographic Atrophy
- Occult Choroidal Neovascularization
- Vascularized Pigment Epithelial Detachment
- Retinal Angiomatous Proliferation
- Retinal Pigment Epithelium Tear
- Subretinal Hemorrhage
- Disciform Scar

Age-related macular degeneration (ARMD) is the leading cause of irreversible severe vision loss among the elderly in Western populations.[1] The cause of ARMD remains elusive and complex, with both environmental and genetic contributions.[2,3] ARMD has 2 distinct forms known as *dry* (non-neovascular) and *wet* (neovascular). Neovascular ARMD evolves from non-neovascular ARMD and represents a late stage of the disease. Neovascular ARMD gets its name from the formation of choroidal neovascularization (CNV) under the macula or the formation of intraretinal neovascularization or a combination of both processes. Most of the severe vision loss in ARMD is caused by neovascular ARMD, but neovascular ARMD represents only a minority of ARMD cases. Proven therapies for ARMD treat the neovascular form of the disease and included only thermal laser photocoagulation and verteporfin photodynamic therapy (PDT) in the past. Recent studies have proven that intravitreal ranibizumab and bevacizumab result in significant

improvement in visual acuity.[4,5] Furthermore, 2-year data comparing ranibizumab to verteporfin PDT demonstrated that ranibizumab provided greater clinical benefit than PDT.[6] Intravitreal ranibizumab and bevacizumab now have a leading role in the treatment of neovascular ARMD.

Optical coherence tomography (OCT) allows cross-sectional imaging of the retina with an axial resolution of approximately 5 μm, providing images that permit identification and differentiation of detailed structures within the neurosensory retina including the inner and outer segment (IS/OS) junction, the underlying retinal pigment epithelium (RPE)/Bruch's/choriocapillaris complex, and in some cases, even the deeper choroid. When performed by an experienced technician, OCT provides both qualitative and quantitative information about these structures and allows for the examination of these structures over time to assess disease progression.[7-10] OCT is a noninvasive, dynamic technology ideal for observing the natural course of ARMD. The structural information provided by OCT is becoming a valuable diagnostic adjunct to fluorescein and indocyanine green angiography. The goal of using OCT is to correlate these observed structural changes to changes in visual acuity, not only to better understand the mechanism of vision loss associated with ARMD, but also to understand the mechanism of visual acuity benefits attributed to various treatments. In particular, OCT is a valuable tool for probing the treatment effects associated with PDT as well

Schuman JS, Puliafito CA, Fujimoto JG, Duker JS, eds.
Optical Coherence Tomography of Ocular Diseases,
Third Edition (pp 197-236).
© 2013 SLACK Incorporated.

as periocular and intraocular pharmacologic therapy in neovascular ARMD.

Drusen are a characteristic fundus finding associated with non-neovascular or dry ARMD.[11] Soft drusen are observed as modulations in the external, highly reflective band consistent with the accumulation of material within or beneath Bruch's membrane. The localized elevation of the external band associated with drusen is shallow compared to the more pronounced scatter-free elevation observed with a serous pigment epithelial detachment (PED). Within the elevation associated with drusen, there is a mild backscatter of the signal probably resulting from the accumulated material that forms the drusen.

Geographic atrophy is a late stage of dry ARMD devoid of drusen and resulting from the loss of RPE and underlying choriocapillaris. This stage has a distinctive appearance on OCT,[7,12] with thinning of the overlying retina and the external band, which represents the RPE/Bruch's/choriocapillaris complex. The loss of the choriocapillaris and the resulting scatter caused by the circulating red blood cells permit increased penetration of the light deeper into the choroid, significantly enhancing the reflections from this layer.

Serous PEDs present as localized, dome-shaped elevations of the external high reflective band that appear optically empty with sharp margins. Reflections from the deeper choroid can be appreciated. This ability to visualize the deeper choroid can be attributed to increased penetration of the probe light through the decompensated RPE, a PED containing low reflective serous fluid, and diminished circulation within the choriocapillaris.

Hemorrhagic PEDs are notable for the absence of reflectance from the choroid with loss of the choroidal image due to the scattering of light from the blood under the RPE. The loss of choroidal detail correlates with the thickness of the blood.

Neovascular lesions have a distinct appearance on fluorescein and indocyanine green angiography, and these imaging modalities have served as the standards for assessing lesion types and disease progression or regression.[11] While OCT cannot predict with certainty the angiographic appearance of neovascular lesions, there are characteristic features observed on OCT that complement angiography and may even serve as better predictors of disease status. OCT has the advantage of discriminating small changes in the structure of the retinal layers and subretinal space, allowing for precise anatomic detection of structural changes that may signal progression or regression of the lesions.

Classic CNV is defined by fluorescein angiography as early bright, lacy hyperfluorescence associated with late leakage that typically obscures the initial boundaries of the CNV on the angiogram.[11] OCT imaging of classic CNV lesions may reveal a fusiform enlargement of the RPE/Bruch's/choriocapillaris reflective band with defined borders. The highly reflective band may appear irregular and duplicated, with high backscattering material between the 2 bands. Occasionally, it may be possible to image the membrane above the RPE (type 2 CNV).

Subretinal fluid appears on OCT imaging as an optically clear space adjacent to the presumed CNV. This space represents a collection of fluid that can be evaluated quantitatively with OCT. Visual acuity may be reduced by causes other than the presence of subretinal fluid, such as macular edema.

Macular edema can be focal, such as cystoid macular edema, or diffuse macular edema, and can be easily missed when interpreting fluorescein angiography images alone due to the overwhelming fluorescence arising from the CNV. OCT has demonstrated the presence of macular edema in 46% of eyes with subfoveal CNV from ARMD, and there is a strong association between cystoid macular edema and classic CNV.[8] In contrast to fluorescein angiography, OCT is a reliable technique for distinguishing between macular edema, persistent leakage from CNV, or fibrotic scarring as the cause of vision loss. In the future, the ability to distinguish between these causes of vision loss may help in determining which treatment may be beneficial, when treatment should be initiated, and when retreatment should be offered. In particular, OCT may prove to be a valuable tool in assessing patients for retreatment with PDT, but it should be emphasized that the decision to retreat with verteporfin therapy should be based on the fluorescein angiographic findings alone until a formal clinical study using OCT alone is performed.

Occult CNV is defined by fluorescein angiography as a fibrovascular PED or as late leakage of an undetermined source.[11] A fibrovascular PED is described as an irregular elevation of the RPE that corresponds on fluorescein angiography with early stippled hyperfluorescence (usually within the first 1 to 2 minutes) going on to fluorescein leakage from CNV in the late phase. OCT imaging of fibrovascular PEDs includes a well-defined RPE elevation of the external band with a deeper area of mild backscattering corresponding to fibrous proliferation. Late leakage of an undetermined source represents speckled fluorescein leakage at the RPE level in the late phase of the angiogram without a corresponding source of leakage in the early phase. The choroidal reflection may be enhanced on the OCT image due to increased light penetration secondary to degenerative changes in the RPE/Bruch's/choriocapillaris complex. During the natural course of macular degeneration, or as the result of treatment, the configuration of the neovascular complex can change over time.

RPE tears can be identified early in their evolution by observing a PED with an undulating or corrugated external band. This may signal the development of an evolving RPE tear that may or may not be obvious on fluorescein angiography. This appearance may evolve so that the PED appears more elevated, less dome-shaped with a steeper contour, and discontinuous along the highly reflective external band at the edge of the RPE tear. The missing RPE results in increased penetration of the light deeper into the choroid, significantly enhancing the reflections from this layer. OCT can image the evolution of a tear and often identifies the site of separation and the rolling edge of the tear.

Blood in the subretinal or sub-RPE space can be distinguished using OCT imaging. Blood in the subretinal space shows an elevated and often edematous retina with a highly reflective underlying layer that is the blood. This blood causes shadowing of the underlying RPE/Bruch's/choriocapillaris complex, and this external band is not visualized. Blood in the sub-RPE space shows an elevated and intact external band with an underlying area of high reflectivity and shadowing corresponding to the blood. Choroidal details are not observed.

Subretinal fibrosis or disciform scarring is the end stage of neovascular ARMD. This area of scarring consists of white, fibrous tissue under the retina involving the RPE/Bruch's/choriocapillaris complex. This tissue is highly reflective on OCT and is frequently associated with overlying retinal atrophy.

Retinal lesion anastomoses and retinal angiomatous proliferations (RAPs) appear early as small intraretinal hemorrhages. RAPs often have these intraretinal hemorrhages overlying a serous PED.[13] As RAPs evolve, macular edema is associated with multiple intraretinal hemorrhages and the PED. The small intraretinal hemorrhages often correspond to small interruptions in the layers of the neurosensory retina as seen by OCT, often followed by the formation of an intraretinal or subretinal neovascular complex. Later in the course of the disease, the lesion appears to extend into the sub-RPE space. The clinical course of RAPs is somewhat intermediate between the usually rapid, aggressive course of classic CNV and the more insidious, slowly progressive course of occult CNV. While laser photocoagulation might be useful for the initial intraretinal neovascularization stage (Stage I: RAP), thermal laser and verteporfin therapy are not particularly useful for the treatment of later stages (Stage II: subretinal neovascularization and Stage III: CNV). There is no single ideal treatment for RAPs, but encouraging results have been observed using PDT followed by intravitreal steroids and anti-angiogenic therapy in selected cases. RAPs have proven more resistant than choroidal neovascular membrane in treatment with intravitreal antivascular endothelial growth factor agents.

Response to therapy is one of the most important clinical uses of OCT. OCT can be used to quantify changes in central retinal thickness and volume, as well as subretinal fluid. Since the evolution of intravitreal antivascular endothelial growth factor agents in the treatment of neovascular ARMD, the utility of OCT findings has exponentially increased. Although initially OCT was only used as an adjunct to clinical examination and fluorescein angiography, the more recent OCT-guided variable dosing regimen has become common practice.[14] Also, OCT provides useful information when deciding if patients require additional courses of therapy following their initial treatment with verteporfin therapy.[7] OCT, when used in conjunction with fluorescein angiography, is helpful in characterizing changes following verteporfin therapy and in detecting early accumulation of subretinal fluid associated with recurrence of CNV.

The radial scan pattern centered in the fovea allows for detailed characterization of the choroidal neovascular complex. To assess the entire lesion, all 6 scans should be reviewed. The appearance of the retina and the presence and location of subretinal fluid can be quantitatively and qualitatively assessed by comparing similar scans.

Reproducibility of the images between follow-up visits in patients with ARMD requires an experienced OCT technician. The vast majority of patients with wet ARMD do not have good fixation and are unable to see the internal fixation device of the OCT with the affected eye. If the other eye has preserved central vision, external fixation with the good eye can usually be obtained. When there is no fixation, careful attention should be given to the anatomic landmarks visualized in the video image to obtain scans that are at a similar location at every visit. Since the video image does not provide the exact location of the scan, there is no reliable method of ensuring scan reproducibility other than the expertise of the technician. Often, manual relocation of the scan line during the image acquisition process is necessary.

The topographic map of the central 6 mm gives important information about the shape of the central macula. Remodeling of the central macula is observed following treatment or as the result of natural progression of the disease. The algorithm is designed to identify the boundaries of the neurosensory retina and calculate its thickness and volume. Careful comparative analysis of the maps between visits is helpful in determining if thickened areas are in the same previous location, represent new extensions of the neovascular complex to adjacent areas, or signal the occurrence of other related complications like RPE tears or neurosensory detachments. The central thickness value provided by the map often correlates well with the visual acuity. Reproducibility of the central thickness measure in patients with poor fixation is best obtained using the fast map scan pattern. Parallel raster scans or linear pattern scans can be obtained at different levels of a lesion and off-centered from the macula to document eccentric lesions when indicated. When the anatomy of the central 6 mm is severely distorted, the interpretation of the map should proceed with caution since the displayed thickness may not represent the actual thickness of the neurosensory retina, but include areas of RPE detachment, subretinal fluid, or hemorrhages.

References

1. Klein R. Epidemiology. In: Berger JW, Fine SL, Maguire MG, eds. *Age-Related Macular Degeneration*. St. Louis, MO: Mosby; 1999:31-56.

2. Rosenfeld PJ, Gorin MB. Genetics of age-related maculopathy. In: Berger JW, Fine SL, Maguire MG, eds. *Age-Related Macular Degeneration*. St. Louis, MO: Mosby; 1999:69-80.

3. Schick JH, Iyengar SK, Klein BE, et al. A whole-genome screen of a quantitative trait of age-related maculopathy in sibships from the beaver dam eye study. *Am J Hum Genet.* 2003;72(6):1412-1424.

4. Rosenfeld PJ, Brown DM, Heier JS, et al. Ranibizumab for neovascular age-related macular degeneration. *N Engl J Med.* 2006;355(14):1419-1431.

5. Spaide RF, Laud K, Fine HF, et al. Intravitreal bevacizumab treatment of choroidal neovascularization secondary to age-related macular degeneration. *Retina.* 2006;26(4):383-390.

6. Brown DM, Michels M, Kaiser PK, et al. Ranibizumab versus verteporfin photodynamic therapy for neovascular age-related macular degeneration: two-year results of the ANCHOR study. *Ophthalmology.* 2009;116(1):57-65.

7. Rogers AH, Martidis A, Greenberg PB, Puliafito CA. Optical coherence tomography findings following photodynamic therapy of choroidal neovascularization. *Am J Ophthalmol.* 2002;134(4):566-576.

8. Ting TD, Oh M, Cox TA, Meyer CH, Toth CA. Decreased visual acuity associated with cystoid macular edema in neovascular age-related macular degeneration. *Arch Ophthalmol.* 2002;120(6):731-737.

9. Neubauer AS, Priglinger S, Ullrich S, et al. Comparison of foveal thickness measured with the retinal thickness analyzer and optical coherence tomography. *Retina.* 2001;21(6):596-601.

10. Van Kerckhoven W, Lafaut B, Follens I, De Laey JJ. Features of age-related macular degeneration on optical coherence tomography. *Bull Soc Belge Ophthalmol.* 2001;(281):75-84.

11. Macular diseases. In: Berkow JW, Flower RW, Orth DH, Kelley JS, eds. *Fluorescein and Indocyanine Green Angiography—Technique and Interpretation*. San Francisco, CA: American Academy of Ophthalmology; 1997:91-103.

12. Hassenstein A, Ruhl R, Richard G. Optical coherence tomography in geographic atrophy—a clinicopathologic correlation. *Klin Monatsbl Augenheilkd.* 2001;218(7):503-509.

13. Yannuzzi LA, Negrao S, Iida T, et al. Retinal angiomatous proliferation in age-related macular degeneration. *Retina.* 2001;21(5):416-434.

14. Lalwani GA, Rosenfeld PJ, Fung AE, et al. A variable-dosing regimen with intravitreal ranibizumab for neovascular age-related macular degeneration: year 2 of the PRONTO study. *Am J Ophthalmol.* 2009;148:43-58.

Index to Cases

Case 7-1A. Drusen

Clinical Summary

A 93-year-old male presents with no visual complaints. Visual acuity measures 20/40 in the left eye. Dilated fundus examination reveals RPE atrophy in the central macula and soft drusen superior to and within this area (A).

Optical Coherence Tomography

Horizontal OCT scan (B) shows focal hyperreflective irregularities of the RPE. The choroid is diffusely thinned. Intraretinal hyperreflective particles (arrow) are suggestive of intraretinal pigment migration. The RPE map (C) better demonstrates these focal findings superior to the macula.

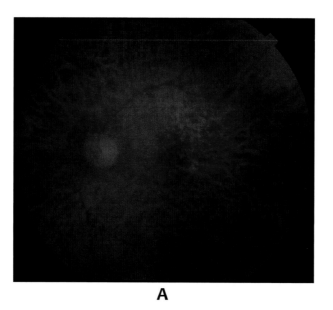

A

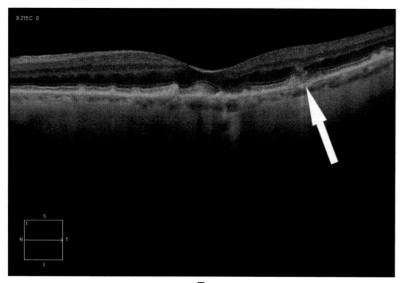

B

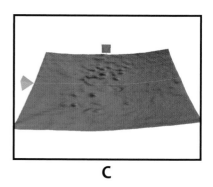

C

Case 7-1B. Drusen

Clinical Summary

A 61-year-old male presents for annual examination with complaints of mild blurring of vision in the right eye. Dilated fundus examination reveals soft, confluent drusen in the central macula (A).

Optical Coherence Tomography

Horizontal OCT scan (B) shows hyperreflective focal irregularities of the RPE, causing elevation of the photoreceptor layer. The RPE map demonstrates these changes more clearly (C).

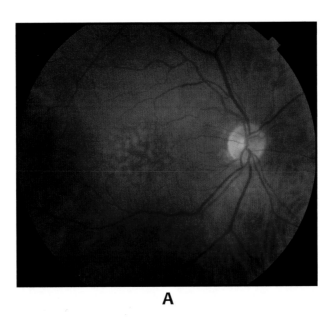

A

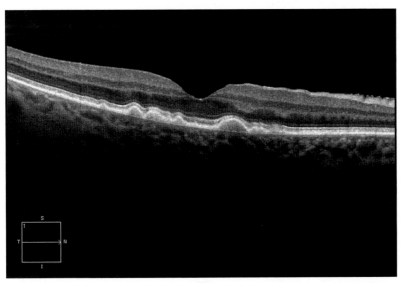

B

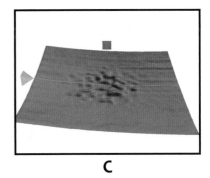

C

Case 7-2. Basal Laminar Drusen

Clinical Summary

A 67-year-old male presents with a decline in vision over the past 6 months. Visual acuity in each eye is 20/70. Dilated fundus exam of each eye reveals an area of central atrophy surrounded by prominent macular drusen (A, B). The inferior margin of the atrophy has a semilunar-shaped area of hyperpigmentation and well-demarcated subretinal fluid in each eye. Fundus autofluorescence confirms the presence of lipofuscin and better demonstrates the drusen (C, D).

Optical Coherence Tomography

Horizontal OCT scan (E, F) of each eye demonstrates focal hyperreflective irregularities beneath the RPE and a hyporeflective cavity beneath the retina, suggestive of fluid or lipofuscin accumulation. The ILM-RPE map of each eye (G, H) reveals the retinal contour. Although a concurrent diagnosis of Best's disease is not confirmed in this patient, it is suspected. Retinal thickness inferior to the fovea is 365 μm in the right eye (I) and 362 μm in the left eye (J).

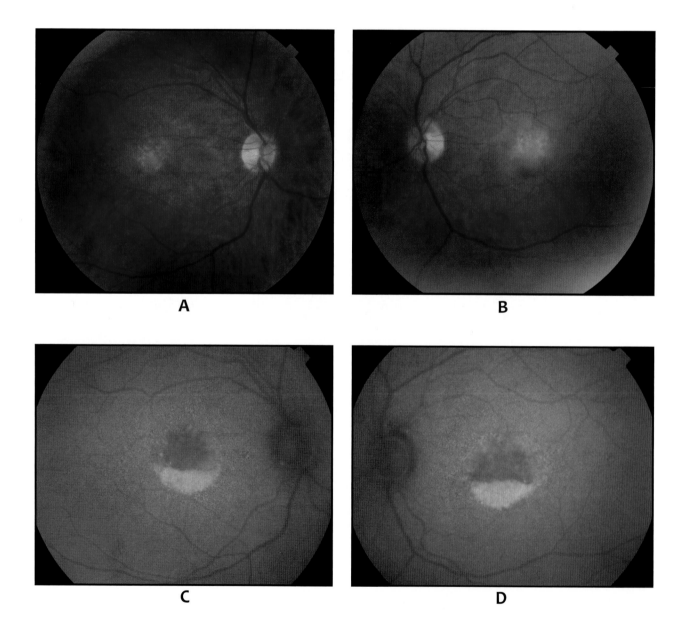

A

B

C

D

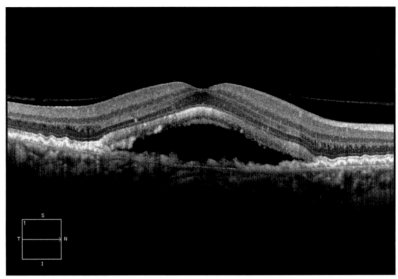

E

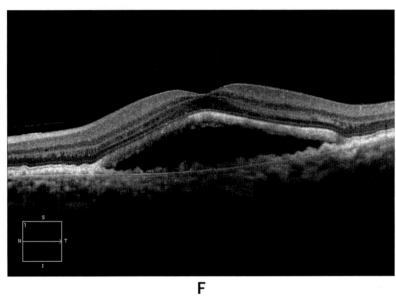

F

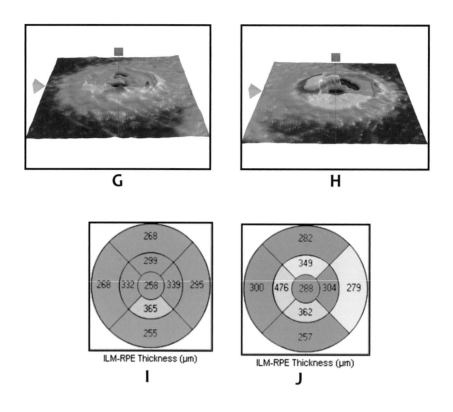

G

H

ILM-RPE Thickness (µm)

I

ILM-RPE Thickness (µm)

J

Case 7-3. Adult Vitelliform Dystrophy

Clinical Summary

A 58-year-old female presents with a decline in vision over 2 years. Her visual acuity measures 20/30 in the right eye and 20/20 in the left eye. Dilated fundus examination of the right eye reveals a minimally elevated, well-circumscribed subretinal yellow lesion (A). Exam of the left eye reveals a focal yellow lesion inferior to the fovea with associated serous fluid along the superior aspect of the lesion and pigment changes (B).

Optical Coherence Tomography

Horizontal OCT scan (C) of the right eye shows accumulation of mildly hyperreflective material originating from the RPE, leading to an elevation of the photoreceptor layer and mild flattening of foveal contour. Horizontal OCT scan (D) of the left eye shows a hyporeflective cavity beneath the pigment epithelium, suggestive of fluid accumulation and flattening of foveal contour. Hyperreflective material in this space may represent pigment epithelium remnants. Central foveal thickness measures 317 μm (E).

The patient did not have an electro-oculogram. Several diagnoses, including late-onset Best's disease and adult vitelliform dystrophy, are in consideration.

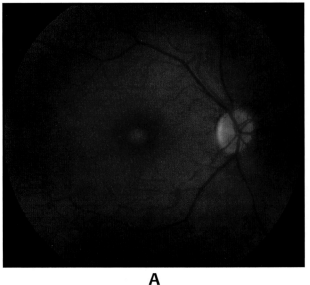

A

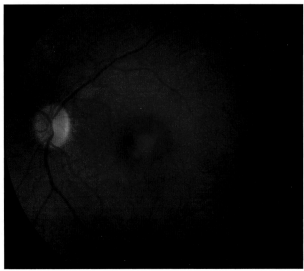

B

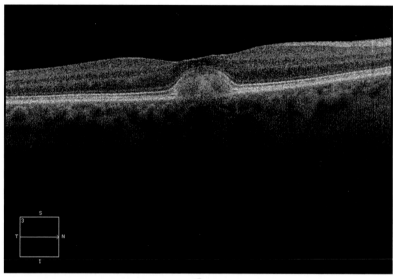

C

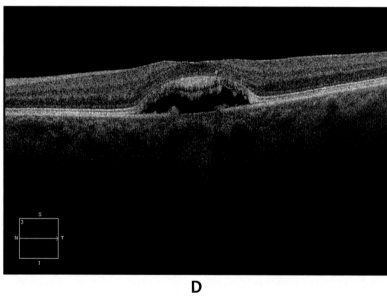

D

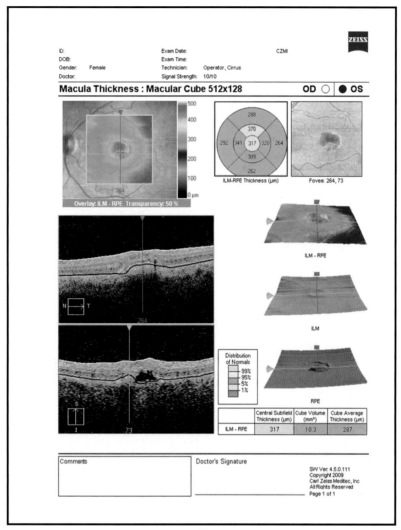

E

Case 7-4A. Geographic Atrophy

Clinical Summary

An 83-year-old female presents with age-related macular degeneration in both eyes. Visual acuity in the right eye is 20/200 and 20/100 in the left eye. Dilated fundus exam shows a central area of geographic atrophy in the left eye (A).

Optical Coherence Tomography

Horizontal OCT scan (B) reveals focal irregularity of the RPE, with thinning nasally and temporally. Intraretinal pigment migration is noted on the scan (arrow).

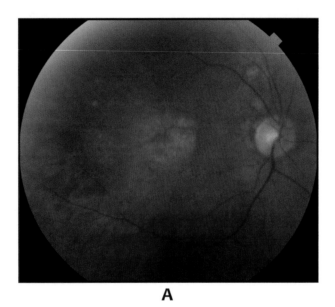

A

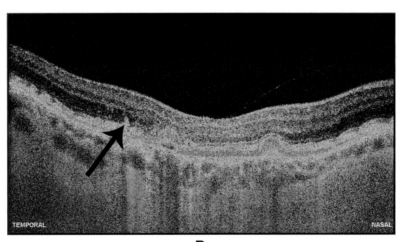

B

Case 7-4B. Geographic Atrophy

Clinical Summary

An 87-year-old female presents for an annual eye exam. She has no visual complaints. Visual acuity in the right eye is 20/40 and 20/50 in the left eye. Dilated fundus exam of the right eye (A) and left eye (B) reveals well-circumscribed geographic atrophy with drusen and RPE mottling.

Optical Coherence Tomography

Horizontal OCT scan of the right eye (C) demonstrates absence of the RPE temporal to and beneath the fovea. Within this area, there is notable thinning of the outer retinal layers. Hyperreflective choroidal structures are seen due to the absence of RPE. Irregular, thickened Bruch's membrane is noted elsewhere. The ILM-RPE map (D) demonstrates retinal contour. Horizontal OCT scan of the left eye (E) reveals areas of RPE absence. In these areas, thinning of the outer retina and hyperreflectivity of the choroidal structures are noted. Again, the ILM-RPE map (F) illustrates the retinal contour.

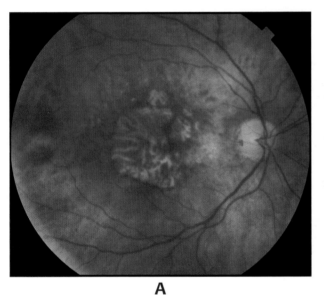

A

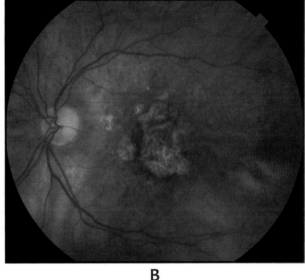

B

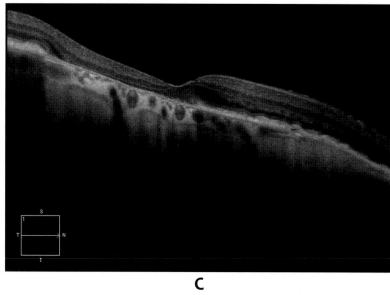

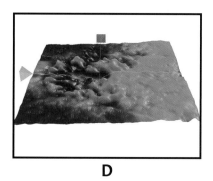

C

D

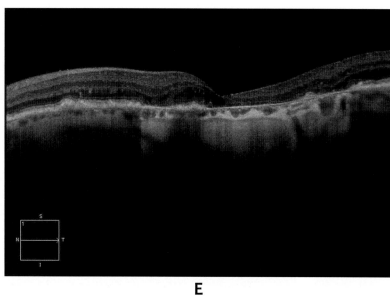

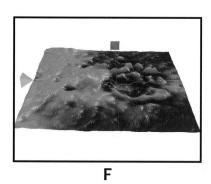

E

F

Case 7-5. Occult Choroidal Neovascularization

Clinical Summary

An 82-year-old female with a 15-year history of age-related macular degeneration and stable visual acuity of 20/40 in the right eye complained of distortion and blurry vision for 4 months. Visual acuity in this eye decreased to 20/200. Fundus examination (A) of the right eye reveals retinal thickening, drusen, and pigmentary changes in the central macula. Fluorescein angiography shows early stippled hyperfluorescence (B) and diffuse late leakage (C) characteristic of an occult choroidal neovascularization. The patient is observed.

Optical Coherence Tomography

A vertical scan through the macula (D) shows an irregular foveal contour associated with intraretinal and subretinal fluid. The thin layer of subretinal fluid extends beneath the center of the fovea. The highly reflective external band appears diffusely thickened and irregular.

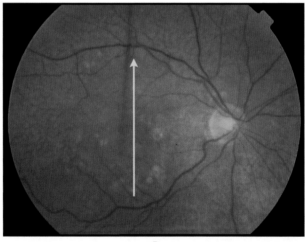

A

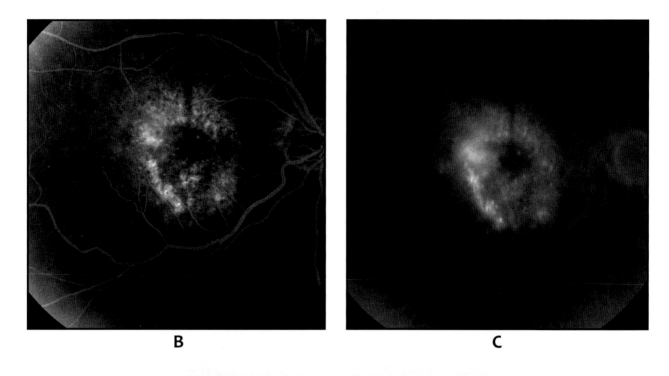

B

C

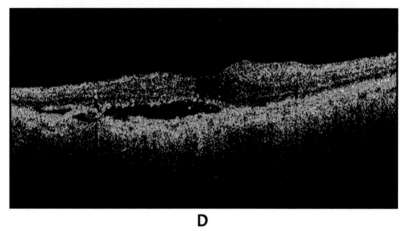

D

Case 7-5. Occult Choroidal Neovascularization (continued)

Continuation of Clinical Summary

Five months later, her vision has decreased to 20/300. Fundus examination (E) reveals persistence of the retinal thickening. Fluorescein angiography (F) shows a small area of early hyperfluorescence temporal to the foveal center surrounded by stippled fluorescence. In the late phase (G), there is diffuse leakage from these areas.

Follow-Up
Optical Coherence Tomography

Repeat vertical scan through the foveal center (H) reveals a diffusely thickened retina. The foveal contour is preserved, but the outer retinal layers appear highly disorganized, likely accounting for the decreased vision. The external highly reflective band appears diffusely thickened and irregular. There is a small amount of fluid beneath the fovea.

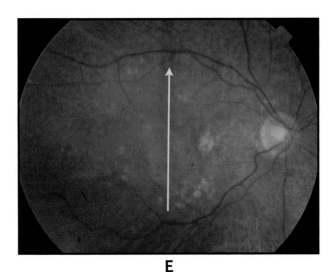

E

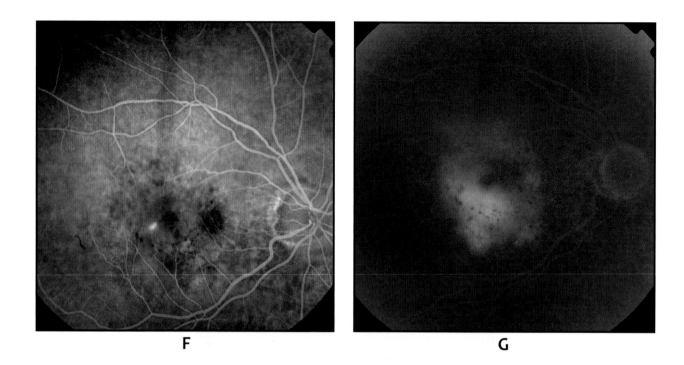

F

G

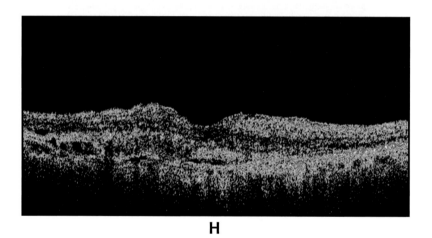

H

Case 7-6. Vascularized Pigment Epithelial Detachment

Clinical Summary

A 79-year-old male with a history of decreased vision has a visual acuity of 20/50 in the left eye. Fundus examination of the left macula (A) reveals pigment mottling and a PED. Fluorescein angiography (B, C) shows the outline of a well-demarcated serous PED with a notch in the nasal edge. Indocyanine angiography (D, E) shows a classic PED with some areas of reticular pigment and a hot spot in the area of the notch.

Optical Coherence Tomography

A horizontal scan through the foveal center (F) shows a dome-shaped elevation of the highly reflective external band with low reflectivity underlying this band consistent with a serous PED. Low reflectance from the choroid underlying the PED is observed secondary to shadowing. The overlying retina appears relatively normal, and the layered architecture of the neurosensory retina overlying the PED is preserved. A small amount of subretinal fluid is present surrounding the PED.

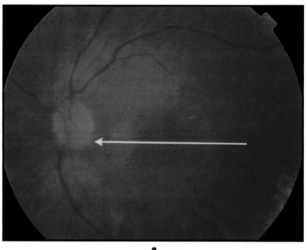

A

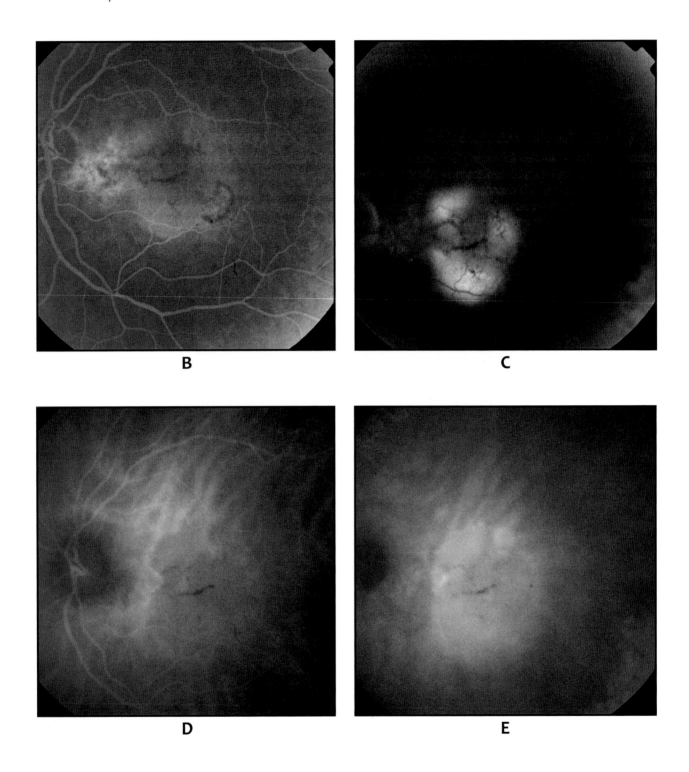

B

C

D

E

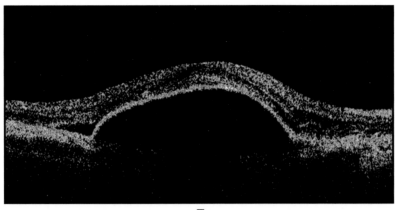

F

Case 7-7A. Retinal Angiomatous Proliferation

Clinical Summary

A 93-year-old female is referred for sudden decline in vision of the right eye 5 days prior. The visual acuity measures 20/60 in the right eye. Dilated fundus exam reveals macular and extramacular drusen, RPE atrophy, calcified drusen, and an area superotemporal to the fovea of intraretinal hemorrhage, subretinal fluid, with an associated retinal angiomatous proliferative lesion (A). Fluorescein angiography reveals a focal hyperfluorescence in the corresponding area, which subsequently leaks (B).

Optical Coherence Tomography

Horizontal OCT scan (C) shows hyporeflective spaces within the retina, beneath the retina, and beneath the RPE, highly suggestive of fluid accumulation in the respective spaces. Central foveal thickness is 355 μm (D). The ILM-RPE overlay illustrates the focal areas of retinal thickening (E).

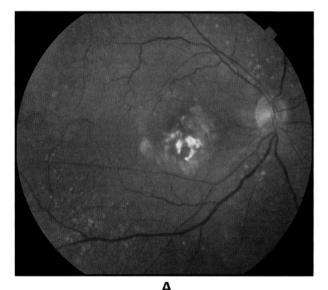

A

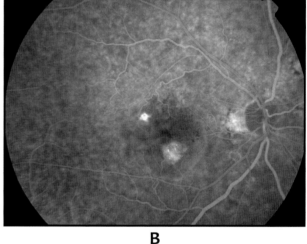

B

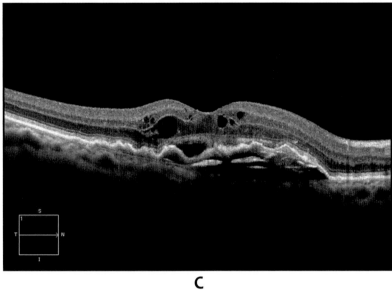

C

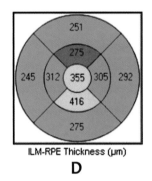

ILM-RPE Thickness (µm)

D

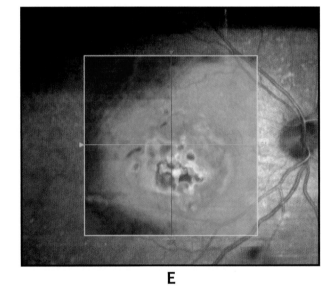

E

Case 7-7B. Retinal Angiomatous Proliferation

Clinical Summary

A 79-year-old male complains of decreased vision in his right eye. Visual acuity is 20/60. Fundus examination (A) of the right eye reveals a large PED centered in the macula with a focal intraretinal hemorrhage inferior to the foveal center. Fluorescein angiography (B, C) shows a focal fluorescent area adjacent to the hemorrhage identified as an early retinal angiomatous proliferation with an overlying anastomotic lesion. The PED appears as an early circular hyperfluorescent area with well-defined borders. Indocyanine green angiography shows a well-defined PED with a hot spot, confirming the subretinal component of the angiomatous proliferation (D, E).

Optical Coherence Tomography

A vertical scan through the foveal center (F) shows elevation of the highly reflective external band in the area of the serous PED. Intraretinal cystic edema is seen overlying the PED. Subretinal fluid is present around the PED inferiorly (left side of the scan).

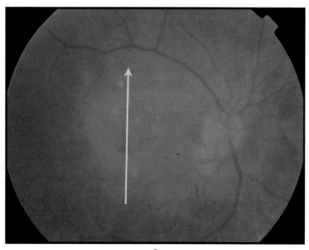

A

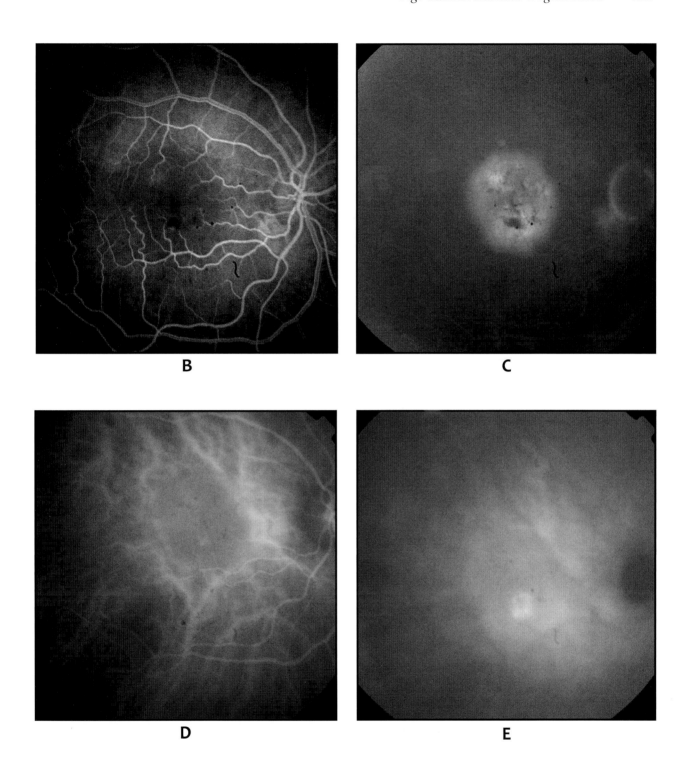

B

C

D

E

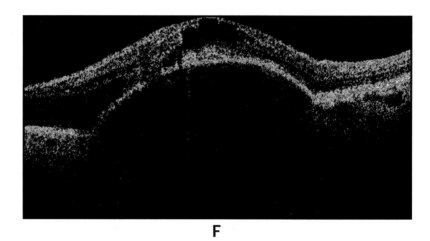

F

Case 7-8A. Retinal Pigment Epithelium Tear

Clinical Summary

A 71-year-old male presents with complaints of a decline in vision in the left eye 2 weeks following an intravitreal antivascular endothelial growth factor injection for a history of age-related macular degeneration. Visual acuity measures 20/60 in the left eye. Dilated fundus exam reveals a large central RPE detachment, of which the temporal edge is highly pigmented, suggestive of rolled RPE in a rip (A).

Optical Coherence Tomography

Horizontal OCT scan (B) reveals a large hyporeflective cavity beneath the neurosensory retina, with elevation of the neurosensory retina. Irregular hyperreflective pigment epithelium is visible temporal to the fovea, which appears fragmented at the temporal edge of the PED. In the subfoveal region, the RPE ends abruptly. An absence of pigment epithelium is noted nasal to the fovea. Vertical OCT scan (C) similarly reveals a large elevation of the neurosensory retina. The inferior scan shows the presence of pigment epithelium, which ends at the base of the neurosensory elevation and is present along the superior scan. Subretinal hyperfluorescent substance may represent a choroidal neovascular membrane, present at the base of the lesion. The RPE map (D) better illustrates the RPE rip.

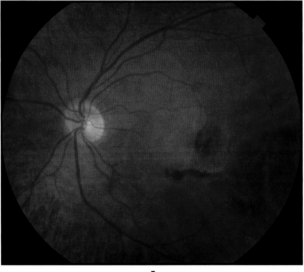

A

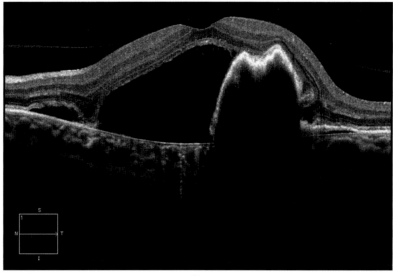

B

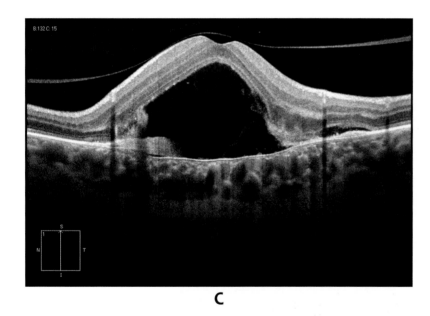

C

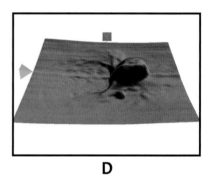

D

Case 7-8B. Retinal Pigment Epithelium Tear

Clinical Summary

A 72-year-old male presents for examination of age-related macular degeneration. He had undergone intravitreal antivascular endothelial growth factor injection in the left eye 5 weeks prior. He denies changes in vision. Visual acuity is 20/30 in the right eye and 20/400 in the left eye. Dilated fundus exam of the left eye (A) shows fine drusen, detachment of the RPE, and a small area of missing RPE with adjacent scrolled RPE temporal to the fovea.

Optical Coherence Tomography

Horizontal OCT scan (B) reveals a hyporeflective space beneath the RPE and several within the retina, suggestive of an RPE detachment and intraretinal fluid, respectively. Temporally, the choroid appears hyperreflective due to a lack of RPE in the region of the rip. The retinal contour is illustrated by the ILM-RPE map (C).

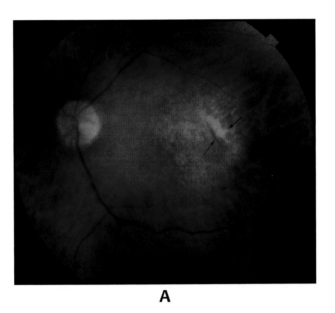

A

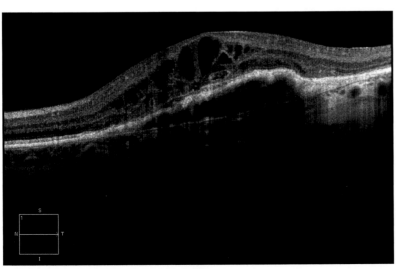

B

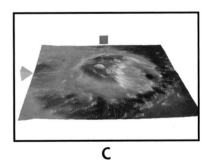

C

Case 7-9A. Subretinal Hemorrhage

Clinical Summary

A 79-year-old male presents with a sudden decline in vision in the right eye. Visual acuity measures 20/100 in the right eye. He has a prior history of photodynamic therapy for choroidal neovascularization in both eyes. Dilated fundus examination of the right eye reveals a hazy view due to nuclear sclerosis, peripapillary atrophy, geographic atrophy, and a subretinal hemorrhage (A).

Optical Coherence Tomography

Horizontal OCT scan (B) demonstrates a concave contour, consistent with high myopia. A hyporeflective band in the subretinal space with elevation of the neurosensory retina corresponds to the subretinal hemorrhage. An epiretinal membrane is noted on the surface of the retina. Thinning of choroidal and near absence of RPE structures are noted. Central foveal thickness is 345 µm (C). The ILM-RPE map (D) demonstrates the area of irregularity.

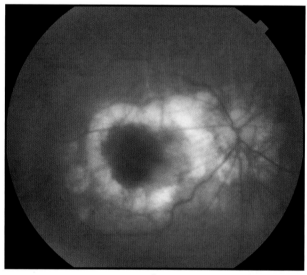

A

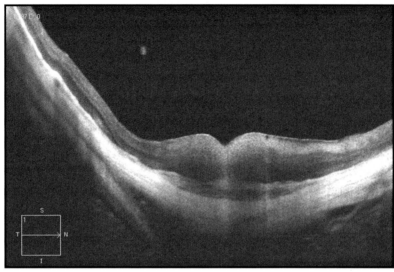

B

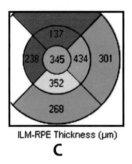

ILM-RPE Thickness (μm)

C

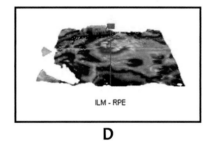

ILM - RPE

D

Case 7-9B. Subretinal Hemorrhage

Clinical Summary

A 69-year-old male presents with a sudden "dark spot" in the central vision of the right eye. Prior history is significant for age-related macular degeneration, treated with multiple intravitreal antivascular endothelial growth factor injections and photodynamic therapy. Visual acuity is 20/200 in the right eye. Dilated fundus examination reveals a large subretinal hemorrhage within the macula and superior to the nerve and 2 hypopigmented fibrotic lesions in the central macula (A).

Optical Coherence Tomography

Horizontal OCT scan (B) shows a large hyporeflective space temporal to the fovea beneath the RPE, suggestive of a hemorrhagic pigment epithelium detachment. A focal hyperreflective area nasal to the fovea represents intraretinal/subretinal fibrosis. Few hyporeflective spaces indicate intraretinal fluid. The ILM-RPE overlay better demonstrates areas of retinal thickness (C). Central foveal thickness is 219 μm (D).

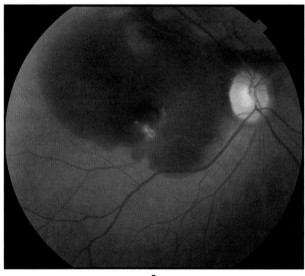

A

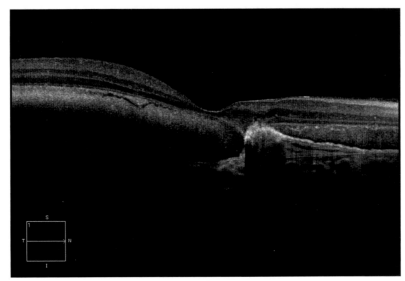

B

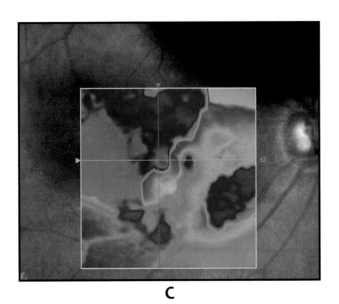

C

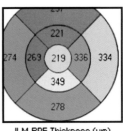

ILM-RPE Thickness (µm)

D

Case 7-10A. Disciform Scar

Clinical Summary

A 79-year-old male was referred for complaints of poor vision in the right eye for several years. Dilated fundus exam of the right eye reveals a large area in the central and superior macula of subretinal fibrosis in the pattern of a disciform scar, mild pigment along the inferior border (A).

Optical Coherence Tomography

Horizontal OCT scan (B) shows diffuse elevation, irregularity, and intraretinal migration of a hyperreflective layer at the level of the RPE. This likely represents fibrosis and leads to an irregular foveal contour. Few hyporeflective spaces within the retina are suggestive of fluid accumulation. Loss of normal linear contour is noted, as well as an anastamosis between the choroidal and retinal architecture. Central foveal thickness is 18 µm (C). The ILM-RPE map demonstrates the irregular macular contour (D).

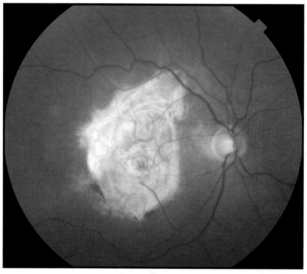

A

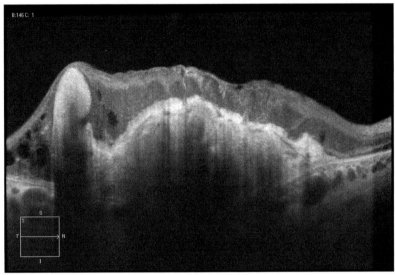

B

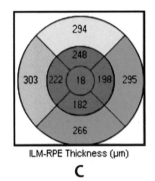

ILM-RPE Thickness (µm)

C

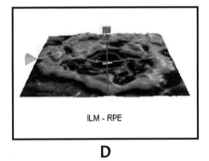

ILM - RPE

D

Case 7-10B. Disciform Scar

Clinical Summary

A 78-year-old female presents for follow-up of age-related macular degeneration. Visual acuity in the right eye is 20/800. Dilated fundus exam of the right eye (A) reveals subretinal fibrosis along the superior macula extending centrally and atrophy of the RPE.

Optical Coherence Tomography

Horizontal OCT scan (B) of the right eye demonstrates a hyperreflective thickened substance beneath the neurosensory retina and hyporeflective spaces within the retina, indicating subretinal fibrosis and intraretinal fluid, respectively. Loss of outer retinal layer architecture is noted. The ILM-RPE map (C) illustrates retinal contour. Foveal thickness superior to the fovea is increased to 450 μm (D).

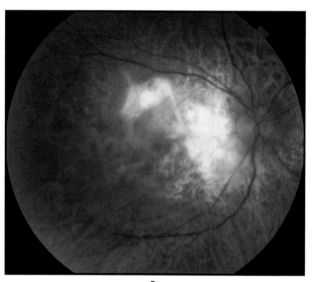

A

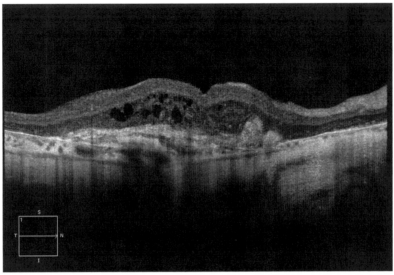

B

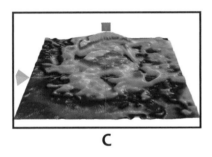

C

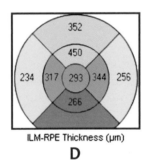

ILM-RPE Thickness (µm)

D

Chapter 8

Miscellaneous Macular Degenerations

Heeral R. Shah, MD; Elias C. Mavrofrides, MD;
Carmen A. Puliafito, MD, MBA; and Jay S. Duker, MD

- Pathologic Myopia
- Angioid Streaks
- Choroidal Neovascular Membrane
- Idiopathic Central Serous Chorioretinopathy With Choroidal Neovascularization
- Juxtafoveal Retinal Telangiectasis With Choroidal Neovascularization
- Presumed Ocular Histoplasmosis

In addition to age-related macular degeneration (ARMD), numerous conditions have been associated with the development of choroidal neovascularization (CNV). These conditions, which primarily affect younger patients, include pathologic myopia, angioid streaks, presumed ocular histoplasmosis, inflammatory chorioretinopathies, hereditary maculopathies, and trauma.[1] Abnormalities of the retinal pigment epithelium (RPE) and Bruch's membrane predispose to the development of CNV in these conditions. In some cases, an underlying cause for the CNV cannot be identified, and these are termed *idiopathic*.

CNV in association with these conditions often differs from neovascularization due to ARMD. Gass described 2 patterns of neovascularization: type 1 growth of new vessels beneath the pigment epithelium and type 2 growth of vessels above the RPE in the subretinal space.[2] Type 2 neovascularization is more readily identified ophthalmoscopically and usually has a "classic" appearance on fluorescein angiography. ARMD most commonly exhibits type 1

neovascularization, while these miscellaneous macular degenerations usually show type 2.[2] CNV in these miscellaneous macular degenerations is also typically smaller, more likely to regress spontaneously, and has a better prognosis than ARMD.

As with ARMD, optical coherence tomography (OCT) can be a valuable tool in the evaluation of patients with these conditions. The CNV in these cases usually appears as a highly reflective mass protruding above the RPE signal into the subretinal space. This appearance is consistent with the type 2 CNV as described by Gass.[2] The overlying retina is usually thickened with hyporeflective cystic spaces indicating intraretinal fluid accumulation.[3-6] In some cases of myopic CNV, intraretinal fluid accumulation does not occur, and the overlying retina may actually appear thinner than the adjacent tissue.[4] Subretinal fluid is also frequently identified around these lesions and appears on the OCT image as a nonreflective space beneath the neurosensory retina. Shadowing of the choroid beneath the CNV varies depending on the density/reflectivity of the lesion.

Several authors have described changes in the appearance of the CNV lesion on the OCT image as activity decreases and scarring develops.[4-6] Histopathologically, the regressing vessels are enveloped by RPE cells and become more fibrotic. As these changes occur, the CNV lesion often exhibits increased reflectivity on the OCT image and may become more fusiform in shape. These changes often make the lesion less distinct from the adjacent

Schuman JS, Puliafito CA, Fujimoto JG, Duker JS, eds.
Optical Coherence Tomography of Ocular Diseases,
Third Edition (pp 237-258).
© 2013 SLACK Incorporated.

RPE signal. The most definitive sign of membrane regression, however, is resolution of the associated subretinal and intraretinal edema.

Less frequently, CNV in these conditions adopts a type 1 growth pattern. The OCT image shows changes similar to CNV associated with ARMD (see Chapter 7). These changes typically include disruption and elevation of the RPE with associated subretinal and intraretinal fluid accumulation. Because there is less penetration of the signal beneath the RPE, the neovascularization is usually not well defined on the OCT image in these instances.

Large subretinal hemorrhages can also occur in association with CNV in these conditions. Visualization of the neovascular lesion can initially be prevented by the hemorrhage. Because the reflectivity of the retina and blood can be similar, the separation between these 2 layers on OCT may be indistinct. Shadowing of the underlying RPE and choroid signal depends on the degree of elevation of the subretinal blood. Usually, penetration of the signal is adequate enough to define the position of the RPE and confirm the subretinal (versus sub-RPE) location of the blood. With subsequent resolution of the hemorrhage, the OCT can then help define the extent and activity of the associated neovascular complex.

The utility of OCT imaging in these conditions is not only characterization of the lesion but also using this information to direct management and monitor response. As mentioned previously, these lesions may regress spontaneously without significant visual alteration. OCT can be useful in confirming and/or monitoring spontaneous regression of the lesion, thus obviating the need for intervention.

In many cases, however, intervention is beneficial for active lesions. The Macular Photocoagulation Study has shown the benefit of focal laser treatment for extrafoveal and juxtafoveal lesions in presumed ocular histoplasmosis syndrome and idiopathic CNV.[7] Photodynamic therapy has subsequently been used for the treatment of subfoveal CNV in many of these conditions.[8-11] Recent small studies reveal the benefits of using intravitreal bevacizumab in the treatment of presumed ocular histoplasmosis syndrome,[12] pathologic myopia,[13] angioid streaks,[14] and idiopathic and CNV secondary to central serous chorioretinopathy.[15] Identification of active or progressive CNV and the status of intraretinal and subretinal fluid on OCT imaging can help establish the need for further treatment.

OCT can then be used to monitor tissue response to these treatments and thus direct further management. Involution of the subretinal lesion with resolution of the associated edema indicates adequate treatment response and the need for observation. Increases in the size of the lesion or the amount of surrounding edema can indicate persistent activity of the neovascularization and the need for additional intervention.

The role of OCT in the surgical removal of subfoveal CNV has also been evaluated.[16,17] Patients with type 2 CNV appear to have better outcomes after surgical removal than those with type 1 lesions. OCT can thus be used to define the anatomic location of the lesion to determine eligibility for surgical intervention.[16] Other lesion characteristics on the OCT image, such as well-defined edges, may also be important in predicting visual outcome after surgery.[17]

References

1. Cohen SY, Laroche A, Leguen Y, Soubrane G, Coscas GJ. Etiology of choroidal neovascularization in young patients. *Ophthalmology.* 1996;103:1241-1244.
2. Gass JDM. Biomicroscopic and histopathologic considerations regarding the feasibility of surgical excision of subfoveal neovascular membranes. *Am J Ophthalmol.* 1994;118:285-289.
3. Hee MR, Baumal CR, Puliafito CA, et al. Optical coherence tomography of age-related macular degeneration and choroidal neovascularization. *Ophthalmology.* 1996;103:1260-1270.
4. Baba T, Ohno-Matsui K, Yoshida T, et al. Optical coherence tomography of choroidal neovascularization in high myopia. *Acta Ophthalmol Scand.* 2002;80:82-87.
5. Fukuchi T, Takahashi K, Ida H, Sho K, Matsumura M. Staging of idiopathic choroidal neovascularization by optical coherence tomography. *Graefes Arch Clin Exp Ophthalmol.* 2001;239:424-429.
6. Iida T, Hagimura N, Sato T, Kishi S. Optical coherence tomographic features of idiopathic submacular choroidal neovascularization. *Am J Ophthalmol.* 2000;130:763-768.
7. Ho AC. Miscellaneous macular degenerations. In: Regillo CD, Brown GC, Flynn HW JR, eds. *Vitreoretinal Diseases—The Essentials.* New York, NY: Thieme Medical Publishers Inc; 1999:241-253.
8. Verteporfin in Photodynamic Therapy Study Group. Photodynamic therapy of subfoveal choroidal neovascularization in pathologic myopia with verteporfin: 1 year results of a randomized clinical trial—VIP report no 1. *Ophthalmology.* 2001;108:841-852.
9. Sickenberg M, Schmidt-Erfurth U, Miller JW, et al. A preliminary study of photodynamic therapy using verteporfin for choroidal neovascularization in pathologic myopia, ocular histoplasmosis syndrome, angioid streaks, and idiopathic causes. *Arch Ophthalmol.* 2000;118:327-336.
10. Karacorlu M, Karacorlu S, Ozdemir H, Mat C. Photodynamic therapy with verteporfin for choroidal neovascularization in patients with angioid streaks. *Am J Ophthalmol.* 2002;134:360-366.
11. Spaide RF, Martin ML, Slakter J, et al. Treatment of idiopathic subfoveal choroidal neovascular lesions using photodynamic therapy with verteporfin. *Am J Ophthalmol.* 2002;134:62-68.

12. Schadlu R, Blinder KJ, Shah GK, et al. Intravitreal bevacizumab for choroidal neovascularization in ocular histoplasmosis. *Am J Ophthalmol.* 2008;145(5):875-878.

13. Parodi MB, Lacono P, Papayannis A, Sheth S, Bandello F. Laser photocoagulation, photodynamic therapy, and intravitreal bevacizumab for the treatment of juxtafoveal choroidal neovascularization secondary to pathologic myopia. *Arch Ophthalmol.* 2010;128(4):437-442.

14. Wiegand TW, Rogers AH, McCabe F, Reichel E, Duker JS. Intravitreal bevacizumab (Avastin) treatment of choroidal neovascularization in patients with angioid streaks. *Br J Ophthalmol.* 2009;93(1):47-51.

15. Chan WM, Lai TY, Liu DT, Lam DS. Intravitreal bevacizumab (Avastin) for choroidal neovascularization secondary to central serous chorioretinopathy, secondary to punctate inner choroidopathy, or of idiopathic origin. *Am J Ophthalmol.* 2007;143(6):977-983.

16. Giovannini A, Amato GP, Mariotti C, Scassellati-Sforzolini B. OCT imaging of choroidal neovascularization and its role in the determination of patients' eligibility for surgery. *Br J Ophthalmol.* 1999;83:438-442.

17. Brindaeu C, Glacet-Bernard A, Coscas F, Mimoun G, Coscas G, Soubrane G. Surgical removal of subfoveal choroidal neovascularization: visual outcome and prognostic value of fluorescein angiography and optical coherence tomography. *Eur J Ophthalmol.* 2001;11:287-295.

Index to Cases

Case 8-1A. Pathologic Myopia

Clinical Summary

A 68-year-old male presents with mild, progressive decline in vision of the right eye over several years. Visual acuity measures 20/50 in the right eye and 20/20 in the left eye. Dilated fundus examination of the right eye reveals peripapillary atrophy with a posterior staphyloma and a horizontal lacquer crack through the fovea with mottling changes (A).

Optical Coherence Tomography

Horizontal OCT scan (B) of the right eye reveals diffuse thinning of the choroid with the exception of a subfoveal and juxtafoveal focal loss of choroidal architecture.

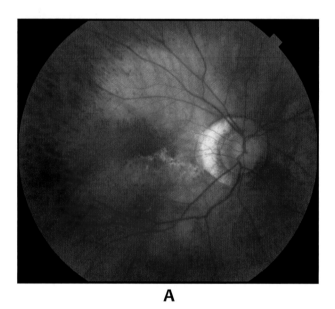

A

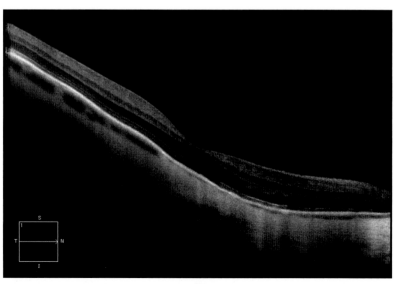

B

Case 8-1B. Pathologic Myopia

Clinical Summary

A 48-year-old female presents for follow-up exam. She denies a change in vision. Visual acuity in the left eye is 20/25. Dilated fundus exam reveals peripapillary atrophy, areas of RPE atrophy in the retina, and a central fibrotic choroidal neovascular membrane (A).

Optical Coherence Tomography

Horizontal OCT scan of the left eye (B) demonstrates a myopic contour, thin choroid, and hyper-reflective substance beneath the retina, likely representing the choroidal neovascular membrane. The ILM-RPE map (C) illustrates the retinal contour. Central foveal thickness is 222 µm (D).

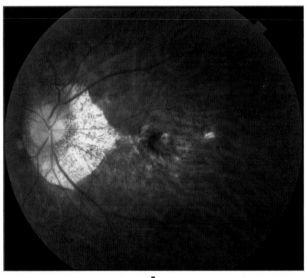

A

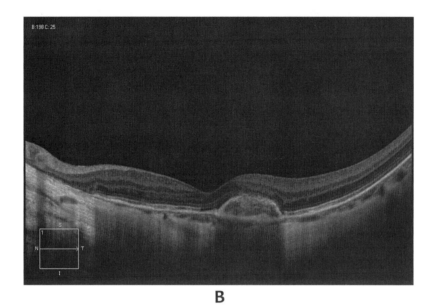

B

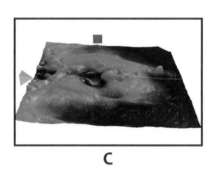

C

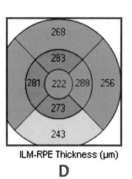

ILM-RPE Thickness (μm)

D

Case 8-2. Pathologic Myopia With Choroidal Neovascularization

Clinical Summary

A 60-year-old female with a history of high myopia complains of a dark spot in the central visual acuity of her left eye for 4 months. Her visual acuity is 20/40 in this eye, and there is central metamorphopsia on Amsler grid testing. Dilated fundus examination (A) shows peripapillary and macular pigmentary atrophy consistent with pathologic myopia. There is a large neovascular complex in the macula with extensive overlying edema. Fluorescein angiography (B) confirms a large classic neovascular lesion that extends under the fovea and leaks in the late phase of the study.

Optical Coherence Tomography

The OCT image (C) shows the neovascularization as a fusiform area of moderate reflectivity extending above the RPE signal into the subretinal space. This lesion shows slightly more intense reflectivity than the overlying retina but is slightly less intense than the adjacent RPE signal. The overlying retina is thickened with intraretinal cystic edema. The retina around the lesion does not show evidence of edema, and there is no associated subretinal fluid. The RPE signal does not show evidence of disruption, although there is mild shadowing beneath the choroidal neovascularization.

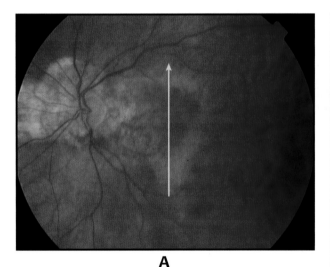

A

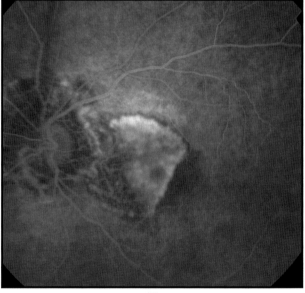

B

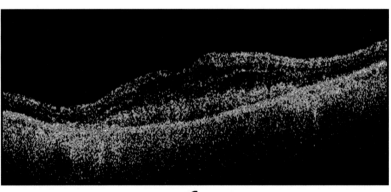

C

Case 8-2. Pathologic Myopia With Choroidal Neovascularization (continued)

Continuation of Clinical Summary

Photodynamic therapy is performed at the initial visit. She returns 1 month later and reports improvement in her distortion. Her visual acuity in this eye is now 20/30. Dilated fundus examination (D) shows pigmentary mottling but no evidence of active neovascularization or edema. On fluorescein angiography (E), there is now a large area of hypofluorescence in the area of previous neovascularization.

Follow-Up Optical Coherence Tomography

The previously identified neovascular lesion is no longer evident on the post-treatment OCT image (F). There has also been resolution of the retinal edema with normalization of the retinal contour. These changes confirm involution of the choroidal neovascularization after the photodynamic therapy treatment.

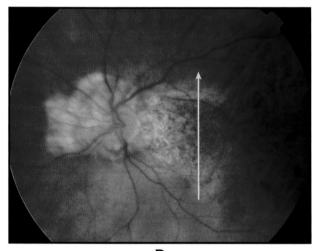

D

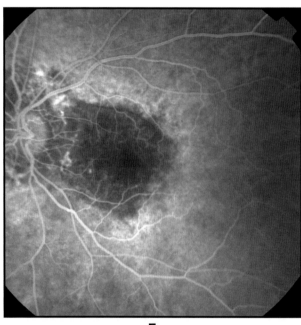

E

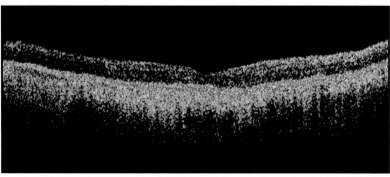

F

Case 8-3. Angioid Streaks

Clinical Summary

A 58-year-old female presents with new onset of blurry vision in the left eye for several days. She has a prior history of submacular surgery in the right eye for subretinal hemorrhage 4 years prior and proliferative diabetic retinopathy with panretinal photocoagulation in both eyes. Visual acuity measures 20/800 in the right eye and 20/40 in the left eye. Dilated fundus examination of the left eye shows a subretinal hemorrhage surrounded by subretinal fluid in the superior macula, angioid streaks radiating from the nerve, and laser scars in the periphery (A). The patient receives intravitreal ranibizumab every 4 months over 16 months. At 16-month follow-up, dilated fundus exam shows focal subretinal fibrosis in the superior macula, surrounded by atrophy and mottling of the RPE in the superior papillomacular bundle (B).

Optical Coherence Tomography

Horizontal OCT scan (C) shows diffuse thinning of the RPE, absence of an intact photoreceptor layer, and disruption of the retinal architecture nasal to the fovea. Diffuse thickening of the RPE and Bruch's membrane is noted. Central foveal thickness is 238 μm (D). The ILM-RPE overlay better illustrates the area of retinal thickening (E).

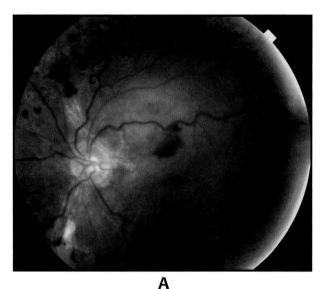

A

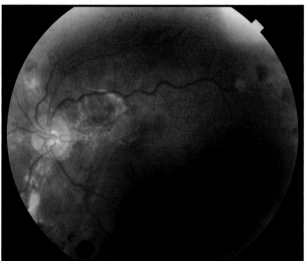

B

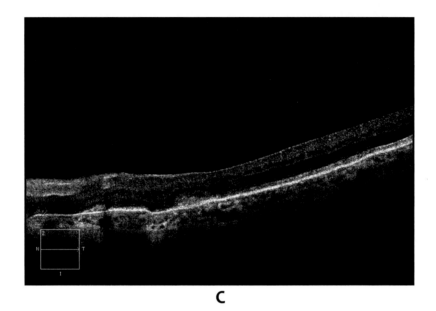

C

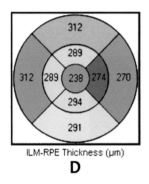

ILM-RPE Thickness (μm)

D

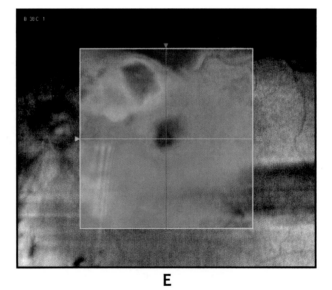

E

Case 8-4. Choroidal Neovascular Membrane—Idiopathic

Clinical Summary

A 79-year-old female presents complaining of a "gray film over my right eye." She received focal laser treatment for a peripapillary choroidal neovascular membrane 2 years prior. Her visual acuity measures 20/30 in the right eye. Dilated fundus exam shows subretinal fluid and hemorrhage adjacent to the prior juxtapapillary laser scar (A). She is treated with one dose of intravitreal bevacizumab. On 2-month follow-up, visual acuity remains 20/30. Dilated fundus exam shows reduced subretinal hemorrhage and fluid. The patient is retreated with intravitreal bevacizumab. On 1-month follow-up, visual acuity has improved to 20/25. Dilated fundus exam shows no persistent subretinal fluid or hemorrhage.

Optical Coherence Tomography

The initial horizontal OCT scan (B) shows a large hyporeflective space, indicating foveal subretinal fluid. Also noted is subretinal fibrosis with one intraretinal cyst in the nasal quadrant, suggestive of a choroidal neovascular membrane in this area. Two months following intravitreal bevacizumab, horizontal OCT scan (C) reveals shallow, persistent subretinal fluid. Following a second intravitreal bevacizumab injection, horizontal OCT scan (D) at the 4-week follow-up reveals no subretinal fluid.

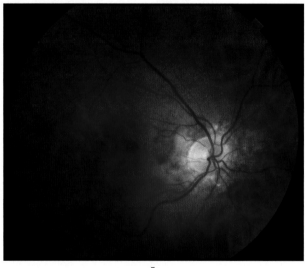

A

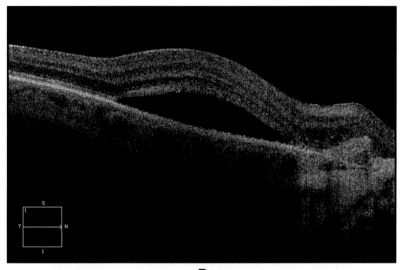

B

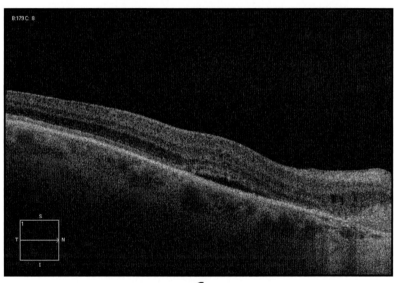

C

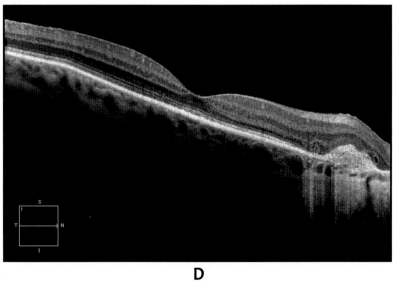

D

Case 8-5. Choroidal Neovascular Membrane—
Age-Related Macular Degeneration

Clinical Summary

An 87-year-old female presents for routine follow-up exam of previously dry age-related macular degeneration. She has no complaints. Visual acuity in the right eye is 20/50 and the left eye is 20/25. Dilated fundus exam of the right eye (A) reveals RPE changes and mild intraretinal fluid.

Optical Coherence Tomography

Horizontal OCT scan (B) reveals a hyporeflective space beneath the retina, suggestive of subretinal fluid. Hyperreflective material adjacent to this space may represent a choroidal neovascular membrane. The ILM-RPE overlay (C) reveals the retinal contour. Central foveal thickness is 257 μm (D).

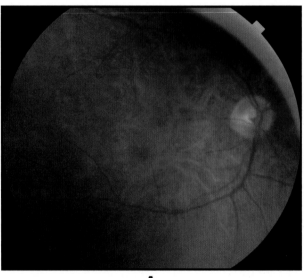

A

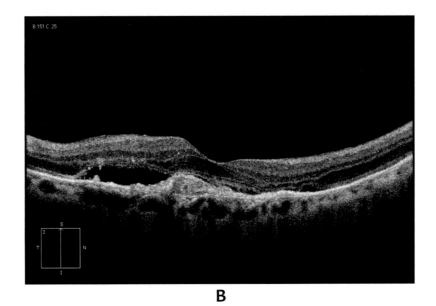

B

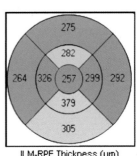

C

ILM-RPE Thickness (μm)

D

Case 8-6. Idiopathic Central Serous Chorioretinopathy With Choroidal Neovascularization

Clinical Summary

An 80-year-old male complains of decreased visual acuity in the right eye for 1 month. He has a history of idiopathic central serous chorioretinopathy and underwent laser treatment to the right eye 20 years earlier. He reports good visual acuity without recurrence after the laser treatment in this eye. His visual acuity is 20/200, and dilated fundus exam (A) reveals extensive pigmentary mottling in the macular region. There is a hyperpigmented lesion with surrounding edema beneath the fovea. Fluorescein angiography (B) shows a well-defined area of hyperfluorescence that progressively leaks consistent with choroidal neovascularization.

Optical Coherence Tomography

The OCT image (C) shows the neovascularization as a dome-shaped lesion with high reflectivity that protrudes into the subretinal space. There is a large nonreflective space over the lesion corresponding to an intraretinal cystic cavity. Smaller intraretinal cysts are also present, and the retinal tissue in this area is thickened. There is no evidence of subretinal fluid on this tomogram.

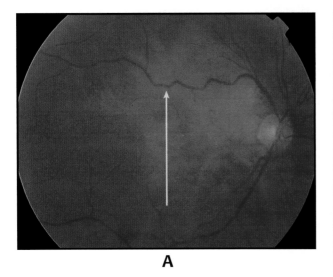

A

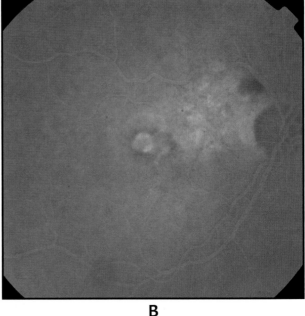

B

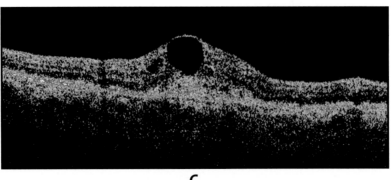

C

Case 8-7. Juxtafoveal Retinal Telangiectasis With Choroidal Neovascularization

Clinical Summary

A 67-year-old male complains of worsening vision in both eyes over the past year. His visual acuity is 20/60 in the right eye. The dilated fundus examination (A) shows telangiectatic vessels temporal to the fovea in this eye. Fluorescein angiography (B) demonstrates hyperfluorescence surrounding the fovea.

Optical Coherence Tomography

The OCT image (C) shows a clear, nonreflective space within the retina at the fovea. There is blunting of the foveal pit, but the retina is otherwise normal in thickness and contour. The high-intensity RPE signal is relatively uniform in appearance without evidence of disruption or thickening. This retinal configuration on OCT is consistent with juxtafoveal telangiectasis.

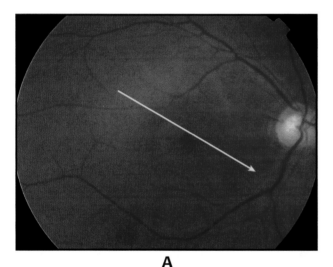

A

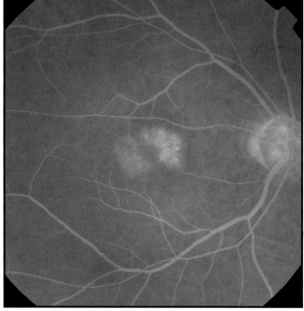

B

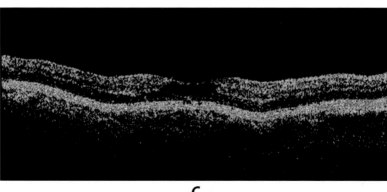

C

Case 8-7. Juxtafoveal Retinal Telangiectasis
With Choroidal Neovascularization (continued)

Clinical Summary

The visual acuity in his left eye is 20/70. The dilated fundus examination (D) shows a localized area of pigmentary mottling with associated edema adjacent to the fovea. Telangiectatic vessels, similar to those in the other eye, are also present in this area. Fluorescein angiography (E) reveals a well-defined area of early hyperfluorescence with late leakage indicating choroidal neovascularization.

Optical Coherence Tomography

OCT images taken through this area (F, G) show a small oval area of thickening along the RPE signal that corresponds to the neovascularization. This lesion can be seen better on the processed image (G) than the scanned image (F). There is mild thickening of the retina but no evidence of subretinal fluid around this lesion. Intraretinal cystic spaces consistent with juxtafoveal telangiectasis are also identified in this eye.

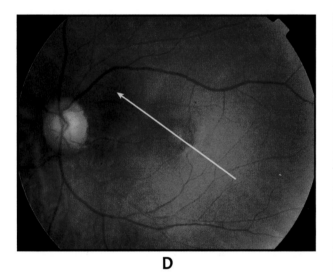

D

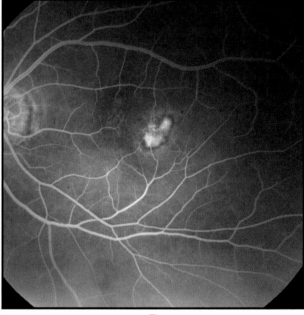

E

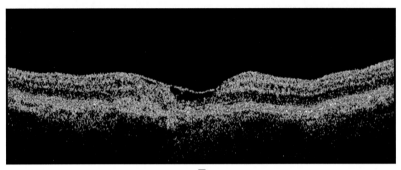

F

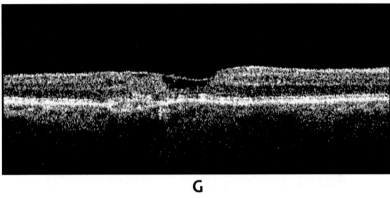

G

Case 8-8. Presumed Ocular Histoplasmosis

Clinical Summary

A 39-year-old female has a diagnosis of ocular histoplasmosis. She has undergone 2 laser treatments in her right eye for choroidal neovascularization in the past. She has been stable for the past 5 years, until 1 month ago when she started noticing decreased vision in her right eye. Her visual acuity in this eye was 20/30 at her last exam 4 months ago but has now declined to 4/200. Retinal examination shows a hypopigmented scar with focal RPE hyperplasia inferior to fixation (A). The foveal edge of the scar appears blurry, indicating the presence of subretinal fluid. Fluorescein angiography reveals a mottled hyperfluorescence in the early phases (B) with late leakage (C) consistent with choroidal neovascularization.

Optical Coherence Tomography

An oblique scan is taken through the scar and fovea (D). As the scan passes through the atrophic scar (left side of the image), the OCT image shows increased intensity of the choroidal signal. This results from the enhanced penetration and reflectivity of the signal through the area of atrophy. The overlying retina appears thinned and irregular. Adjacent to the scar in the fovea (center of the image), there is a small reflective lesion extending above the RPE signal into the subretinal space. This corresponds to the neovascularization. The retina overlying this lesion is edematous with small intraretinal cysts.

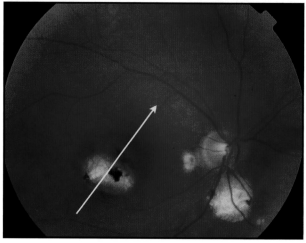

A

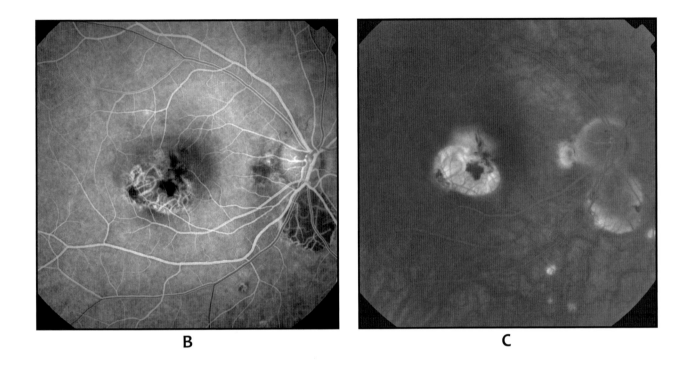

B

C

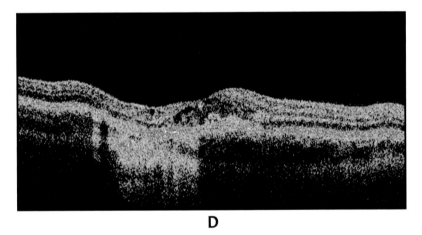

D

Chapter 9

Chorioretinal Inflammatory Diseases

Heeral R. Shah, MD; Natalia Villate, MD; Elias C. Mavrofrides, MD;
Janet Davis, MD; and Jay S. Duker, MD

- Idiopathic Retinal Vasculitis and Neuroretinitis
- Multifocal Choroiditis and Panuveitis
- Posterior Scleritis With Subretinal Fluid
- Sympathetic Ophthalmia
- Birdshot Chorioretinopathy
- Toxoplasmosis
- Intermediate Uveitis With Cystoid Macular Edema
- Sarcoidosis With Choroidal Granulomas
- Vogt-Koyanagi-Harada Disease
- Cytomegalovirus Retinitis

Uveitis is classified according to anatomic location and secondarily to the underlying cause. Location, etiology, duration, and severity determine the extent of damage to intraocular tissues. Complications secondary to uveitis are similar to those observed in other retinal diseases: cystoid macular edema (CME), choroidal neovascularization (CNV), and chorioretinal scarring. Optical coherence tomography (OCT) provides an effective means of quantifying reflectivity, location, and extent of these secondary complications of uveitis.[1] It may also have relevance in imaging inflammatory lesions that are specific to particular types of uveitis that affect the posterior segment.[2]

OCT produces high-resolution cross-sectional imaging of the retina that directly measures the z-plane, with a theoretical axial resolution of 10 to 14 µm. A high degree of reproducibility in measur-

ing macular thickness in normal individuals and diabetic patients has been described.[3] Therefore, it is well suited to repeated measurements of macular status in uveitis patients in whom management decisions are required longitudinally.

The use of OCT in the precise depiction of CME is perhaps its most practical use in the management of ocular inflammatory diseases. CME is the most common sight-threatening complication of uveitis and has the potential for long-term visual morbidity. When compared to fluorescein angiography,[4] OCT is effective in detecting CME. It has the advantage of being noninvasive and without risk for the patient. Furthermore, OCT can provide reliable information in patients with moderate vitreous opacities or small pupils resulting from posterior synechiae, both common findings in uveitis patients that can prevent acceptable stereoscopic fluorescein angiography.

In chronic CME, retinal thickness, size and location of cysts, and subretinal fluid accumulation can be monitored by OCT in order to determine results of, or need for, therapy.[5] Sequential OCT scans of CME can demonstrate anatomic changes from persistence of CME. In the late stages, CME may be associated with lamellar or full-thickness macular hole formation. OCT may help distinguish between holes and large central cysts. Detection of vitreomacular traction or an epiretinal membrane by OCT may lead to consideration of membrane peeling to release traction on the macula.[1] In contrast, retinal thinning in the aftermath of CME may lead the clinician to

Schuman JS, Puliafito CA, Fujimoto JG, Duker JS, eds.
Optical Coherence Tomography of Ocular Diseases,
Third Edition (pp 259-286).
© 2013 SLACK Incorporated.

conclude that vision loss is irreversible and further therapy is not indicated.

CNV is an uncommon complication of uveitis, but one that is uniquely suited to imaging with OCT. OCT has the potential to help distinguish between inflammatory lesions and adjacent CNV in some cases, such as neovascularization arising from toxoplasmic chorioretinitis. In eyes with subfoveal neovascular membranes secondary to multifocal choroiditis, a hyperreflective band anterior to the retinal pigment epithelium (RPE) and an optically clear separation zone underneath the RPE have been associated with a good postoperative outcome after subretinal surgery to remove the CNV.[6]

The use of OCT for the examination of posterior inflammatory lesions is largely untested. Hypothetically, inflammation would increase optical reflectivity because infiltrates of inflammatory cells would increase the optical scattering. However, tissue swelling from inflammation may decrease optical reflectivity, and inflammatory infiltrates may cause shadowing of posterior structures. Careful interpretation of OCT images is therefore required along with clinical and angiographic correlation.[2] It seems likely that OCT will help localize inflammatory infiltrates to specific retinal and inner choroidal layers and thereby provide information regarding the pathophysiology of posterior uveitis.

We have selected cases that demonstrate the OCT appearance of either ocular complications of uveitis or posterior inflammatory lesions. OCT data on both topics will likely accrue rapidly in the future.

References

1. Hassenstein A, Bialasiewicz AA, Richard G. Optical coherence tomography in uveitis patients. *Am J Ophthalmol.* 2000;130(5):669-670.
2. Wang RC, Zamir E, Dugel PU, et al. Progressive subretinal fibrosis and blindness associated with multifocal granulomatous chorioretinitis: a variant of sympathetic ophthalmia. *Ophthalmology.* 2002;109(8):1527-1531.
3. Hee MR, Puliafito CA, Wong C, et al. Quantitative assessment of macular edema with optical coherence tomography. *Arch Ophthalmol.* 1995;113(8):1019-1029.
4. Antcliff RJ, Stanford MR, Chauhan DS, et al. Comparison between optical coherence tomography and fundus fluorescein angiography for the detection of cystoid macular edema in patients with uveitis. *Ophthalmology.* 2000;107(3):593-599.
5. Antcliff RJ, Spalton DJ, Stanford MR, Graham EM, Ffytche TJ, Marshall J. Intravitreal triamcinolone for uveitic cystoid macular edema: an optical coherence tomography study. *Ophthalmology.* 2001;108(4):765-772.
6. Zolf R, Glacet-Bernard A, Benhamou N, Mimoun G, Coscas G, Soubrane G. Imaging analysis with optical coherence tomography: relevance for submacular surgery in high myopia and in multifocal choroiditis. *Retina.* 2002;22(2):192-201.

Index to Cases

Case 9-1. Idiopathic Retinal Vasculitis and Neuroretinitis

Clinical Summary

A 36-year-old Haitian female presents complaining of snowflakes in each eye that last several minutes. Her visual acuity measures 20/25 in the right eye and 20/20 in the left eye. Dilated fundus exam of the right eye reveals disc edema, venous sheathing, inferior branch retinal artery occlusion, and cotton-wool spots (A). Exam of the left eye demonstrates mild epiretinal membrane, disc edema, and an aneurysm of the optic nerve (B). Early fluorescein angiography reveals occlusion of the inferior branch retinal artery and aneurysm of the left optic nerve (C). She is treated with panretinal photocoagulation. She returns several months later with a decline in visual acuity in her right eye to 20/50 secondary to a large subhyaloid hemorrhage along the inferior arcade (D). She is treated with further panretinal photocoagulation followed by a 23-gauge pars plana vitrectomy. She returns 12 days later with a visual acuity measuring 20/80 in the right eye. Fundus examination reveals clear media, absence of subhyaloid hemorrhage, resolution of traction, and good panretinal photocoagulation (E).

Optical Coherence Tomography

Horizontal OCT scan (F) during the first decline in vision reveals thickening of the retina. Hyporeflective cavities are suggestive of fluid accumulation, likely created by traction on the retina. Central foveal thickness is 475 μm (G). Horizontal OCT scan (H) after partial resolution of the subhyaloid hemorrhage reveals persistent thickening of the fovea. A hyperreflective linear density inserting near the fovea suggests remaining posterior hyaloid. A hyporeflective cavity at the fovea represents fluid accumulation, likely as a result of traction from the posterior hyaloid. Final horizontal OCT (I) following pars plana vitrectomy reveals a decrease in foveal thickness. Hyperreflective tufts at the retinal surface are suggestive of focal retinal tissue elevation, caused by peeling of the internal limiting membrane. A hyporeflective subfoveal cavity beneath the photoreceptor layer likely represents fluid accumulation. Central foveal thickness is 312 μm (J). Final ILM-RPE overlay (K) best illustrates the macular contour.

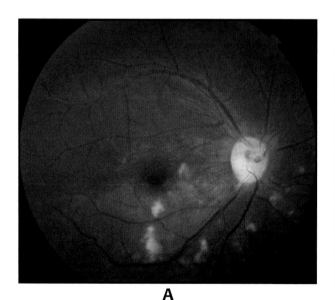

A

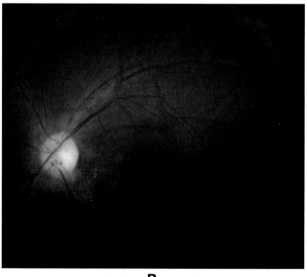

B

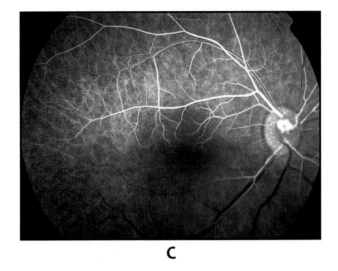

C

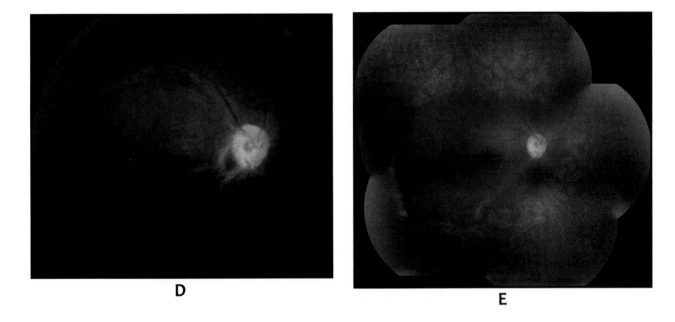

D

E

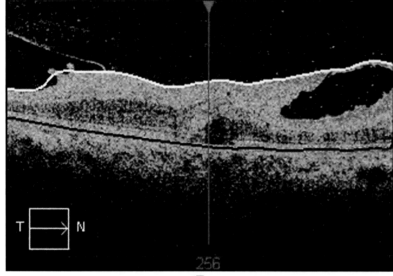

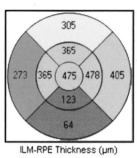

ILM-RPE Thickness (μm)

G

F

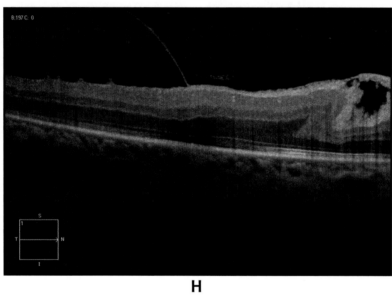

H

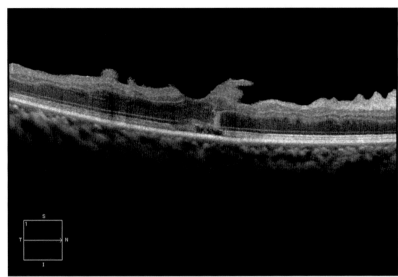

I

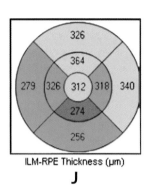

ILM-RPE Thickness (µm)

J

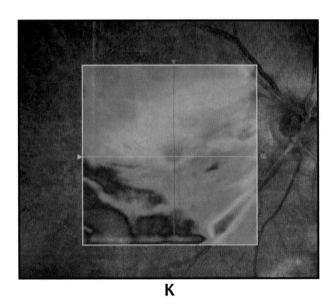

K

Case 9-2. Multifocal Choroiditis and Panuveitis

Clinical Summary

A 17-year-old female presents with complaints of episodes of photophobia and blurry vision. Visual acuity measures 20/30 in the right eye and 20/20 in the left eye. Dilated fundus exam reveals mild vitreous cell in the right eye, 360 degrees of multiple, punched-out, linear, hypopigmented choroidal lesions in a circumferential pattern (A).

Optical Coherence Tomography

OCT scans parallel to the lesions (B, C) show focal photoreceptor and RPE atrophy with associated hyperreflective choroidal structures. Perpendicular OCT scans to the choroidal lesions (D, E) similarly show focal areas of photoreceptor and retinal pigment irregularities corresponding to the choroidal lesion.

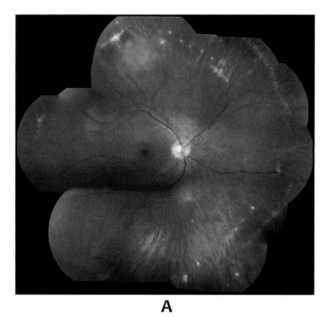

A

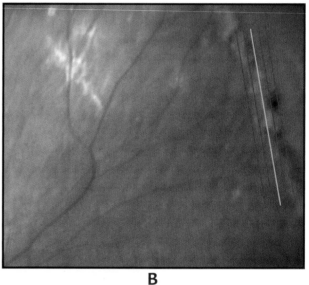

B

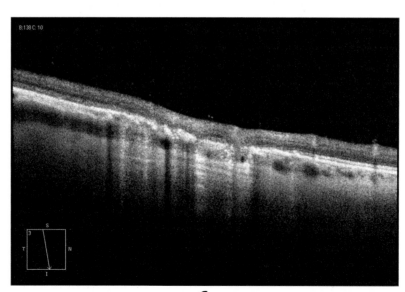

C

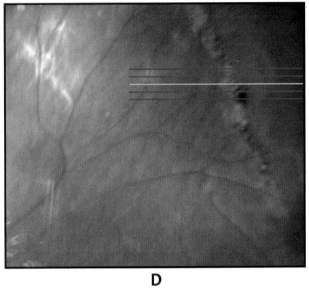

D

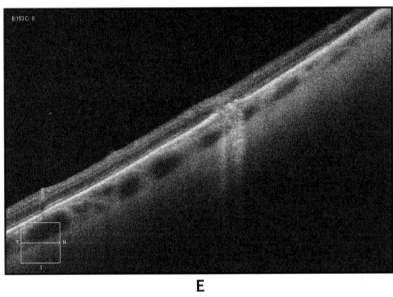

E

Case 9-3. Posterior Scleritis With Subretinal Fluid

Clinical Summary

A 29-year-old female presents with eye pain and edema with a decline in vision of the left eye for 2 weeks. She was previously diagnosed with biopsy-proven orbital pseudotumor. Visual acuity measures 20/20 in the right eye and counts fingers at 7 feet in the left eye. Dilated fundus exam demonstrates an area of subretinal fluid involving and nasal to the fovea in the left eye (A). Late fluorescein angiography reveals pinpoint hyperfluorescent leakage temporal to the nerve (B).

Optical Coherence Tomography

Horizontal OCT scan (C) of the left eye demonstrates a small hyporeflective subretinal cavity, leading to a larger hyperreflective subretinal cavity with elevation of the neurosensory retina, suggestive of subretinal fluid. Central foveal thickness is 725 µm (D). The ILM-RPE overlay (E) demonstrates the contour of macular thickness.

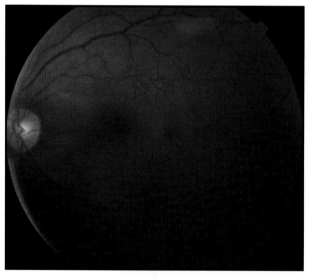

A

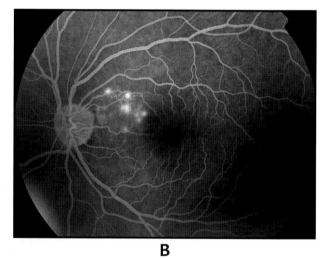

B

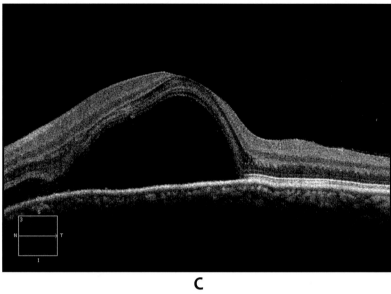

C

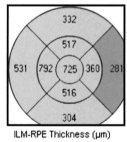

ILM-RPE Thickness (μm)

D

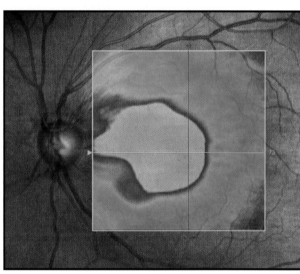

E

Case 9-4. Sympathetic Ophthalmia

Clinical Summary

A 63-year-old male presents with a 6-day history of decline in vision in the right eye. Four months prior, he had undergone a penetrating keratoplasty with synechiolysis of the left eye and subsequently developed anterior chamber inflammation with a white cataract. He then had phacoemulsification with intraocular lens implantation of the left eye. Visual acuity in the right eye is 20/70. Dilated fundus exam reveals mild RPE mottling and subretinal fluid within the macula (A).

Optical Coherence Tomography

Horizontal OCT scan of the right eye (B) reveals a hyporeflective cavity beneath the retina, indicative of subretinal fluid. Linear structures connecting the RPE to the outer retina may represent fibrin. Central retinal thickness is 403 μm (C). The ILM-RPE map reveals the retinal contour (D).

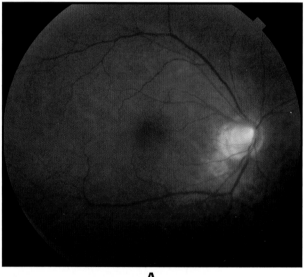

A

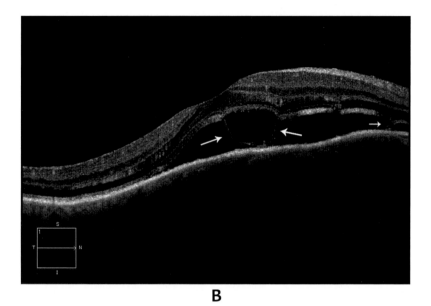

B

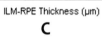

ILM-RPE Thickness (μm)

C

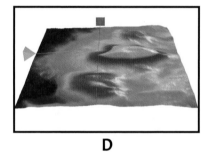

D

Case 9-5. Birdshot Chorioretinopathy

Clinical Summary

A 76-year-old male presents with a decline in vision in both eyes. Visual acuity measures 20/30 in both eyes. Dilated fundus exam findings include hypopigmented choroidal lesions extending from the optic nerve in a radial pattern and macular drusen (A, B).

Optical Coherence Tomography

Horizontal OCT scan (C) of the right eye reveals focal hyperreflective elevation of the RPE and mild irregularity of the pigment epithelium. Horizontal OCT scan (D) of the left eye similarly demonstrates a focal hyperreflective elevation of the RPE.

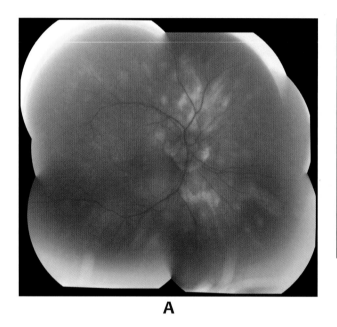

A

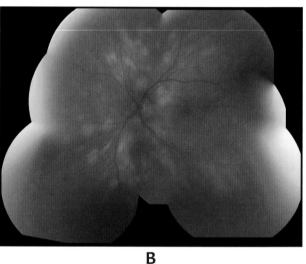

B

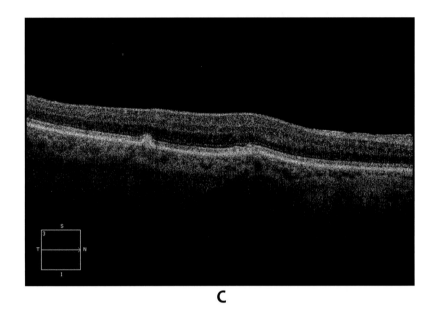

C

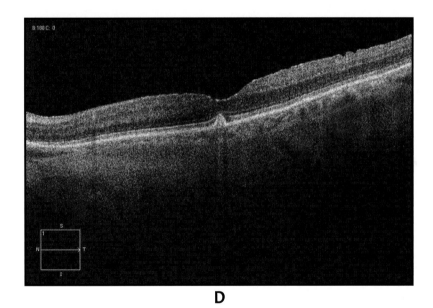

D

Case 9-6. Toxoplasmosis

Clinical Summary

A 30-year-old Brazilian male presents with a decline in vision in the left eye over 1 week and mild ocular pain. Visual acuity measures 20/20 in the right eye and 20/40 in the left eye. Dilated fundus exam of the left eye reveals mild anterior vitreous cells, sheathing along inferior arcade vessels, and a 3-disc diameter, white, elevated choroidal lesion in the inferotemporal periphery (A). Magnified photograph demonstrates cellular aggregates in the vitreous anterior to and surrounding the lesion (B).

Optical Coherence Tomography

Horizontal OCT scan through the lesion (C, D) reveals hyperreflective particles in the vitreous anterior to the lesion and at the vitreous-retina interface, likely representing cellular aggregates. Retinal and choroidal thickening with an increase in diffuse hyperreflectivity is evident compared to adjacent normal retina.

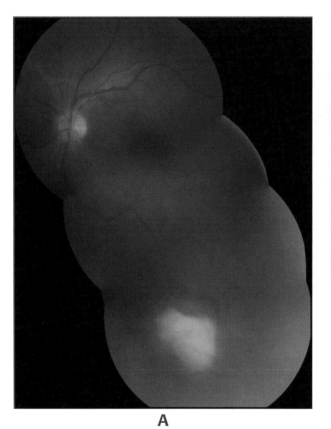

A

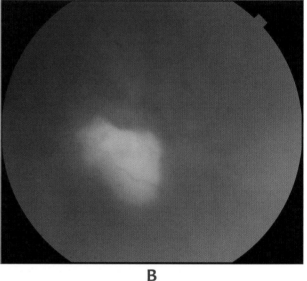

B

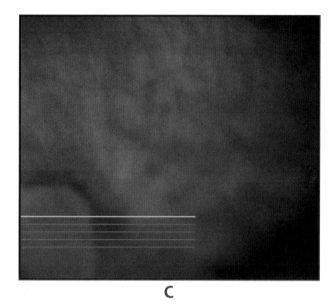

C

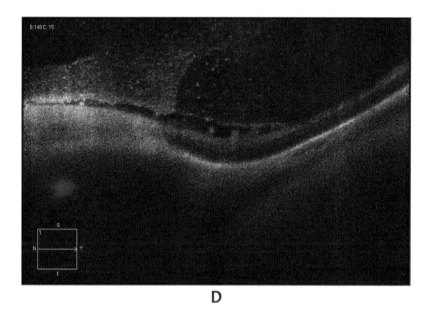

D

Case 9-7. Intermediate Uveitis With Cystoid Macular Edema

Clinical Summary

A 50-year-old African American female has a 3-year history of chronic bilateral intermediate uveitis. Systemic work-up is negative. She had received focal laser treatment for macular edema in both eyes by her previous physician. Best-corrected visual acuity is 20/50 in both eyes. On examination, she has persistent low-grade inflammation. Fundus exam of the right eye (A) reveals pigment mottling and macular thickening. Fluorescein angiography shows early mottled hyperfluorescence in the posterior pole (B) with late diffuse leakage in a cystoid pattern (C). Of note is the presence of a nonfilling central cyst.

Optical Coherence Tomography

An oblique scan through the macula (D) reveals partial loss of the foveal contour with large cystic cavities within the retina. A neurosensory detachment is observed directly beneath the fovea. Tissue bands separate the fluid-filled cavities, probably representing stretched Müller cells. The central retinal elevation is 541 μm, including both the thickened retina and the subretinal fluid. The retinal map (E) depicts a 3-mm area of marked elevation centered on the fovea with moderate elevation in the 6-mm area of the map. The "nonfilling cyst" seen on fluorescein angiography may correspond to the lack of pooling in the neurosensory detachment.

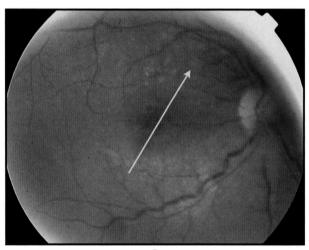

A

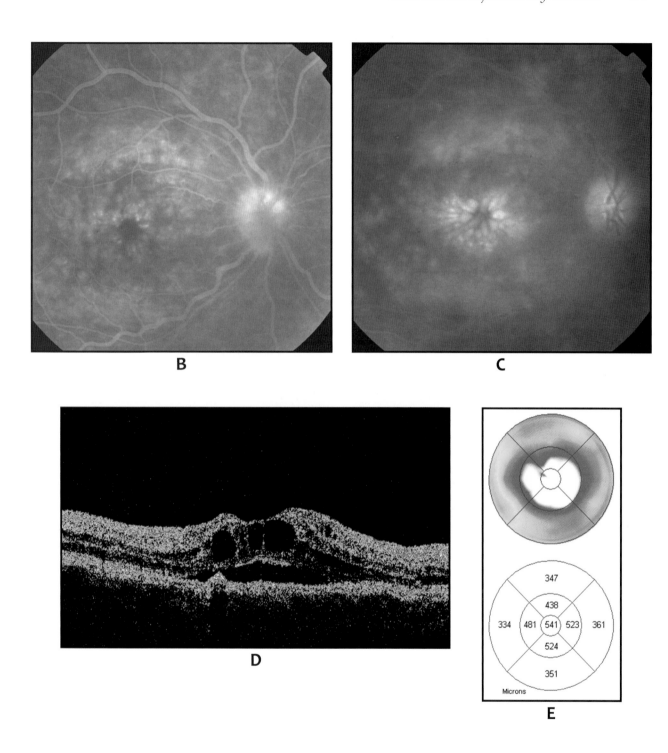

B

C

D

E

Case 9-7. Intermediate Uveitis With Cystoid Macular Edema (continued)

Clinical Summary

The left eye shows similar findings (F). A late petalloid pattern of cystoid macular edema with a filled center and diffuse macular leakage are evident on fluorescein angiography (G).

Optical Coherence Tomography

A vertical scan through the center of the fovea (H) shows loss of foveal contour with flattening and irregularity of the inner retinal surface. The central elevation is increased to 547 μm (I), and there are cystic cavities occupying the center of the fovea. No subretinal fluid is detected in the central macula, corresponding to the filled center on fluorescein angiography.

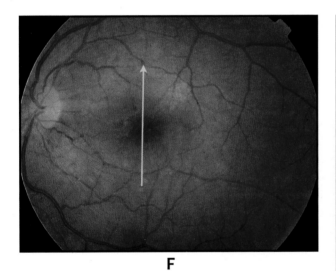

F

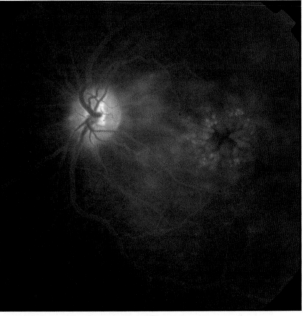

G

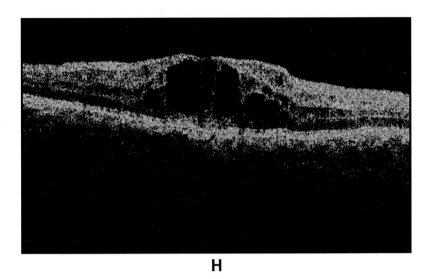

H

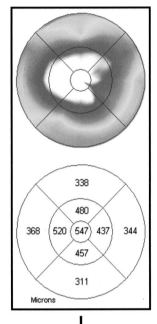

I

Case 9-8. Sarcoidosis With Choroidal Granulomas

Clinical Summary

A 51-year-old female presents with acute anterior granulomatous uveitis in her right eye and visual acuity of 20/60. Systemic work-up reveals a positive angiotensin-converting enzyme test and hilar adenopathy. A diagnosis of sarcoidosis is made. The anterior segment inflammation resolves on topical corticosteroids. Subsequently, slightly elevated, pale choroidal lesions are noted in the macular area as shown in the color fundus photograph (A). Similar lesions are also visible in the midperiphery of the right eye. These indistinct, slightly elevated choroidal lesions appear hypofluorescent in the early phases of the angiogram (B) and stain faintly in the late phases (C).

Optical Coherence Tomography

A vertical scan through the macula (D) shows a preserved foveal contour and normal central thickness. There are 2 oval-shaped, well-demarcated low reflective areas localized in the choroid, causing mild elevation of the overlying high reflective band. Since the retinal map measures thickness from the inner retinal surface to the outer high reflective band, the elevation caused by the choroidal change is not evident on the map (E).

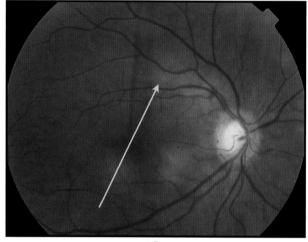

A

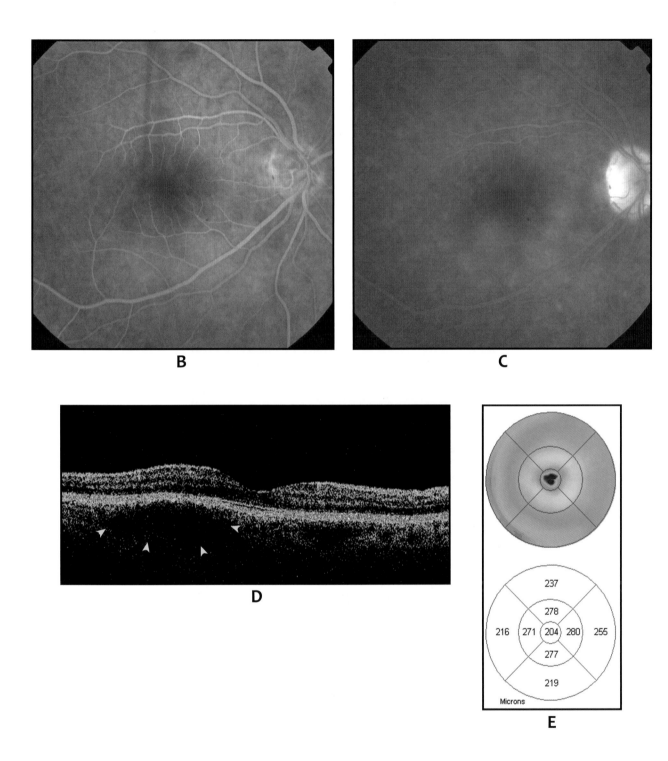

B

C

D

E

Case 9-8. Sarcoidosis With
Choroidal Granulomas (continued)

Continuation of Clinical Summary

The patient is treated with oral prednisone for 3 weeks. Visual acuity in the right eye returns to 20/40. Retinal examination (F) reveals flattening of the lesions with a persistent discoloration of the area inferior to the foveal center.

Follow-Up
Optical Coherence Tomography

Repeat scan through the macula (G) shows resolution of the hyporeflective lesions beneath the RPE and flattening of the red band. The choroidal backscattering signal has returned to normal with visualization of the lumen of choroidal vessels.

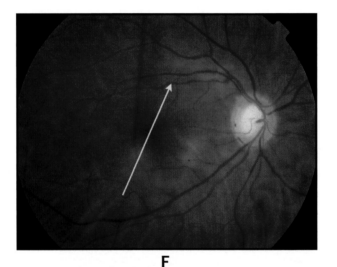

F

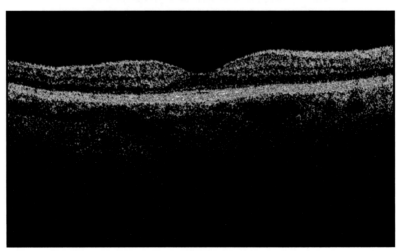

G

Case 9-9. Vogt-Koyanagi-Harada Disease

Clinical Summary

A 31-year-old female presents with loss of vision in both eyes to the 20/400 level for 3 days. Fundus evaluation (A) of the right eye reveals serous retinal detachment involving the macula. Fluorescein angiography (B) shows multiple punctate hyperfluorescent lesions at the level of the RPE. Pooling of the dye under the areas of serous detachment is observed in the late frames of the angiogram (C).

Optical Coherence Tomography

A horizontal scan through the macula (D) shows extensive elevation of the neurosensory retina. The inner retinal layers are relatively well preserved, and the foveal contour can still be identified. There appears to be complex infolding of the outer retinal layers, creating variably sized cystic cavities. Although some of the fluid is clearly subretinal, in other areas it is difficult to differentiate subretinal from intraretinal location of the fluid. The fluid in these spaces shows a moderate amount of backscattering signal, probably indicating higher protein content. The retinal map (E) confirms elevation of the central macula to a peak of 727 µm.

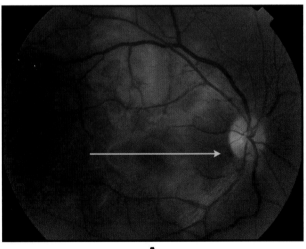

A

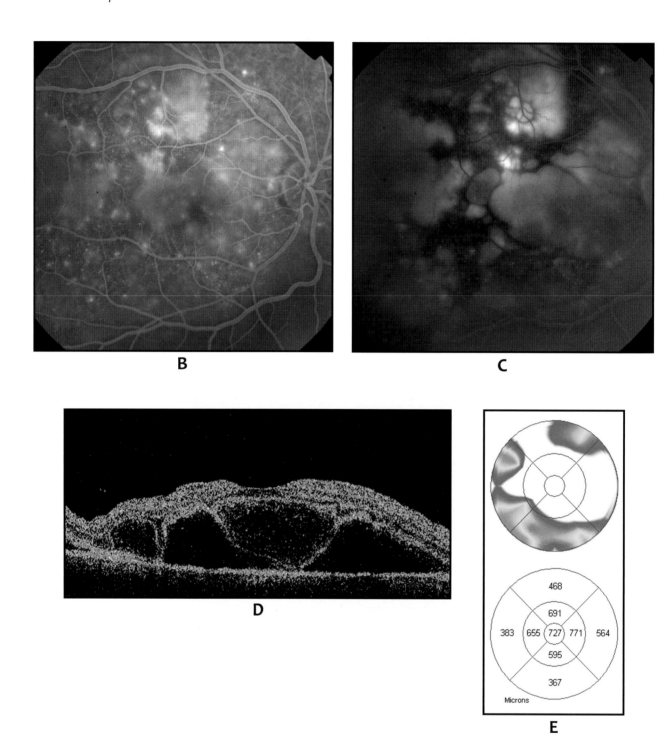

B

C

D

E

Case 9-10. Cytomegalovirus Retinitis With Immune Recovery Vitreitis and Cystoid Macular Edema

Clinical Summary

A 31-year-old male had cytomegalovirus retinitis successfully treated 5 years before. After starting on highly active antiretroviral therapy, he had no further reactivations but developed chronic anterior uveitis. He complains of persistent decrease in vision and floaters in both eyes. Best-corrected visual acuity is 20/60 in the right eye. Anterior segment examination reveals trace cellular reaction. There is mild vitreous inflammation with vitreous strand formation. Retinal examination of the right eye (A) shows extensive areas of healed retinitis extending into the macula. Pigment abnormalities and focal thickening are noted in the foveal region. He is diagnosed with immune recovery uveitis.

Optical Coherence Tomography

A vertical scan through the foveal center of the right eye (B) shows vitreous opacities parallel to the inner retina. These may represent focal cellular infiltrates on the posterior hyaloid surface. There is a mild increase in central thickness with cystoid macular edema. The superior aspect of the scan cuts through an area of healed retinitis, where the retinal tissue is compacted and highly reflective.

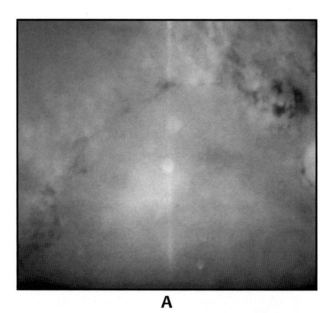

A

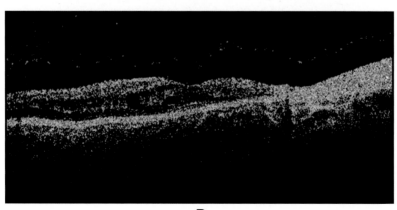

B

Case 9-10. Cytomegalovirus Retinitis With Immune Recovery Vitreitis and Cystoid Macular Edema (continued)

Clinical Summary

Best-corrected visual acuity is 20/50 in the left eye. There is mild cellular reaction in the anterior chamber and vitreous cavity of this eye. Retinal examination (C) shows peripheral scarring from the previous retinitis. There is extensive cystoid macular edema in this eye.

Optical Coherence Tomography

A vertical scan through the fovea of the left eye (D) also shows vitreous opacities lying above the retinal surface. There is a suggestion of focal attachment to the foveal center with possible traction. There is loss of the foveal contour with intraretinal thickening. Cystoid macular edema is seen as nonreflective cavities within the retina.

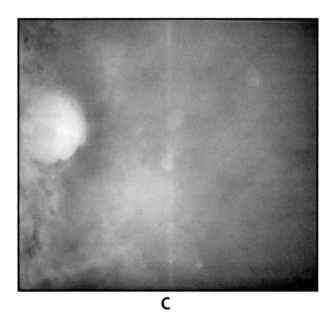

C

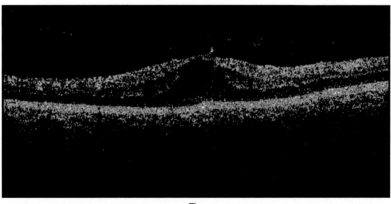

D

Chapter 10

Retinal Dystrophies

Heeral R. Shah, MD; Vanessa Cruz-Villegas, MD; Philip J. Rosenfeld, MD, PhD; Carmen A. Puliafito, MD, MBA; and Jay S. Duker, MD

- Retinitis Pigmentosa
- Stargardt's Disease
- Best's Disease
- Pattern Dystrophy

Optical coherence tomography (OCT) plays a pivotal role in diagnosing, monitoring, and assessing treatment benefit in different macular conditions such as diabetic and cystoid macular edema (CME), epiretinal membranes, macular holes, vitreomacular traction syndrome, and macular edema secondary to retinal vein occlusions. This noninvasive diagnostic tool can also help in the clinical evaluation and management of hereditary retinal disorders.[1] OCT contributes to our understanding of the histopathology of these disorders by providing high-resolution cross-sectional imaging of the retina and retinal pigment epithelium (RPE)/choriocapillaris.

Retinitis Pigmentosa

Retinitis pigmentosa is one of the most common hereditary retinal disorders seen in clinical practice. Patients with retinitis pigmentosa typically experience nyctalopia and peripheral vision loss. Clinical findings include pale optic nerve heads; attenuated retinal vessels; peripheral pigmentary changes; or bone-spicule formation and peripheral atrophy of the retina, RPE, and choriocapillaris. CME is a common, potentially treatable cause of central visual loss in retinitis pigmentosa. OCT can detect the presence of CME in a noninvasive way and quantify the response to treatment to acetazolamide.[1,2] CME is visualized in OCT as cystic intraretinal spaces of reduced optical reflectivity. In retinitis pigmentosa or rod-cone dystrophies, thinning of the affected neurosensory retina and RPE/choriocapillaris complex may be observed by OCT.[3,4] This atrophy or thinning of the neurosensory retina allows better penetration of light, and hence, enhanced reflectivity from the choroid is evident in these cases.[3] The pigmented lesions are seen as hyperreflective areas.[3]

Stargardt's Disease

Stargardt's disease is also a common hereditary condition that usually affects individuals in their first or second decade of life. Individuals with this disease may present with bilateral yellowish flecks at the level of the RPE and macular atrophic changes. Histopathologic studies reveal accumulation of lipofuscin-like material at the RPE level and loss of RPE and photoreceptor cells.[5] OCT findings correlate with these descriptions and provide an in vivo evaluation of the histopathology of this condition. Patients with Stargardt's disease may show thinning of the affected retina and disorganization and loss of the outer nuclear layer in OCT. Atrophy of the neurosensory retina and RPE allows better light penetration, resulting in increased choroidal reflectivity.

Schuman JS, Puliafito CA, Fujimoto JG, Duker JS, eds.
Optical Coherence Tomography of Ocular Diseases,
Third Edition (pp 287-318).
© 2013 SLACK Incorporated.

Best's Disease

Best's disease is an inherited macular dystrophy characterized by the presence of bilateral subretinal vitelliform lesions. These vitelliform lesions may progress and evolve over time to an atrophic end stage. It is not unusual to observe choroidal neovascularization (CNV) in patients with this disorder. Histopathologic reports reveal degeneration of photoreceptors, accumulation of lipofuscin at the level of the RPE, and sub-RPE fibrillar material deposition.[6] Unfortunately, there are no histopathology reports describing the vitelliform stage. OCT contributes to our knowledge of this macular dystrophy by providing high-resolution in vivo imaging of the retina and RPE/choriocapillaris complex. OCT findings seen in Best's disease vary depending on the stage of the condition. The findings described in the literature include elevation and/or splitting of the RPE/choriocapillaris complex. A hyporeflective space is sometimes visualized between the split layers of this complex.[7] Also, central neurosensory retinal detachments like the ones observed in idiopathic central serous chorioretinopathy may be observed.[7,8] Since Best's disease is a dynamic macular dystrophy that evolves into different stages, OCT findings disclose the changing and variegated nature of the disorder. In addition, OCT not only provides insight into the nature of the disease, it also helps to follow the evolution of the condition. This is particularly important in cases of CNV in which OCT may assist in the assessment of treatment response.[9]

Pattern Dystrophy

Pattern dystrophy is a dominantly inherited macular condition characterized by yellowish deposits at the level of the RPE in the macular region. The configuration of the foveal lesions may present in different patterns, including vitelliform round or oval lesions, reticular, and triradiate or butterfly lesions.[10] OCT findings seen in this condition correlate with the diversity of the clinical presentation. Thickening at the level of the RPE[8] as well as hyperreflective deposits under the neurosensory retina overlying the RPE have been described in the literature.[11] Also, thinning of the neurosensory retina and photoreceptor loss may be observed in the macular area.

References

1. Stanga PE, Downes SM, Ahuja RM, et al. Comparison of optical coherence tomography and fluorescein angiography in assessing macular edema in retinal dystrophies: preliminary results. *Int Ophthalmol*. 2001;23(4-6):321-325.
2. Rumen F, Souied E, Oubraham H, Coscas G, Soubrane G. Optical coherence tomography in the follow up of macular edema treatment in retinitis pigmentosa. *J Fr Ophthalmol*. 2001;24(8):854-859.
3. Hamada S, Yoshida K, Chihara E. Optical coherence tomography images of retinitis pigmentosa. *Ophthalmic Surg Lasers*. 2000;31(3):253-256.
4. Jacobson SG, Buraczynska M, Milam AH, et al. Disease expression in X-linked retinitis pigmentosa caused by a putative null mutation in the RPGR gene. *Invest Ophthalmol Vis Sci*. 1997;38(10):1983-1997.
5. Birnbach CD, Jarvelainen M, Possin DE, Milam AH. Histopathology and immunocytochemistry of the neurosensory retina in fundus flavimaculatus. *Ophthalmology*. 1994;101(7):1211-1219.
6. Frangieh GT, Green WR, Fine SL. A histopathologic study of Best's macular dystrophy. *Arch Ophthalmol*. 1982;100(7):1115-1121.
7. Pianta MJ, Aleman TS, Cideciyan AV, et al. In vivo micropathology of Best macular dystrophy with optical coherence tomography. *Exp Eye Res*. 2003;76(2):203-211.
8. Pierro L, Tremolada G, Introini U, Calori G, Brancato R. Optical coherence tomography findings in adult-onset foveomacular vitelliform dystrophy. *Am J Ophthalmol*. 2002;134(5):675-680.
9. Andrade RE, Farah ME, Cardillo JA, Hofling-Lima AL, Uno F, Costa RA. Optical coherence tomography in choroidal neovascular membrane associated with Best's vitelliform dystrophy. *Acta Ophthalmol Scand*. 2002;80(2):216-218.
10. Gass JDM. *Stereoscopic Atlas of Macular Diseases*. 4th ed. St. Louis, MO: CV Mosby; 1997:314-325, 374-376.
11. Benhamou N, Souied EH, Zolf R, Coscas F, Coscas G, Soubrane G. Adult-onset foveomacular vitelliform dystrophy: a study by optical coherence tomography. *Am J Ophthalmol*. 2003;135(3):362-367.

Index to Cases

Case 10-1A. Retinitis Pigmentosa

Clinical Summary

A 70-year-old female presents with a known diagnosis of retinitis pigmentosa. Visual acuity in each eye is 20/400. Dilated fundus exam of each eye reveals waxy nerve pallor, vascular attenuation, and bony spicules (A, B).

Optical Coherence Tomography

Ultrahigh horizontal OCT scan of the right eye (C) demonstrates diffuse loss of the photoreceptor layer. Ultrahigh horizontal OCT scan of the left eye (D) reveals diffuse photoreceptor loss, epiretinal membrane over the nasal retina with trace thickening, and an irregular foveal contour.

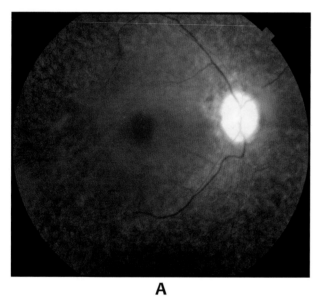

A

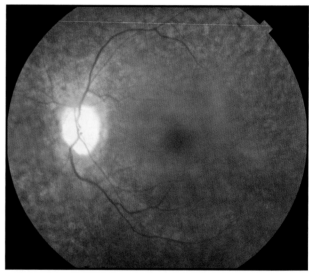

B

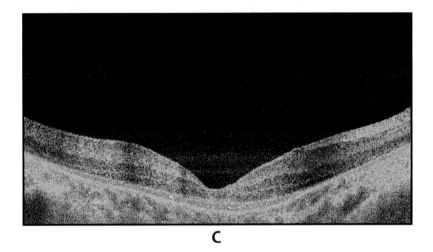

C

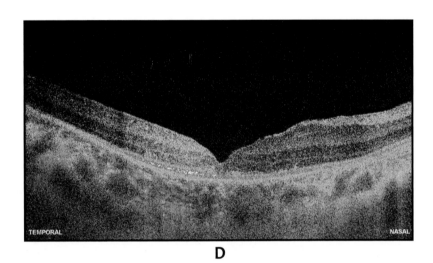

D

Case 10-1B. Retinitis Pigmentosa

Clinical Summary

A 63-year-old female presents for an annual examination. She complains of progressive decline in vision in both eyes. Visual acuity is counts fingers at 3 feet in the right eye and counts fingers at 5 feet in the left eye. Dilated fundus examination of each eye (A, B) reveals waxy nerve pallor, attenuated vessels, bony spicules, patches of RPE atrophy, and RPE mottling in the central macula.

Optical Coherence Tomography

Horizontal OCT scan of each eye (C, D) reveals diffuse retinal thinning, an absence of the photoreceptor layer, and a mildly abnormal foveal contour. Central retinal thickness of the right eye is 216 µm (E). Central retinal thickness of the left eye is 172 µm (F). The ILM-RPE color maps of each eye (G, H) illustrate the general retinal contour.

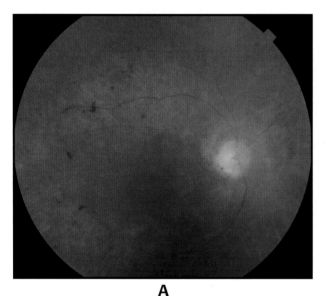

A

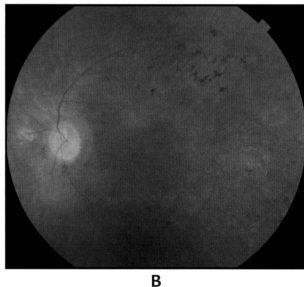

B

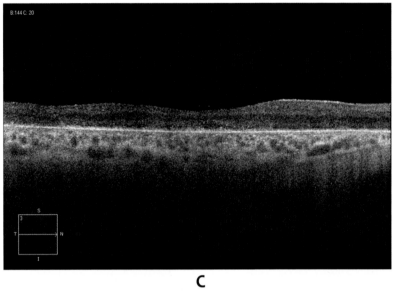

C

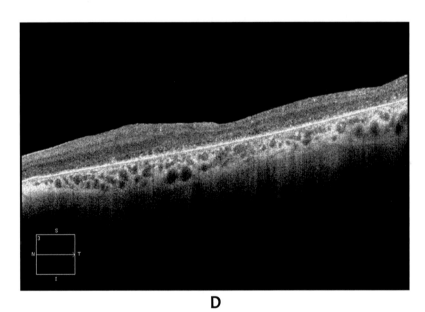

D

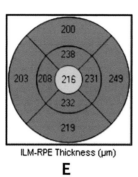

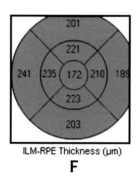

ILM-RPE Thickness (µm)

E

ILM-RPE Thickness (µm)

F

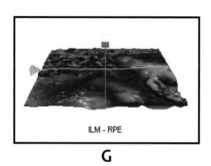

ILM - RPE

G

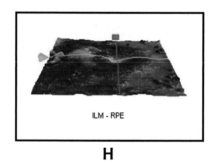

ILM - RPE

H

Case 10-2. Stargardt's Dystrophy

Clinical Summary

A 56-year-old female presents with a presumed diagnosis of Stargardt's macular dystrophy. Dilated fundus exam shows well-demarcated RPE atrophy in the central macula, with a ring of subretinal yellow lesions temporal to this area of atrophy (A). Fundus exam of the left eye shows a ring of RPE atrophy, surrounded by a ring of subretinal yellow lesions (B).

Optical Coherence Tomography

Horizontal OCT scan of the right eye (C) shows thinning and irregularity of the RPE and thinning of the outer retinal layers, including the photoreceptor layer, all in the area corresponding to RPE atrophy. The hyperreflectivity of the choroid likely represents an unusually large amount of light passing through an abnormally thin retina and RPE. Horizontal OCT scan of the left eye (D) similarly shows thinning of the outer retinal layers and photoreceptor layer in the area corresponding to the ring of RPE atrophy. Mild change in foveal contour is noted.

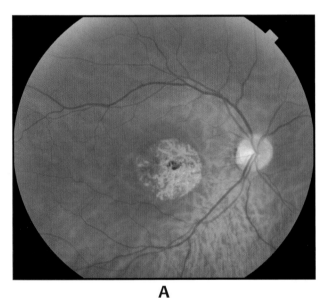

A

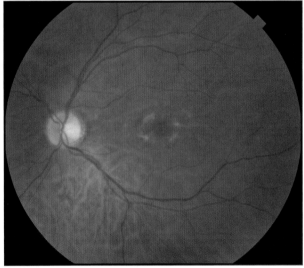

B

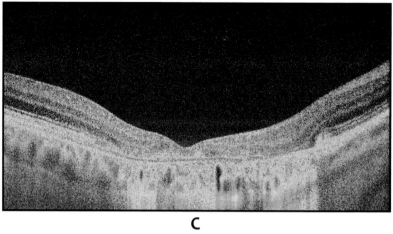

C

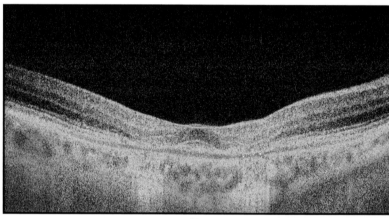

D

Case 10-3. Stargardt's Macular Dystrophy RTVue-100

Clinical Summary

A 47-year-old male presents for routine follow-up examination. He denies a recent change in vision. Visual acuity is 20/200 in each eye. Dilated fundus exam of each eye (A, B) reveals a central area of RPE atrophy and changes and peripheral retinal flecks.

Optical Coherence Tomography

Horizontal OCT scan of each eye (C, D) demonstrates diffuse RPE and retinal thinning. Retinal thickness of each eye (E, F) is revealed by the respective thickness maps.

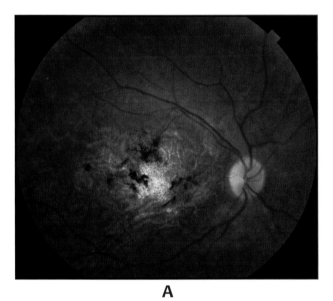

A

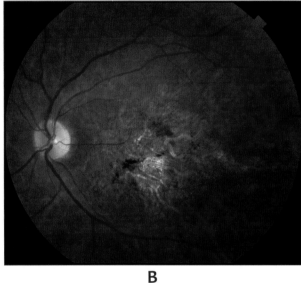

B

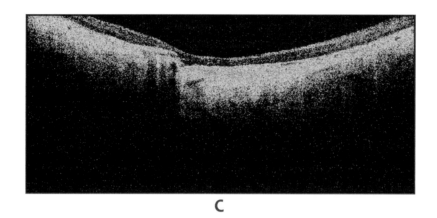

C

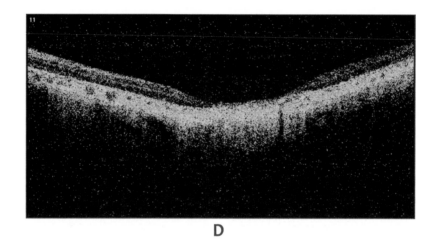

D

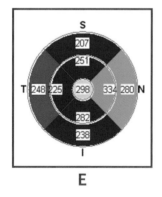

E

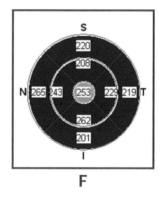

F

Case 10-4A. Best's Disease—Unilateral

Clinical Summary

An 8-year-old male is referred for a macular lesion in the right eye. He denies visual changes. Visual acuity in the right eye is 20/30 and the left eye is 20/25. Dilated fundus exam of the right eye reveals a 300-μm, round, yellow subretinal lesion (A). Fundus exam of the left eye is normal (B). Autofluorescence of the right eye (C) reveals the lipofuscin accumulation.

Optical Coherence Tomography

Horizontal OCT scan (D) shows a focal, hyper-reflective, subfoveal lesion originating from the RPE, leading to an elevation of the photoreceptor layer and mild change in foveal contour. Central foveal thickness is 245 μm (E). The ILM-RPE overlay (F) demonstrates the central macular contour.

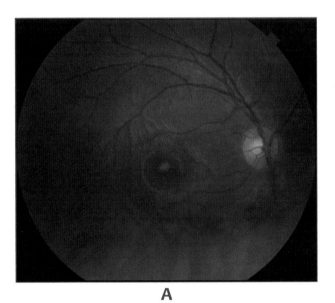

A

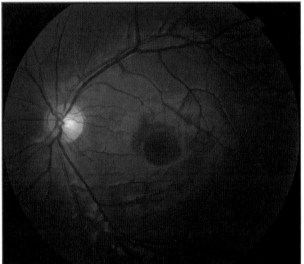

B

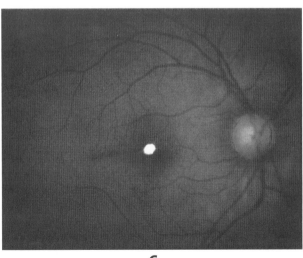

C

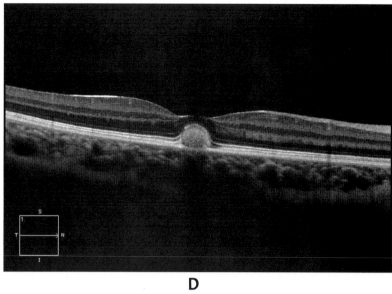

D

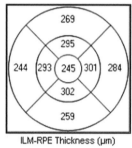

ILM-RPE Thickness (µm)

E

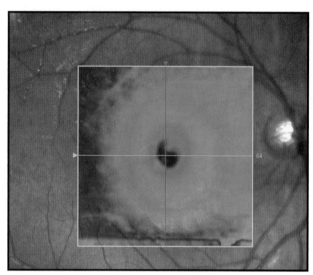

F

Case 10-4B. Best's Disease

Clinical Summary

A 9-year-old male is referred for macular lesions. Ocular history involves a prior diagnosis of Best's macular dystrophy and intravitreal bevacizumab 2 years prior for presumed choroidal neovascular membrane in the left eye. Family history is significant for Best's macular dystrophy in the mother and maternal aunt. Visual acuity is 20/100 in the right eye and 20/200 in the left eye. Fundus examination of the right eye reveals a yellow, fibrotic, pigmented scar involving and inferior to the fovea (A). Examination of the left eye demonstrates an elevated yellow subretinal lesion with surrounding pigment changes (B).

Optical Coherence Tomography

Vertical OCT scan (C) obtained through the vitelliform lesion shows an elevated hyperreflective thickening, beginning at the level of RPE and protruding into subretinal space. Elevation of the neurosensory retina is present, but without subretinal or intraretinal fluid accumulation. Hyporeflective cavities at the base of the lesion may represent accumulation of fluid or material beneath the RPE. Central foveal thickness is 220 µm (D). The ILM-RPE map (E) demonstrates the retinal contour. Horizontal OCT scan (F) through the vitelliform lesion in the left eye reveals highly reflective material splitting Bruch's membrane and the RPE at its margins and protruding into subretinal and intraretinal space. The apex of the fovea shows one hyporeflective space consistent with intraretinal fluid accumulation. Another hyporeflective space at the base of the subretinal material suggests either accumulation of material or the presence of subretinal fluid beneath the RPE. Central foveal thickness is 318 µm (G). The ILM-RPE map (H), again, illustrates the retinal contour.

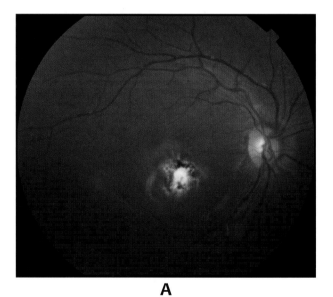

A

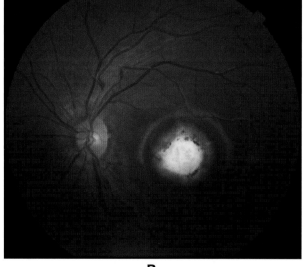

B

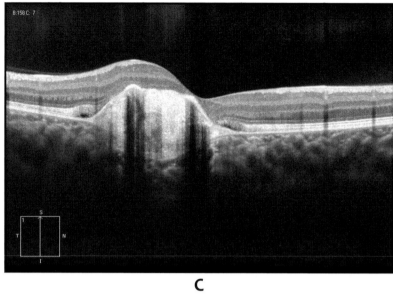

C

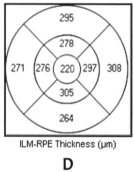

ILM-RPE Thickness (μm)

D

ILM - RPE

E

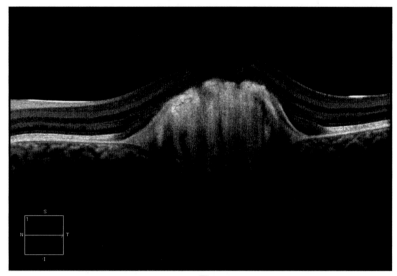

F

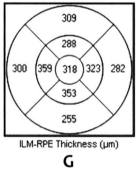

ILM-RPE Thickness (µm)

G

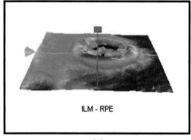

ILM - RPE

H

Case 10-5. Pattern Dystrophy

Clinical Summary

A 37-year-old female presents with complaints of metamorphopsia in the right eye. Visual acuity measures 20/70 in the right eye and 20/30 in the left eye. Dilated fundus exam of both eyes reveals prominent cruciate RPE changes in each macula (A, B).

Optical Coherence Tomography

Horizontal OCT scan (C) of the right eye reveals subfoveal elevated hyperreflective material beneath the RPE, corresponding to the center of the cruciate. Nasally, thickened RPE is evident; this scan overlies one arm of the pattern dystrophy. The ILM-RPE map (D) demonstrates the abnormality. Horizontal OCT scan (E) of the left eye shows diffuse subfoveal sub-RPE thickening. A central hyperreflective pinpoint area is present at the retinal surface.

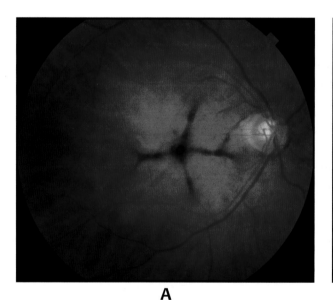

A

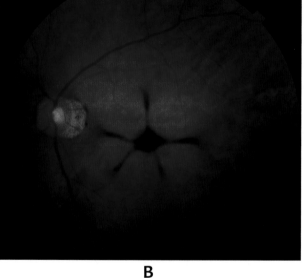

B

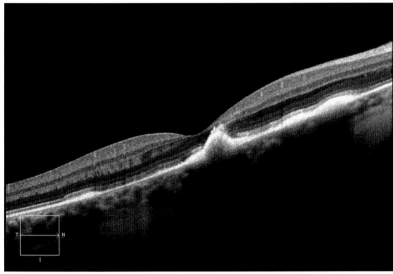

C

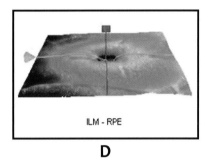

ILM - RPE

D

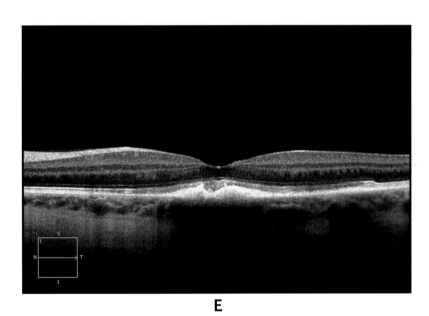

E

Case 10-6. Plaquenil Toxicity

Clinical Summary

A 40-year-old female is referred for use of hydroxychloroquine. She denies visual complaints. Late fluorescein angiography of the right eye (A) reveals hypofluorescence in the central macula, surrounded by a late staining in a ring pattern. These findings are more notable on late fluorescein angiography of the left eye (B).

Optical Coherence Tomography

Horizontal ultrahigh-resolution OCT scan of the right eye (C) reveals absence of the photoreceptor layer in the temporal and nasal aspects, with preservation beneath the fovea. Horizontal ultrahigh-resolution OCT scan of the left eye (D) shows near-complete absence of the photoreceptor layer.

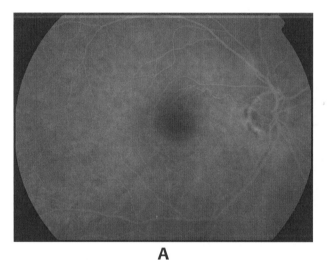

A

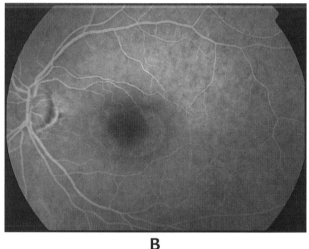

B

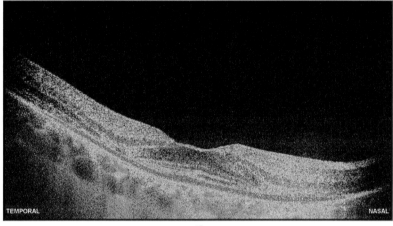

C

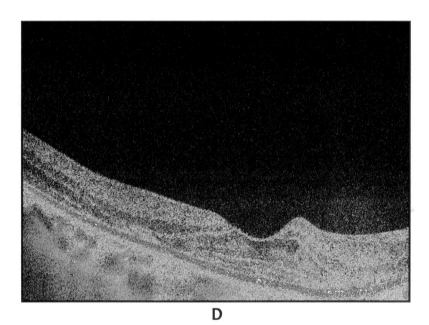

D

Case 10-7. Retinitis Punctata Albescens

Clinical Summary

A 10-year-old female with a history of retinitis punctata albescens is examined. Her visual acuity is 20/25 in the right eye. Retinal examination of the right eye reveals wrinkling of the ILM in the posterior pole and cystoid macular changes (A). Mottling and patchy atrophic alterations are visualized throughout the midperiphery and periphery. White dots are observed scattered throughout the fundus (B-D).

Optical Coherence Tomography

OCT (E) depicts loss of the normal foveal contour and cystic areas of reduced reflectivity at the level of the outer plexiform layer consistent with cystoid macular edema. The central macular thickness measures 362 µm in this eye (F).

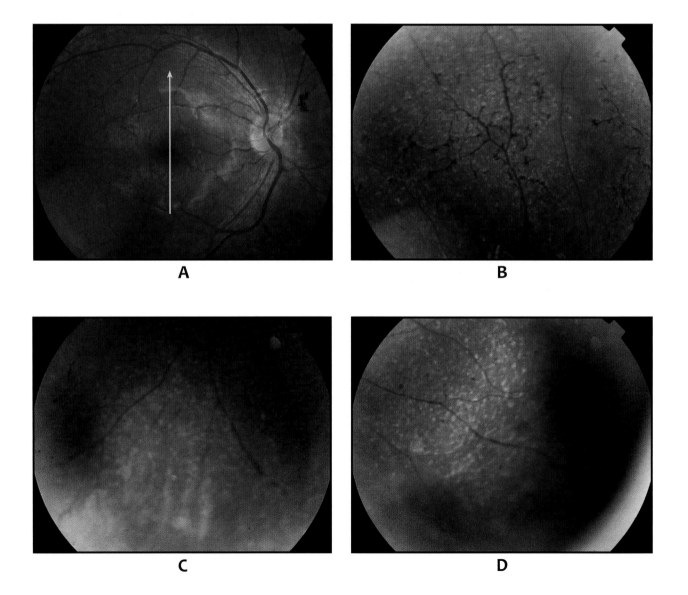

A

B

C

D

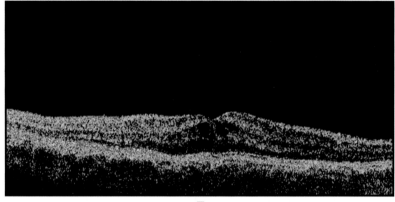

E

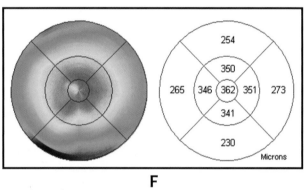

F

Case 10-7. Retinitis Punctata Albescens (continued)

Clinical Summary

Evaluation of the patient's left eye reveals the same clinical findings (G-J). Visual acuity measures 20/20 in this eye.

Optical Coherence Tomography

An OCT scan obtained through the fovea (K) shows tiny low reflective cystic spaces representing cystoid macular edema. The foveal thickness measures 322 μm (L).

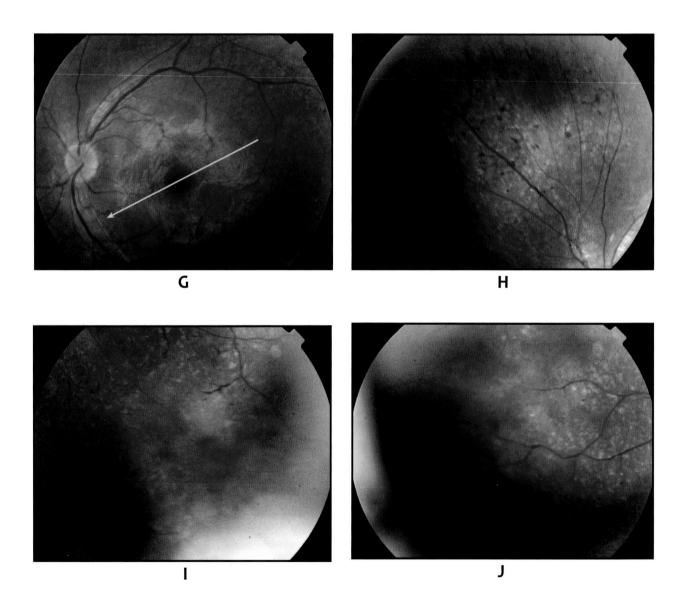

G

H

I

J

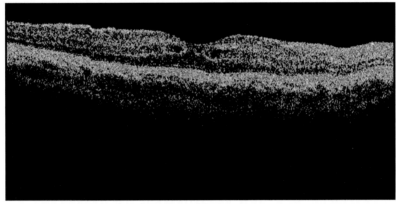

K

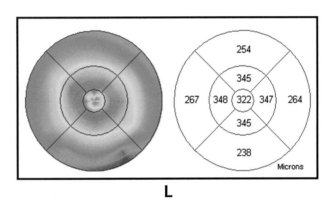

L

Case 10-8. Rod-Cone Dystrophy

Clinical Summary

A 47-year-old male was diagnosed with rod-cone dystrophy. His visual acuity is 20/50 in the right eye. Retinal examination of this eye reveals a slight optic nerve pallor, attenuation of retinal vessels, and RPE atrophy more prominently seen in the macular area. The macula also shows some cystic alterations (A). Fluorescein angiography (B) shows staining and window defects corresponding to the areas of RPE atrophy.

Optical Coherence Tomography

Despite the fact that no obvious dye leakage was appreciated in fluorescein angiography, a horizontal OCT scan (C) shows cystic spaces of reduced reflectivity in the outer retinal layers consistent with cystoid macular edema. The perifoveal area surrounding the central cystic fovea shows enhanced reflectivity of the choroid due to increased optical penetration in this atrophic area. The central macular thickness is 409 μm. The perifoveal area is thin, with a thickness ranging from 188 to 232 μm (D).

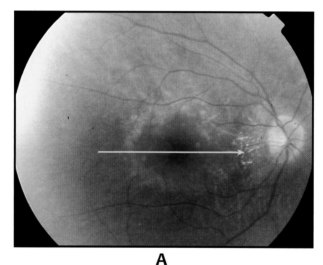

A

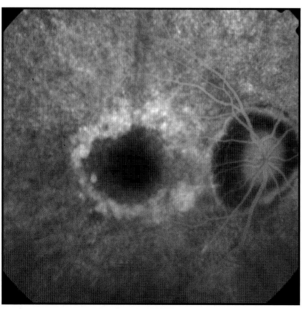

B—early

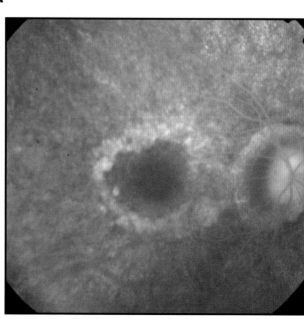

B—late

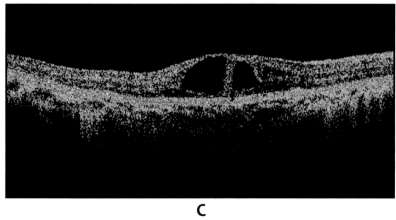

C

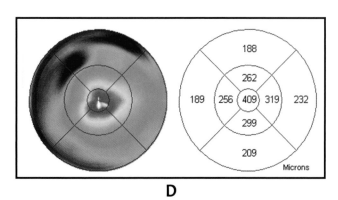

D

Case 10-8. Rod-Cone Dystrophy (continued)

Clinical Summary

The left eye shows similar findings (E). Visual acuity is 20/40 in this eye. Fluorescein angiography (F) reveals window defects consistent with RPE atrophy in the macular area but no apparent leakage.

Optical Coherence Tomography

A horizontal OCT scan (G) obtained through the fovea reveals intraretinal fluid accumulation represented by cystic spaces of reduced reflectivity. Enhanced choroidal reflectivity secondary to increased light penetration is appreciated in the perimacular area, which correlates with the aforementioned atrophic alterations. The retinal map analysis shows a central foveal thickness of 351 μm. The perimacular ring measures from 196 to 241 μm in thickness (H).

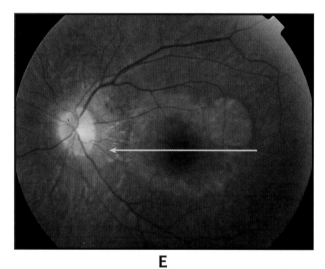

E

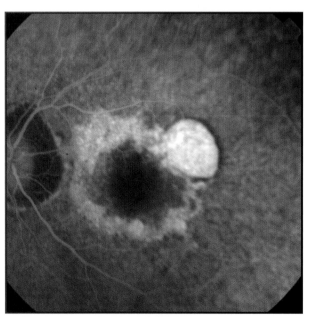

F—early

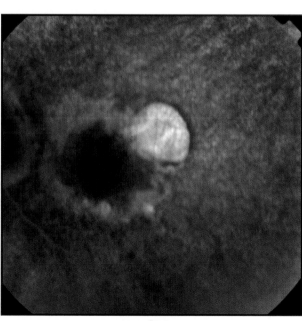

F—late

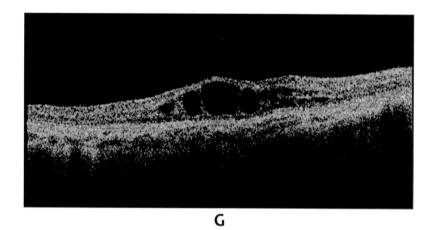

G

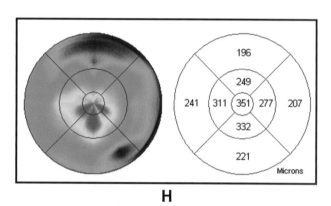

H

Case 10-9. X-Linked Juvenile Retinoschisis

Clinical Summary

An 8-year-old male with a history of X-linked juvenile retinoschisis is examined. His visual acuity is 20/60 in the right eye. Retinal examination shows a stellate maculopathy and a peripheral schisis extending from the inferotemporal quadrant toward the inferotemporal arcade in the posterior pole. Retinal pigment alterations are also noticed (A).

Optical Coherence Tomography

A vertical OCT scan obtained through the fovea (B) confirms the presence of the foveal cystic alterations predominantly in the outer layers. Cleavage or splitting in the retinal tissue at the level of the nerve fiber layer and bridging retinal elements are noticeable inferior to the fovea where the peripheral schisis cavity is observed.

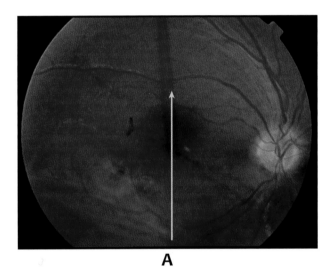

A

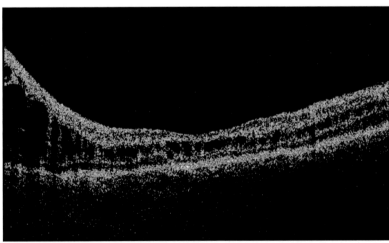

B

Case 10-10. Retinoschisis

Clinical Summary

A 51-year-old male is referred for "progression" of a retinoschisis cavity in the right eye. He denies visual changes. Visual acuity is 20/20 in each eye. Dilated fundus exam of the right eye reveals retinoschisis inferotemporal to the macula. No inner or outer holes are present (A). Fundus exam of the left eye reveals peripheral retinoschisis in the superotemporal periphery.

Optical Coherence Tomography

Obliquely oriented OCT scan (inferotemporal to superonasal) of the right eye retinoschisis cavity (B) shows initial absence of inner retinal layers, leading to the presence of a hyperreflective linear density from the vitreous cavity forming the inner retinal layers. Hyporeflective spaces in the superonasal quadrant of the scan may represent cystic degeneration in the nerve fiber layer.

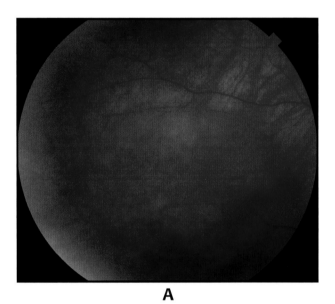

A

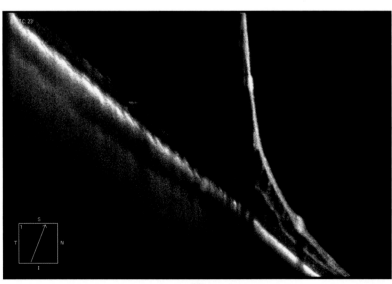

B

Chapter 11

Miscellaneous Retinal Diseases

Heeral R. Shah, MD; Elias C. Mavrofrides, MD; Vanessa Cruz-Villegas, MD; Carmen A. Puliafito, MD, MBA; and Jay S. Duker, MD

- Cystoid Macular Edema
- Rhegmatogenous Retinal Detachment
- Posterior Segment Trauma
- Optic Nerve Pit

Optical coherence tomography (OCT) can be useful in the evaluation of a broad range of retinal conditions. This chapter provides additional examples of the application of OCT in various clinical situations.

Cystoid Macular Edema

One of the most powerful applications of OCT is in the evaluation and management of patients with cystoid macular edema (CME) regardless of the underlying etiology. CME appears as retinal thickening with intraretinal cavities of reduced reflectivity on OCT.[1] The use of OCT for CME caused by diabetic retinopathy, retinal vein occlusion, choroidal neovascularization, inflammatory conditions, and retinal dystrophies has been detailed in other chapters.

CME can also occur in many other clinical settings, most notably following intraocular surgery. Clinically significant CME is estimated to occur in 1% to 2% of patients undergoing cataract extraction and is likely more common after other types of intraocular surgery.[2] Establishing the diagnosis by fundus examination alone can be difficult, and fluorescein angiography is often needed for confirmation. OCT appears to be equally effective as angiography in establishing the diagnosis but is far less invasive and significantly quicker. OCT also has the advantage of providing a quantitative assessment of macular thickness, which can be used to monitor the clinical course. Repeated quantitative evaluations with OCT can be invaluable in therapeutic decision making. Resolution of the edema without improvement of visual acuity can prompt evaluation for other factors contributing to vision loss. Persistent edema unresponsive to initial therapy (ie, topical medications) can establish the need for more invasive intervention (ie, steroid injection or vitrectomy).

Rhegmatogenous Retinal Detachment

As with other types of retinal detachment, OCT can be useful in the evaluation of patients with rhegmatogenous retinal detachments. OCT is extremely sensitive in identifying elevation of the neurosensory retina because of the distinct difference in optical reflectivity between the retina and underlying retinal pigment epithelium (RPE)/choroid. Detachment of the neurosensory retina can be seen as nonreflective space between the elevated retinal signal and the underlying high-intensity RPE/choroidal band.

In patients with rhegmatogenous retinal detachment, OCT can confirm the presence of shallow

Schuman JS, Puliafito CA, Fujimoto JG, Duker JS, eds.
Optical Coherence Tomography of Ocular Diseases,
Third Edition (pp 319-344).
© 2013 SLACK Incorporated.

subretinal fluid that may be difficult to identify on ophthalmoscopy. OCT can also help distinguish true retinal detachment from other entities in the differential, such as retinoschisis.

Following retinal detachment repair, there is a great deal of variability in the degree and time course of visual recovery. OCT has been used to identify the presence of shallow subretinal fluid beneath the fovea in patients with delayed visual recovery after successful detachment surgery.[3,4] This shallow fluid could not be identified on clinical exam or fluorescein angiography. As a result, OCT can provide important information about visual outcomes and prognosis after retinal detachment repair.

Posterior Segment Trauma

Several characteristics make OCT an effective tool in the management of patients with posterior segment trauma. OCT is usually more comfortable for the traumatized patient than other examination techniques since it is noninvasive and uses infrared illumination.[5] OCT images can often be obtained even when the view to the retina is limited since only a small aperture is needed for effective imaging. OCT is also highly sensitive in identifying small anatomic changes, such as a traumatic macular hole, that may be difficult to confirm clinically.

Post-traumatic retinal alterations, such as edema or inflammation, manifest as changes in the contour and reflectivity of neurosensory retina on OCT. Retinal atrophy can be seen as thinning of the retinal signal, while scarring usually results in increased reflectivity.

Hemorrhage, a common finding in trauma, results in relatively high reflectivity with shadowing of the underlying layers on the OCT image. The degree of shadowing depends on the thickness and density of the hemorrhage. In some cases, the reflectivity of the hemorrhage may be similar to the retina, making distinction of these 2 layers slightly difficult.

Changes in the RPE and choroid following trauma can also be seen on the OCT image. Detachment of the RPE can be seen as elevation of the high-intensity outer band with shadowing of the underlying choroidal signal. RPE defects or choroidal rupture allow deeper penetration and increased reflectivity of the signal, resulting in a thick, intense outer band.

Optic Nerve Pit

OCT imaging has also helped our understanding of the retinal changes associated with optic nerve pit. In many cases, OCT shows severe outer retinal edema causing a schisis-like configuration in the macula. This is often associated with the accumulation of subretinal fluid creating bilaminar structure. Fluid appears to pass directly from the optic nerve pit into the retinal stroma and then secondarily into the subretinal space.[6,7] Several authors have subsequently demonstrated the usefulness of OCT in the monitoring of patients who have undergone surgical intervention for this condition.[7-10]

References

1. Hee MR, Puliafito CA, Wong C, et al. Quantitative assessment of macular edema with optical coherence tomography. *Arch Ophthalmol.* 1995;113(8):1019-1029.
2. Nelson ML, Martidis A. Managing cystoid macular edema after cataract surgery. *Curr Opin Ophthalmol.* 2003;14(1):39-43.
3. Hagimura N, Iida T, Suto K, Kishi S. Persistent foveal detachment after successful rhegmatogenous retinal detachment surgery. *Am J Ophthalmol.* 2002;133(4):516-520.
4. Wolfensberg TJ, Gonvers M. Optical coherence tomography in the evaluation of incomplete visual acuity recovery after macula-off retinal detachments. *Graefes Arch Clin Exp Ophthalmol.* 2002;240(2):85-89.
5. Hee MP, Izatt JA, Huang D, et al. Optical coherence tomography of the human retina. *Arch Ophthalmol.* 1995;113:325-332.
6. Rutledge BK, Puliafito CA, Duker JS, Hee MR, Cox MS. Optical coherence tomography of macular lesions associated with optic nerve head pits. *Ophthalmology.* 1996;103(7):1047-1053.
7. Lincoff H, Schiff W, Krivoy D, Ritch R. Optical coherence tomography of pneumatic displacement of optic disc pit maculopathy. *Br J Ophthalmol.* 1998;82(4):367-372.
8. Theodossiadis GP, Theodossiadis PG. Optical coherence tomography in optic disk pit maculopathy treated by the macular buckling procedure. *Am J Ophthalmol.* 2001;132(2):184-190.
9. Konno S, Akiba J, Sato E, Kuriyama S, Yoshida A. OCT in successful surgery of retinal detachment associated with optic nerve head pit. *Ophthalmic Surg Lasers.* 2000;31(3):236-239.
10. Todokoro D, Kishi S. Reattachment of retina and retinoschisis in pit-macular syndrome by surgically-induced vitreous detachment and gas tamponade. *Ophthalmic Surg Lasers.* 2000;31(3):233-235.

Index to Cases

Case 11-1. Pseudophakic Cystoid Macular Edema

Clinical Summary

A 66-year-old female presents 2 months following uncomplicated phacoemulsification with intraocular lens implant of the left eye. Visual acuity measures 20/40 in the operative eye. Dilated fundus examination reveals retinal striae in the fovea (A) with intraretinal cysts (B). The patient was placed on topical corticosteroid and nonsteroidal anti-inflammatory drops for 1 month. Follow-up examination reveals a stable visual acuity.

Optical Coherence Tomography

Horizontal OCT scan (C) shows large hyporeflective cavities in the outer plexiform layer; smaller hyporeflective cavities, likely within the inner plexiform layer; and a subretinal hyporeflective pocket, consistent with macular edema. Hyperreflective material is present within a few of the outer plexiform cavities, suggestive of inflammatory cellular material. Central foveal thickness measures 682 μm (D). The ILM-RPE map reveals the retinal contour (E). Horizontal OCT scan (F) 1 month after topical drops shows a decrease in but persistent hyporeflective cavities, indicating macular edema. Central foveal thickness is reduced to 644 μm (G).

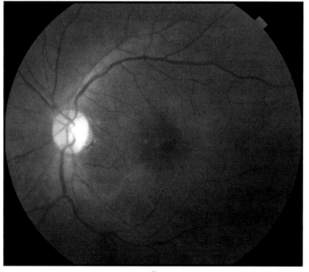

A

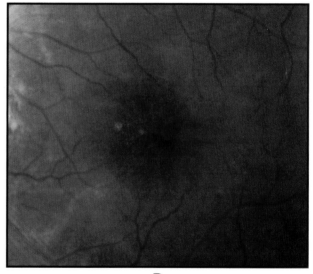

B

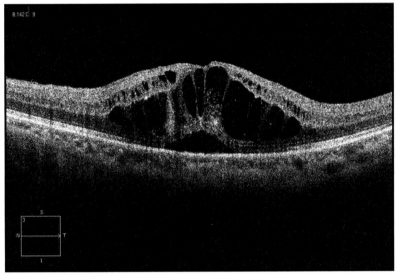

C

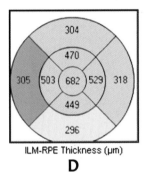

ILM-RPE Thickness (µm)

D

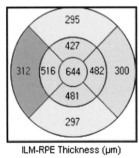

ILM - RPE

E

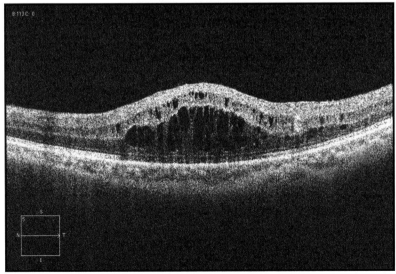

F

ILM-RPE Thickness (µm)

G

Case 11-2. Posterior Segment Trauma

Clinical Summary

A 45-year-old male presents after a sudden change in vision in the left eye. He has a remote history of penetrating injury 22 years ago. A metallic foreign body was later detected in the retrobulbar space. Dilated fundus exam of the left eye (A) demonstrates a focal area of retinal pigment atrophy with mild surrounding pigment hyperplasia, encircled by laser scars.

Optical Coherence Tomography

Obliquely oriented OCT scan through the area (B) reveals a focal absence of retinal tissue with a thickened, hyperreflective, irregular layer from beneath the RPE, suggestive of fibrous tissue. Choroidal pattern is not visible. The vitreous appears adherent and disturbed in this focal area. The ILM-RPE overlay illustrates the retinal contour (C).

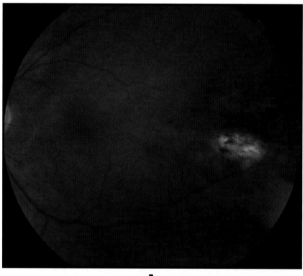

A

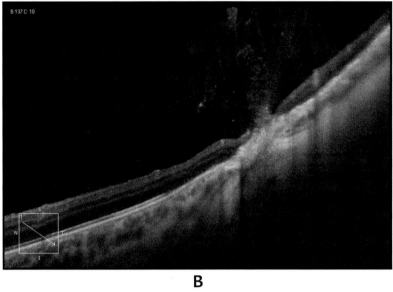

B

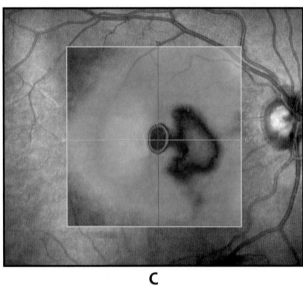

C

Case 11-3. Cystoid Macular Edema Associated With Glaucoma Drops

Clinical Summary

A 58-year-old female is referred for evaluation of macular edema in the left eye. She has a history of glaucoma and underwent tube shunt placement in the left eye 6 months earlier. She currently uses multiple glaucoma drops, including a prostaglandin analog in both eyes, for persistent elevation of IOP. Her visual acuity is 20/60 in the left eye, and dilated fundus exam (A) reveals macular edema.

Optical Coherence Tomography

The initial OCT image (B) shows extensive thickening of the foveal retina. There are a few small cystic cavities in the inner retinal layers. A larger area of decreased reflectivity in the outer retina indicates extensive cystoid edema. Bridging retinal elements can be seen passing through this area, and a thin layer of retinal tissue is seen at the base of this cavity, confirming the anatomic location as intraretinal. Central foveal thickness measures 479 μm and reaches a peak of 536 μm superior to the fovea (C).

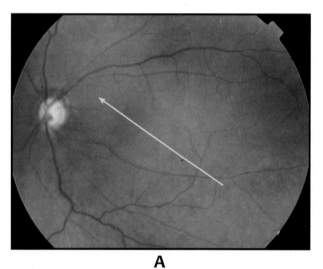

A

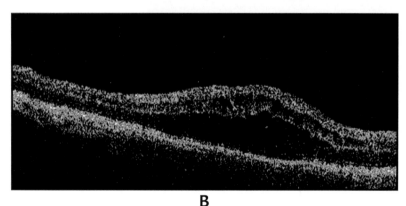

B

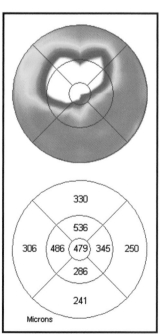

	330	
	536	
306	486 (479) 345	250
	286	
	241	

Microns

C

Case 11-3. Cystoid Macular Edema Associated With Glaucoma Drops (continued)

Continuation of Clinical Summary

Her prostaglandin analog was discontinued, and she was started on a topical nonsteroidal anti-inflammatory drug. Six weeks later, her visual acuity has improved to 20/40, and there is minimal edema evident on exam.

Follow-Up
Optical Coherence Tomography

Six weeks after changing her medications, there is a significant decrease in retinal thickness on the OCT image (D). A cyst is still present in the fovea, but the large outer retinal cystic cavity has resolved. Central foveal thickness has decreased to 367 μm, and there has been a reduction of retinal thickness throughout the macula (E).

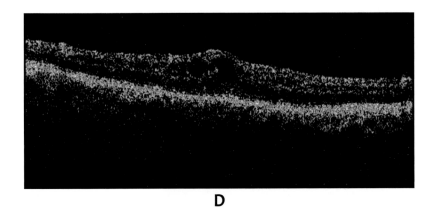

D

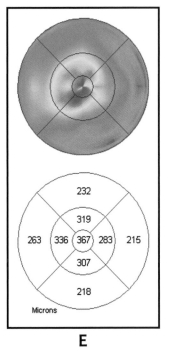

E

Case 11-4. Choroidal Folds

Clinical Summary

A 75-year-old female complains of mild blurring of vision in the left eye. Visual acuity measures 20/25 in the right eye and 20/100 in the left eye. Refractive error is +3.50 spherical equivalent in each eye. Dilated fundus examination of the right eye reveals a faint epiretinal membrane, extramacular drusen, and prominent choroidal folds (A). Examination of the left eye is limited due to dense nuclear sclerotic cataract.

Optical Coherence Tomography

Horizontal OCT scan (B) through the superior macula shows folded RPE, leading to an irregular foveal contour. An intravitreal linear density above the retina is suggestive of a posterior vitreous detachment. The RPE map (C) shows linear folds of the pigment epithelium.

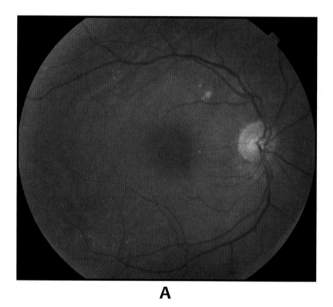

A

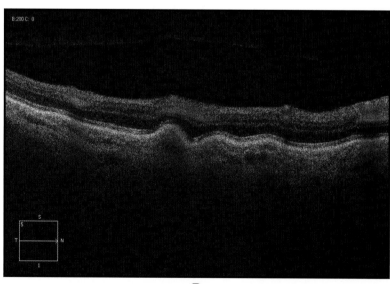

B

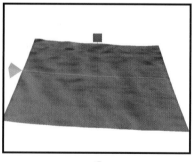

C

Case 11-5. Post-Traumatic Choroidal Rupture

Clinical Summary

A 23-year-old female complains of decreased vision in her left eye after being punched in this eye earlier that evening. Her visual acuity is 20/200. There is extensive periorbital edema and bruising. Dilated fundus examination (A) shows evidence of a choroidal rupture through the macula with associated submacular hemorrhage. The choroidal ruptures are seen as hyperfluorescent window defects on the angiogram (B). Three parallel areas of choroidal rupture can be seen inferotemporal to the fovea.

Optical Coherence Tomography

OCT (C) shows elevation of the fovea from the subretinal hemorrhage. Because the retina and blood have similar reflectivity, it is difficult to precisely differentiate these layers. As the scan passes through the inferotemporal macula (left side of the tomogram), there are 3 areas of increased choroidal reflectivity. These areas result from increased penetration and reflectivity of the signal as it passes through the choroidal ruptures.

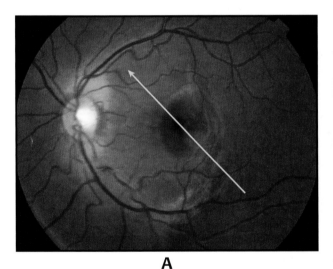

A

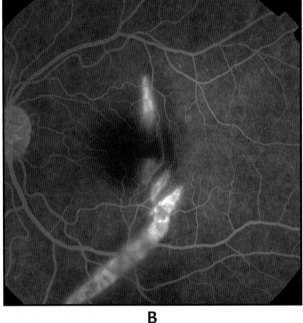

B

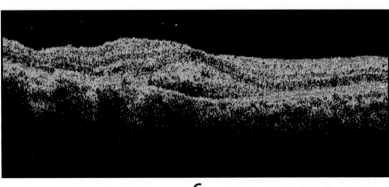

C

Case 11-6. Choroidal Nevus

Clinical Summary

A 60-year-old female is referred for a suspicious nevus. She has no visual symptoms. Dilated fundus exam reveals an approximately 9-mm x 6-mm elevated choroidal lesion with overlying drusen inferior to the fovea (A).

Optical Coherence Tomography

Horizontal OCT scans through the nevus (B) show elevation of the RPE and neurosensory retina. Focal irregularities in the photoreceptor layer at the apex of the nevus are noted. Choroidal architecture is not visible.

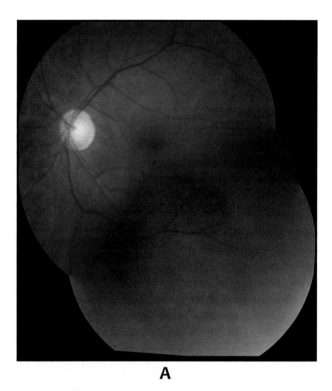

A

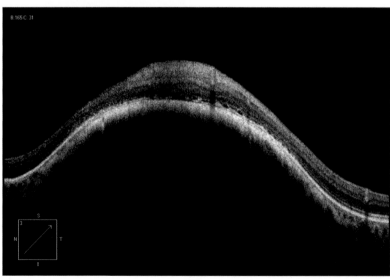

B

Case 11-7. Congenital Hypertrophy of the Retinal Pigment Epithelium

Clinical Summary

A 34-year-old female presents for an exam. She denies visual complaints. Visual acuity is 20/20 in each eye. Dilated fundus examination of the right eye (A, B) reveals a jet-black well-circumscribed flat lesion in the superotemporal periphery.

Optical Coherence Tomography

Vertical OCT scan through the lesion (C, D) reveals an increase in reflectivity of the RPE and shadowing of posterior choroidal structures.

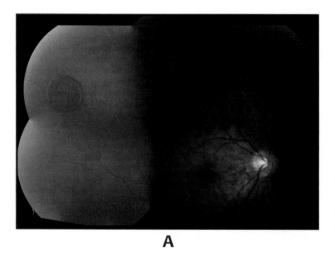

A

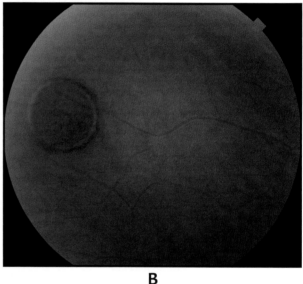

B

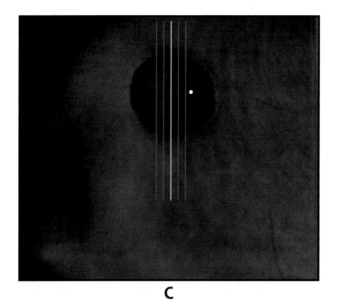

C

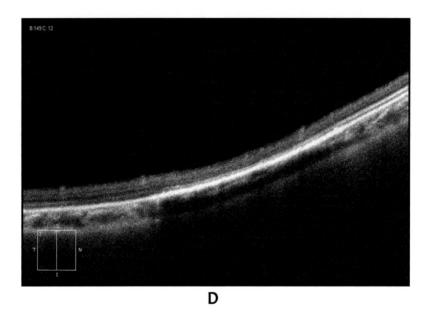

D

Case 11-8. Valsalva Retinopathy

Clinical Summary

A 19-year-old female experienced vision decrease after several episodes of vomiting during her third trimester of pregnancy. Her vision is 20/80 in this eye. Dilated fundus examination shows a subhyaloid hemorrhage involving the foveal center (A).

Optical Coherence Tomography

An OCT scan through the fovea (B) reveals a dome-shaped reflective area consistent with subhyaloid blood beneath a reflective band corresponding to the posterior hyaloid. The neurosensory retina is visualized underneath the blood. The hemorrhage blocks to some degree the optical reflections returning from the retina and RPE/choriocapillaris layers. Scan C shows a region inferonasal to the fovea (right side of the scan) where the subhyaloid hemorrhage is less dense, allowing better light propagation and resulting in adequate visualization of the neurosensory retina as well as the RPE/choriocapillaris.

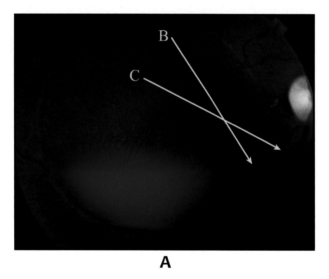

A

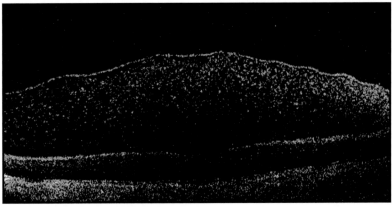

B

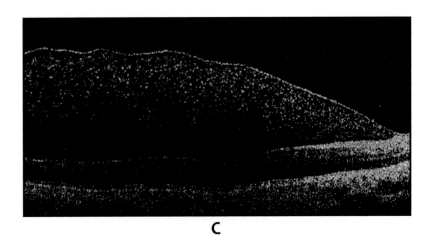

C

Case 11-9. Chorioretinitis Sclopetaria

Clinical Summary

A 24-year-old male suffered a gunshot wound to the left periorbital region 8 months earlier. The bullet entered through the left inferior orbital rim. The patient underwent facial bone reconstruction and complained of poor vision in his left eye. Visual acuity measures 20/200 in this eye. Dilated fundus examination shows extensive chorioretinal scarring and fibrosis involving the macular region (A) and inferior retina (B).

Optical Coherence Tomography

A horizontal OCT scan (C) obtained through the fovea shows thinning of the overlying neurosensory retina in association with irregular thickening of the RPE/choroid layer. A reflective band is visible anterior to the retinal tissue consistent with a posterior vitreous detachment. Another OCT scan (D) shows marked retinal atrophy. The underneath RPE layer shows a highly reflective irregular configuration. Shadowing of the choroidal optical reflections is observed below this highly reflective area. Scan E depicts a region of high backscattering consistent with fibrosis fusing the neurosensory retina and RPE/choroid. A horizontal scan obtained inferior to the optic nerve (F) reveals preretinal fibrosis, seen as a region of increased reflectivity (right side of the scan) in association with a highly reflective and thickened RPE/choroid underneath. The atrophic retina lost its normal architecture. The central macular area measures 177 µm (G).

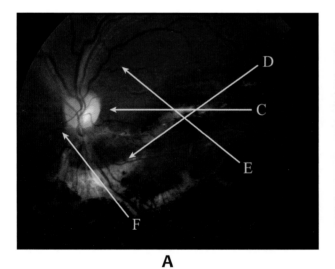

A

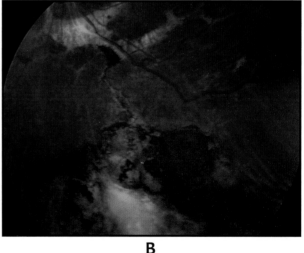

B

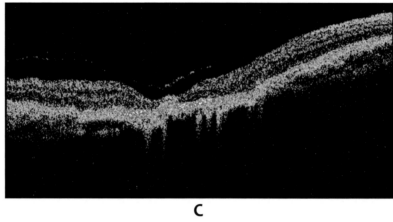

C

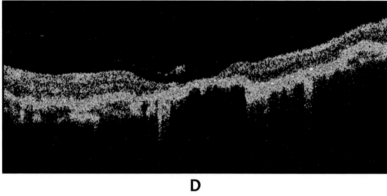

D

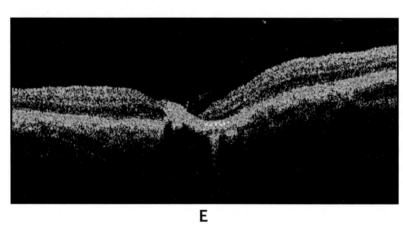

E

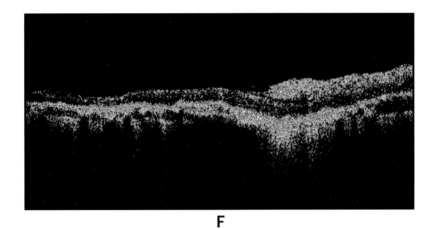

F

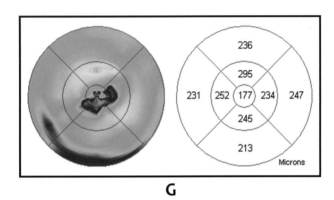

G

Case 11-10A. Optic Nerve Pit

Clinical Summary

A 22-year-old female presents for her annual check-up. Her history is significant for an optic nerve pit in the right eye treated with laser 5 years ago for subretinal fluid. She denies visual changes. Visual acuity is 20/20 in each eye. Dilated fundus examination of the right eye (A) reveals an optic nerve pit at the temporal border, peripapillary RPE atrophy and pigment changes in the area of prior laser, and cystic changes in the central macula.

Optical Coherence Tomography

Horizontal OCT scan (B) reveals hyporeflective spaces within the inner retina, with linear tissue across this area, suggestive of Müller's cells and foveal retinoschisis. The RPE and outer retinal layers are not present in the area corresponding to prior laser. Central foveal thickness is 461 μm (C). The ILM-RPE overlay reveals the area of elevation leading from the optic nerve (D).

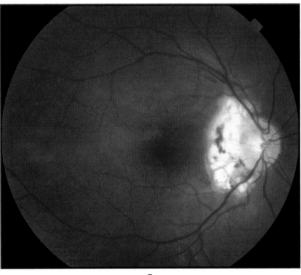

A

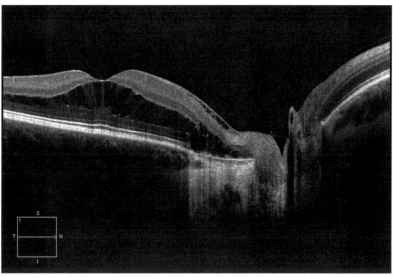

B

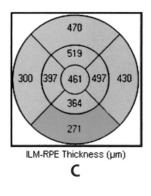

ILM-RPE Thickness (μm)

C

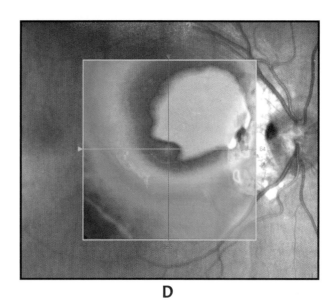

D

Case 11-10B. Optic Nerve Pit

Clinical Summary

A 28-year-old female presents for follow-up examination without new complaints. She had previously undergone several pars plana vitrectomies and lasers for a retinal detachment in the presence of an optic nerve pit in the right eye. Visual acuity is 20/125 in the right eye. Dilated fundus exam of the right eye (A) reveals an optic nerve pit, laser scars in the temporal macula, superior to the nerve, and around the nerve. Shallow fluid is present in the macula with retinal striae.

Optical Coherence Tomography

Horizontal OCT scan (B) demonstrates hyporeflective spaces within the retina and beneath the retina, indicating intraretinal and subretinal fluid, respectively. Loss of retinal architecture is noted. The ILM-RPE map (C) illustrates the retinal contour. Central foveal thickness is 392 μm (D).

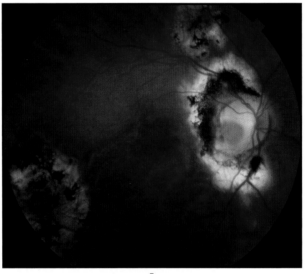

A

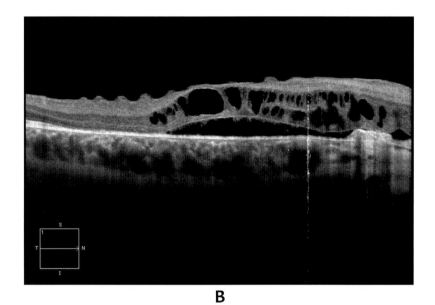

B

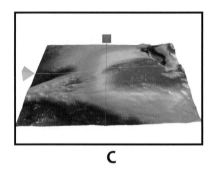

C

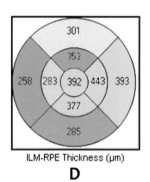

ILM-RPE Thickness (µm)

D

Case 11-11. Myelinated Nerve Fiber Layer

Clinical Summary

A 57-year-old male is referred for an abnormal nerve appearance. He denies visual changes. Dilated fundus exam of the left eye reveals whitening of the nerve fiber layer along the superior border of the disc, with obscuration of some vessels (A).

Optical Coherence Tomography

Vertical OCT scan (B) through the optic nerve reveals an increase in hyperreflectivity in the nerve fiber layer along the superior aspect of the nerve.

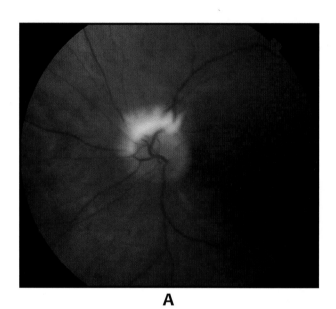

A

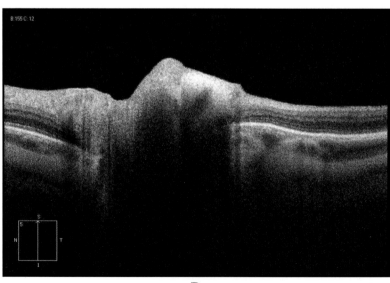

B

Case 11-12. Cancer-Associated Retinopathy

Clinical Summary

A 65-year-old female is referred for evaluation of unexplained vision loss. She complains of progressive dimming of her vision in both eyes over the past 3 months. Her visual acuity is 20/25, and formal visual field testing shows extensive constriction of the peripheral field in both eyes. Dilated fundus exam (A, B) shows mild narrowing of the retinal arterioles but is otherwise unremarkable. Fluorescein angiography shows a mild delay in A-V transit time but is otherwise normal. Full-field electroretinography demonstrates bilateral photoreceptor degeneration. A computed tomography scan of the chest shows a pulmonary mass with hilar lymphadenopathy, and subsequent biopsy confirms small cell lung cancer.

Optical Coherence Tomography

The OCT (C, D) shows thinning of the neurosensory retina in the peripheral macula. The foveal thickness and contour are relatively normal, but the neurosensory retina thins dramatically as the scan passes away from the fovea. This is best demonstrated on the retinal thickness map (E) where the peripheral macular thickness is approximately half normal. This pattern of retinal thinning appears similar to other conditions that result in photoreceptor degeneration (see Chapter 10).

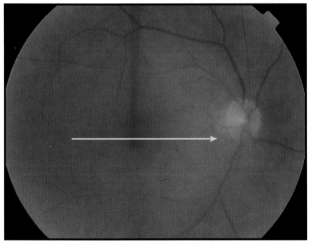

A

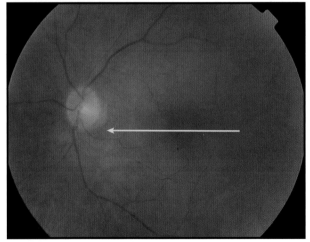

B

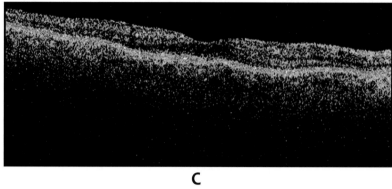

C

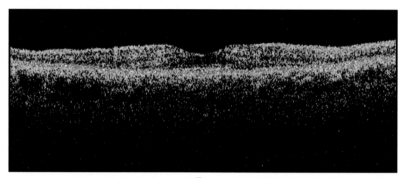

D

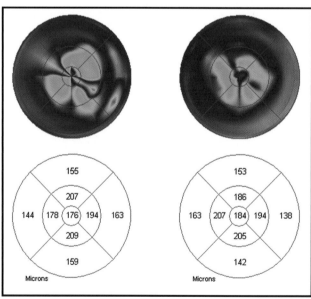

E

Section III

Optical Coherence Tomography in Glaucoma, Neuro-Ophthalmology, and the Anterior Segment

Chapter 12

Optical Coherence Tomography's Clinical Utility in Glaucoma

Gadi Wollstein, MD; Lindsey S. Folio, MS, MBA; Jessica E. Nevins, BS; and Joel S. Schuman, MD

- Normal
- Structure-Function Correspondence
- Structure-Function Disagreement
- Structural Loss Suggests Future Functional Loss
- Utility of Imaging in Longitudinal Glaucoma Assessment

Glaucoma is a progressive optic neuropathy often (but not always) associated with high intraocular pressure (IOP), characterized by irreversible loss of ganglion cell and retinal nerve fiber layer (RNFL) with corresponding typical visual field abnormalities. The morphological changes appearing in glaucoma are evaluated clinically by optic nerve head (ONH) and RNFL assessment. However, qualitative assessment is highly observer dependent and prone to large interobserver variation.[1-4] In addition, longitudinal detection of tissue changes is important for determining the need for treatment or altering ongoing treatment, although this imposes a substantial clinical challenge because of the slowly progressive nature of the disease.

Visual field testing is conventionally used to estimate functional glaucomatous damage. The test is a subjective assessment that requires patient cooperation and often exhibits large intervisit variation. Due to high variability, detection of visual field changes requires several repetitions of the test, thus delaying diagnosis.

Several studies have suggested that glaucomatous field abnormalities may be preceded by structural changes of the ONH[5-7] and RNFL.[8-10] Histological evaluation estimated that up to 50% of the RNFL may be lost prior to the appearance of initial visual field damage.[11] This damage may be detected in 60% of RNFL photographs up to 6 years prior to the appearance of a detectable visual field defect.[10] Detection of early structural damage may help identify patients who require preventive therapy because they are at a high risk for visual loss and may spare patients without damage the cost and morbidity of treatment.

Several imaging devices are commercially available, all aimed at providing objective quantitative measures of posterior segment ocular structures, and are commonly used for glaucoma management.

- **Confocal scanning laser ophthalmoscopy (CSLO)** acquires sequential coronal scans of the ONH at different depths to create a 3-dimensional reconstruction of the imaged tissue. The CSLO is capable of assessing the ONH, and due to the large normal anatomical variability and the structural complexity of this region, the capability of this device to detect glaucomatous damage is limited.
- **Scanning laser polarimetry (SLP)** uses the birefringent properties of the RNFL to estimate the thickness of this layer in the peripapillary region. Confounding may occur due to the birefringence of several ocular tissues, such as lens, cornea, sclera, and retinal pigment epithelium (RPE).

Schuman JS, Puliafito CA, Fujimoto JG, Duker JS, eds.
Optical Coherence Tomography of Ocular Diseases,
Third Edition (pp 347-468).
© 2013 SLACK Incorporated.

- **Optical coherence tomography (OCT)** is a quantitative, high-resolution device capable of scanning the ONH, peripapillary, and macular regions in the posterior segment. The capability to scan all 3 regions improves the ability to detect and confirm the structural involvement.

Structural imaging provided by OCT enables the assessment of structure-function correspondence. It has been suggested that this association is weak at early stages of the disease when deviations in RNFL thickness are present but only minimal visual field abnormalities have occurred.[12] After reaching an RNFL threshold, visual field changes are detectable and the association between structure and function improves. Corresponding structural and functional abnormalities might eliminate the need to repeat visual field testing in order to confirm the presence of a new or subtle defect and allow earlier treatment adjustment.

OCT has become a valuable tool in clinical glaucoma management for disease detection and monitoring glaucoma progression over time.

References

1. Sturmer J, Poinoosawmy D, Broadway DC, Hitchings RA. Intra- and interobserver variation of optic nerve head measurements in glaucoma suspects using disc-data. *Int Ophthalmol.* 1992;16(4-5):227-233.

2. Abrams LS, Scott IU, Spaeth GL, et al. Agreement among optometrists, ophthalmologists, and residents in evaluating the optic disc for glaucoma. *Ophthalmology.* 1994;101(10): 1662-1667.

3. Gaasterland DE, Blackwell B, Dally LG, et al. The Advanced Glaucoma Intervention Study (AGIS): 10. Variability among academic glaucoma subspecialists in assessing optic disc notching. *Trans Am Ophthalmol Soc.* 2001;99:177-84; discussion 84-85.

4. Tielsch JM, Katz J, Quigley HA, et al. Intraobserver and interobserver agreement in measurement of optic disc characteristics. *Ophthalmology.* 1988;95(3):350-356.

5. Sommer A, Pollack I, Maumenee AE. Optic disc parameters and onset of glaucomatous field loss. I. Methods and progressive changes in disc morphology. *Arch Ophthalmol.* 1979;97(8):1444-1448.

6. Pederson J, Anderson D. The mode of progressive disc cupping in ocular hypertension and glaucoma. *Arch Ophthalmol.* 1980;98:490-495.

7. Quigley HA, Katz J, Derick RJ, et al. An evaluation of optic disc and nerve fiber layer examinations in monitoring progression of early glaucoma damage. *Ophthalmology.* 1992;99(1):19-28.

8. Sommer A, Miller NR, Pollack I, et al. The nerve fiber layer in the diagnosis of glaucoma. *Arch Ophthalmol.* 1977;95(12):2149-2156.

9. Sommer A, Quigley H, Robin A. Evaluation of nerve fiber layer assessment. *Arch Ophthalmol.* 1984;102:1766-1771.

10. Sommer A, Katz J, Quigley HA, et al. Clinically detectable nerve fiber atrophy precedes the onset of glaucomatous field loss. *Arch Ophthalmol.* 1991;109(1):77-83.

11. Quigley HA, Addicks EM, Green WR. Optic nerve damage in human glaucoma. III. Quantitative correlation of nerve fiber loss and visual field defect in glaucoma, ischemic neuropathy, papilledema, and toxic neuropathy. *Arch Ophthalmol.* 1982;100(1):135-146.

12. Wollstein G, Kagemann L, Bilonick RA, et al. Retinal nerve fiber layer and visual function loss in glaucoma: the tipping point. *Br J Ophthalmol.* 2012;96:47-52.

Index to Cases

Case 12-1. Normal Visual Field Verified With Normal SD-OCT Imaging of Retinal Nerve Fiber Layer and Macular Region

This case presents the right eye of a 45-year-old healthy male with best-corrected visual acuity of 20/20, IOP of 12 mm Hg, and central corneal thickness of 594 μm. The anterior segment exam shows wide-open angles. The dilated fundus exam reveals a normal ONH with small central cup with no evidence of any RNFL defects (A). Visual field (B) and Heidelberg Retinal Tomography Moorfields regression analysis ([HRT MRA] C) are both normal.

The Table indicates global RNFL thickness measurements from the available devices. All thickness values for this patient remain in the normal range.

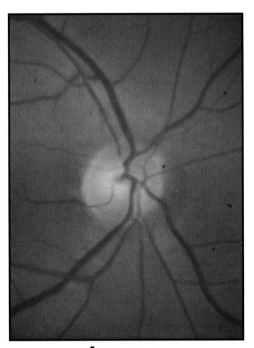

A. Disc photo.

B. Visual field pattern deviation, mean deviation = 1.37 dB.

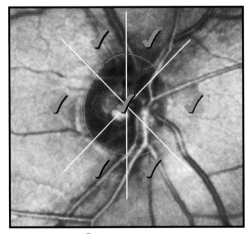

C. HRT MRA.

RNFL Thickness Measurements

Device	RNFL Thickness (μm)
Stratus TD-OCT	99
Cirrus HD-OCT	86
RTVue-100	106

Stratus TD-OCT

Stratus (Carl Zeiss Meditec, Inc, Dublin, CA) TD-OCT imaging reveals a normal RNFL thickness in the circumpapillary region (D-G). The fundus photo (D) shows that the ONH is correctly centered for the scan. E displays the circumpapillary RNFL cross section. The sectoral thickness analysis (F) and the RNFL thickness profile (G) show that the RNFL measurements are all in the normal thickness range. H was acquired from the Fast Mac scan and also shows a normal retinal thickness that is best shown in I. This is a normative distribution for retinal thicknesses of the macula, where the green range indicates measurements within normal limits.

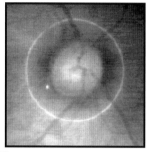

D. Fast RNFL fundus image.

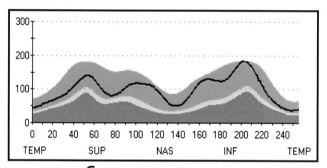

E. RNFL cross-section image.

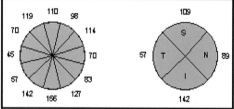

F. RNFL sectoral thickness analysis.

G. RNFL thickness profile.

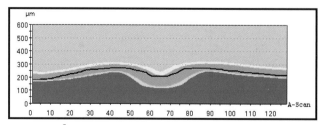

H. Macular cross section.

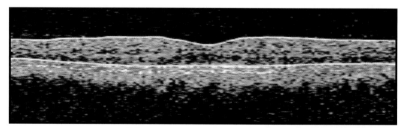

I. Macular retinal thickness profile.

Cirrus HD-OCT

Cirrus (Carl Zeiss Meditec, Inc) HD-OCT imaging reveals a normal circumpapillary RNFL thickness as shown in the 200 x 200 Optic Disc Cube scan (J-L). The thickness distribution remains in the normal region (J), as indicated by the green coloring. No abnormal loss of RNFL thickness occurs in K. L shows the disc (black) and cup (red) margins, with a normal rim thickness. L also shows the 3.4-mm diameter RNFL scanning circle in purple and minimal deviation from normal, shown as yellow spots; however, they present minimal significance because they are small and scattered. The macular cube thickness analysis (M), overlaid on the OCT fundus, and the vertical macular cross-section image (N) also indicate normal retinal thickness. The macular cube ganglion cell analysis (O-Q) indicates normal macular thickness by the thickness map (O), deviation map (P), and in all sectors (Q).

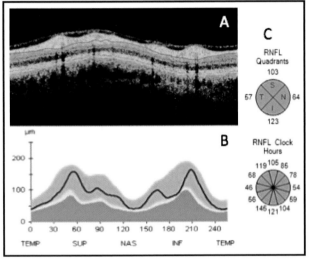

J. Optic Disc Cube scan. (A) Circumpapillary RNFL cross section. (B) RNFL thickness compared to a normative database. (C). RNFL sectoral analysis.

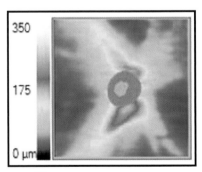

K. RNFL thickness map.

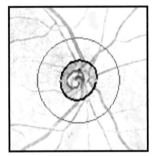

L. RNFL deviation map on en face image with ONH disc and cup margins.

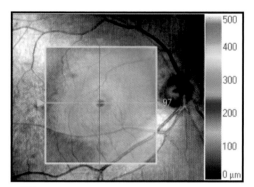

M. Macular cube thickness analysis on LSO image.

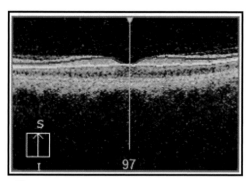

N. Macular vertical cross-section image.

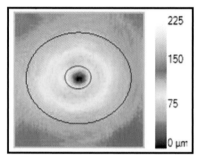

O. Macular cube ganglion cell analysis thickness map.

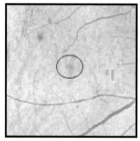

P. Macular cube ganglion cell analysis deviation map.

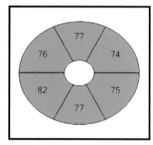

Q. Macular cube ganglion cell analysis sectors.

Spectralis HRA+OCT

The Spectralis HRA+OCT (Heidelberg Engineering, GmbH, Heidelberg, Germany) ONH thickness map (R) shows the regional thicknesses surrounding the ONH. For this normal patient, most of the areas surrounding the ONH are green, with the ONH in red. The ONH 3D view (S) shows the infrared CSLO image paired with the SD-OCT image for direct comparison. T (left) shows the infrared CSLO indicating where the OCT line scan was acquired. T (right) shows the SD-OCT cross-sectional image directly across the ONH. From this scan we see normal cupping of the ONH and a normal RNFL thickness.

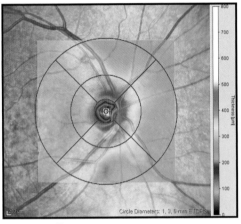

R. ONH thickness map.

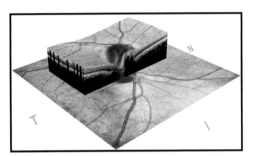

S. SD-OCT ONH scan combined with infrared CSLO image.

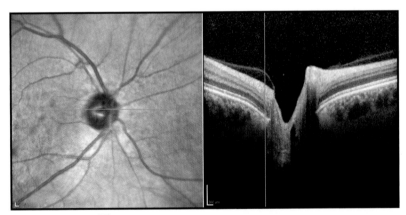

T. (Left) Infrared CSLO image of ONH.
(Right) SD-OCT line scan across ONH.

RTVue-100

RTVue-100 (Optovue, Inc, Fremont, CA) imaging also shows a normal RNFL thickness in the 3.4-mm diameter surrounding the ONH (U-W). U shows the cross-section image acquired on a 3.4-mm circle surrounding the ONH. V and W show the thickness analysis for the circumpapillary region, compared to a normative database of aged-matched healthy patients. The macular region appears normal in both the ganglion cell complex imaging analysis (X) and cross-line (Y) image.

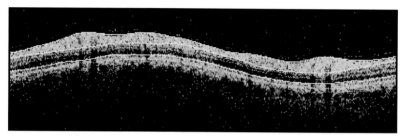

U. Circumpapillary RNFL cross-section image.

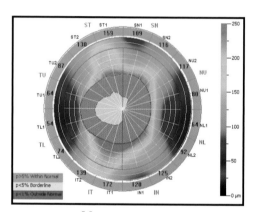

V. ONH analysis.

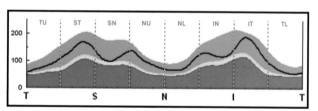

W. Circumpapillary RNFL thickness analysis.

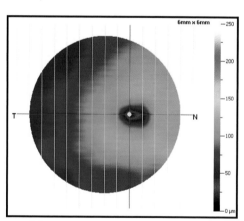

X. Macular ganglion cell complex thickness map.

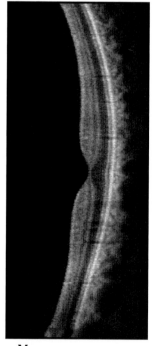

Y. Macular cross-line image.

3D OCT-1000

Imaging with the 3D OCT-1000 (Topcon Medical Systems, Inc, Oakland, NJ) shows a normal thickness for the circumpapillary RNFL scan (Z) as well as small, central, and shallow cupping of the ONH (AA). BB shows the region of cube data that was captured for this patient, and CC shows the horizontal cross-section image of the macula, with a thicker RNFL (uppermost red band) in the nasal aspect of the macula (left side of the image) compared to the temporal aspect.

Comment

This case demonstrates SD-OCT imaging for a healthy patient and will be useful as a comparison for the following cases.

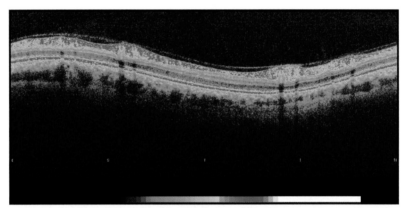

Z. Circumpapillary RNFL cross-section image.

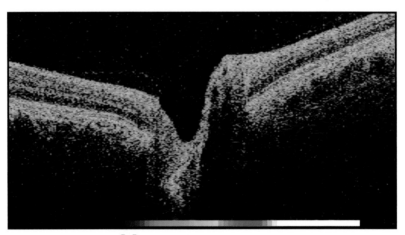

AA. ONH cross-section image.

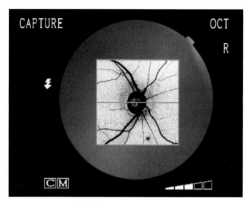

BB. ONH image.

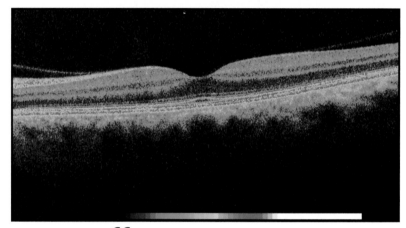

CC. Macular cross-section image.

Case 12-2. Early Damage in Visual Field With Corresponding Defects Shown by SD-OCT Devices

Clinical Summary

This case presents the right eye of a 70-year-old female with primary open-angle glaucoma in both eyes being treated with travoprost. Ocular examination reveals a best-corrected visual acuity of 20/16, IOP of 10 mm Hg, and central corneal thickness of 506 μm. The anterior segment examination shows a moderate nuclear sclerotic cataract. The dilated fundus exam reveals a thin rim with a cup-to-disc ratio of 0.7 (A). Visual field testing reveals an early inferior arcuate scotoma (B). HRT imaging (C) shows abnormalities over the entire rim area.

The Table shows that the mean RNFL thicknesses for Stratus TD-OCT, Cirrus HD-OCT, and RTVue-100 all are in the normal range.

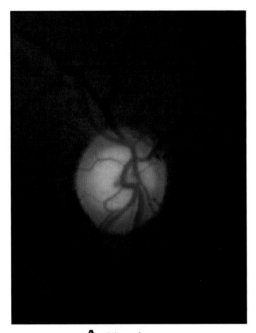

A. Disc photo.

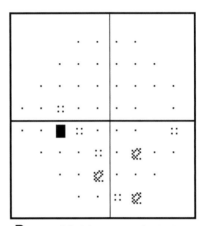

B. Visual field pattern deviation, mean deviation = -1.01 dB.

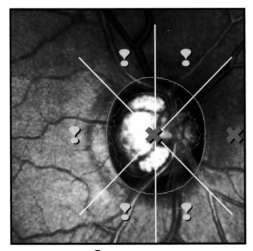

C. HRT MRA.

RNFL Thickness Measurements	
Device	RNFL Thickness (μm)
Stratus TD-OCT	81
Cirrus HD-OCT	83
RTVue-100	94

Cirrus HD-OCT

Cirrus HD-OCT imaging reveals an RNFL thickness in the borderline range, when compared to a normative distribution, in the superonasal region surrounding the ONH (D). This is also displayed by a decrease in the superonasal thickness in E and a borderline thickness wedge defect in F, indicated by the yellow band. The macular scan (G, H) does not show any abnormality. The macular cube ganglion cell analysis (I-K) indicates an early defect mostly in the superior and temporal aspects of the macula. Note the improved diagnostic performance of the ganglion cell analysis compared to the full retinal analysis.

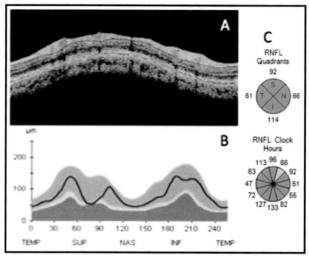

D. Optic Disc Cube scan. (A) Circumpapillary RNFL cross section. (B) RNFL thickness compared to a normative database. (C) RNFL sectoral analysis.

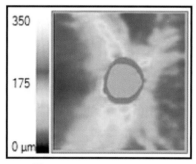

E. RNFL thickness map.

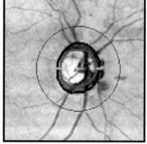

F. RNFL deviation map on en face image with ONH disc and cup margins.

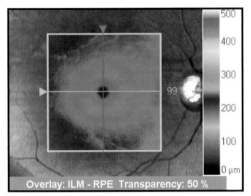

G. Macular cube thickness analysis on LSO image.

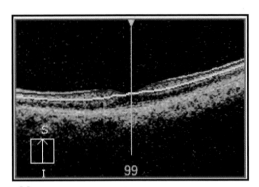

H. Macular vertical cross-section image.

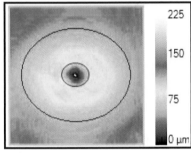

I. Macular cube ganglion cell analysis thickness map.

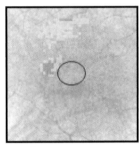

J. Macular cube ganglion cell analysis deviation map.

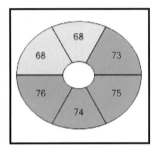

K. Macular cube ganglion cell analysis sectors.

RTVue-100

RTVue-100 circumpapillary RNFL thickness analysis (L, M) indicates a normal thickness. However, the ONH scan analysis (N, O) shows RNFL thickness to be in the borderline range superotemporally, as indicated by the yellow sections. N shows the thin RNFL in the superonasal region (arrows), where the superior hump is flattened. Thinning of the inner retinal layers is evident in the macular cross-line image (P) and better depicted in the ganglion cell complex thickness map (Q) where thinning is mostly noticeable in the superior and superotemporal regions.

Comment

This case demonstrates SD-OCT imaging analysis closely coinciding with the visual field.

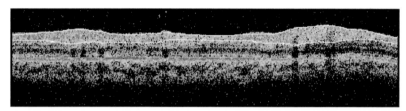

L. Circumpapillary RNFL cross-section image from the RNFL scanning.

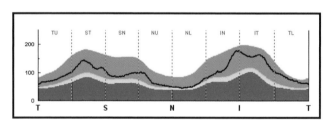

M. Circumpapillary RNFL thickness analysis.

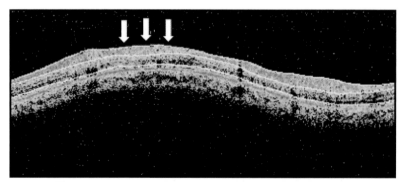

N. Circumpapillary RNFL cross-section image from the ONH scanning pattern.

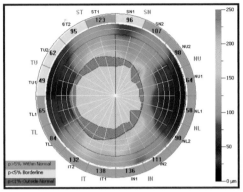

O. ONH analysis.

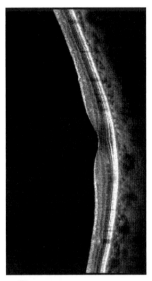

P. Macular cross-line image.

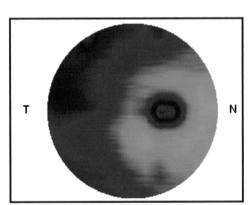

Q. Macular ganglion cell complex thickness map.

Case 12-3. Thin Inferior Retinal Nerve Fiber Layer Shown With Imaging Without a Corresponding Visual Field Deficit

Clinical Summary

This case presents the right eye of an 83-year-old male with primary open-angle glaucoma who has been treated surgically with selective laser trabeculoplasty and endoscopic cyclophotocoagulation performed during a cataract surgery and currently being treated topically with dorzolamide/timolol. Best-corrected visual acuity is 20/20, and IOP is 13 mm Hg. The anterior segment examination shows open angles and a well-centered posterior chamber intraocular lens. The dilated fundus exam reveals an ONH with a cup-to-disc ratio of 0.95 with a neuroretinal rim thinnest inferiorly (A). Humphrey visual field (B) shows a nonspecific superior defect, and HRT MRA (C) shows an abnormality in the inferior temporal region. GDx enhanced corneal compensation (D) also shows reduced birefringence in the inferior temporal region.

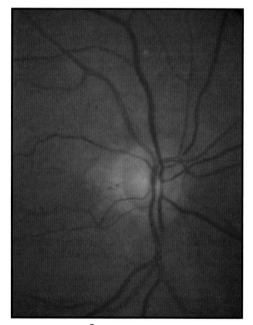

A. Disc photo.

B. Visual field pattern deviation, mean deviation = -0.61 dB.

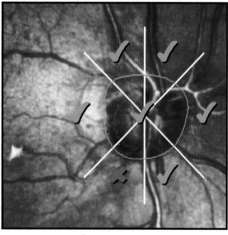

C. HRT MRA.

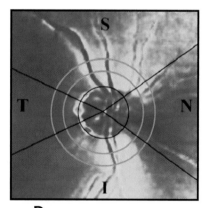

D. GDx enhanced corneal compensation nerve fiber thickness map.

Cirrus HD-OCT

Cirrus HD-OCT imaging shows a thin RNFL in the inferotemporal region (E), where the black thickness line dips into the red region (part B). This is shown in E (part C), where a localized thin RNFL is shown in the sectoral analysis, and in F, where a wedge defect can be detected in the inferotemporal region as a blue sector rather than the normal yellow color. A localized thin RNFL is also noted in the superior nasal region (E, part B), marked as a borderline thickness in the superior quadrant and 1:00 (E, part C). These areas of abnormality are easily observed in the thickness deviation map where the inferotemporal abnormality extends to the inferior macula and is accompanied by a thin inferotemporal rim (G). The macula is also shown to be thin in the corresponding inferior region as shown in H through L. The inferior thinning of the macula is evident in the cross section (I, arrow) along with the deviation map (K) and the sectoral measurement (L).

Comment

This case illustrates a situation where the structural assessment discloses localized abnormalities both in the peripapillary and macular regions, but no corresponding visual field abnormality is present. This might reflect a preperimetric abnormality where the functional involvement will follow in the future.

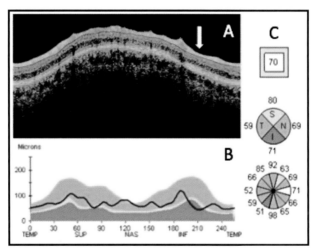

E. Optic Disc Cube scan. (A) Circumpapillary RNFL cross section. (B) RNFL thickness compared to a normative database. (C) RNFL sectoral analysis.

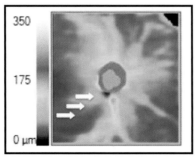

F. RNFL thickness map.

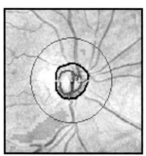

G. RNFL deviation map on en face image with ONH disc and cup margins.

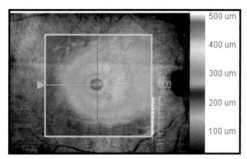

H. Macular cube thickness analysis on LSO image.

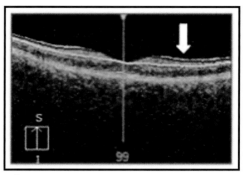

I. Macular vertical cross-section image.

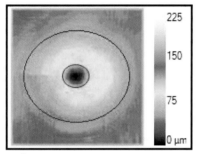

J. Macular cube ganglion cell analysis thickness map.

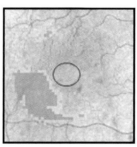

K. Macular cube ganglion cell analysis deviation map.

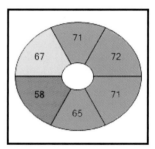

L. Macular cube ganglion cell analysis sectors.

Case 12-4. Localized Wedge Defect Shown in SD-OCT Images

Clinical Summary

This case presents the left eye of a 63-year-old female with normal tension glaucoma treated with selective laser trabeculoplasty. Best-corrected visual acuity is 20/25, IOP is 14 mm Hg, and central corneal thickness is 538 μm. The anterior segment examination shows keratoplasty scars, wide-open angles, and a mild nuclear sclerotic cataract. The dilated fundus exam reveals an ONH with a cup-to-disc ratio of 0.8 and an RNFL wedge defect inferotemporally (A).

Visual field testing exhibits a central scotoma (B). The HRT reflectance image clearly demonstrates the inferotemporal wedge defect, but the MRA analysis (C) shows a borderline abnormality due to the small size of the defect compared to the entire sector.

The Table, however, indicates normal global RNFL thicknesses in all OCT devices. This is due to the localized area of the wedge defect. SD-OCT local analysis is able to determine a thin RNFL in the location of the wedge defect.

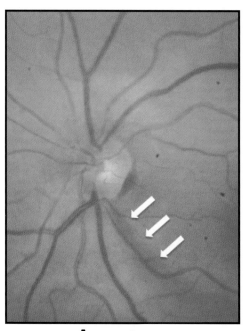

A. Disc photo.

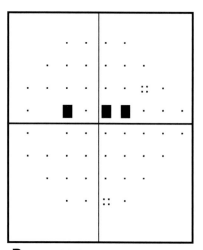

B. Visual field pattern deviation, mean deviation = -0.46 dB.

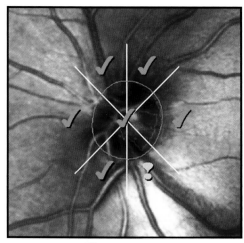

C. HRT MRA.

RNFL Thickness Measurements

Device	RNFL Thickness (μm)
Stratus TD-OCT	88
RTVue-100	96
Spectralis HRA+OCT	86

Spectralis HRA+OCT

Spectralis HRA+OCT CSLO image shows clearly the location of the wedge defect (D) and provides detailed images of the layers of the retina across the wedge defect. A horizontal cross section of the ONH cube scan (green line, D, left) shows a thin RNFL in the area of the defect (D, right). The circumpapillary RNFL scan reveals a normal thickness in all sectors except for the well-demarcated wedge defect sector. This sector, with a thickness of 95 μm, is indicated to be outside normal limits, as shown in E. Note that for all other locations, the thickness profile (black line) is near the mid-range of healthy population as represented by the light blue line (E, right bottom).

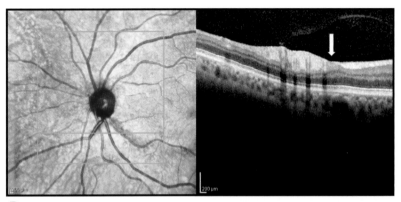

D. (Left) Infrared CSLO image of ONH where green line indicates OCT scan. (Right) SD-OCT line scan across the inferotemporal region.

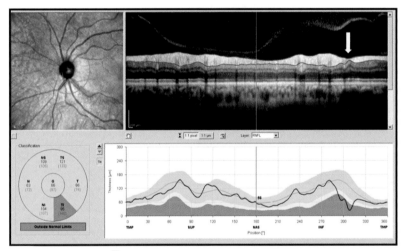

E. Circumpapillary RNFL analysis.

RTVue-100

RTVue-100 imaging indicates a thin RNFL in the inferotemporal region in both the ONH and RNFL scans, as shown in F and G. The cross-sectional image and analysis along the 3.4-mm diameter circle (H, I) show a thickness at the wedge that enters the borderline range. The vertical scan through the fovea demonstrates a perifoveal localized thin RNFL (J). An abnormality in thickness in the ganglion cell complex scan (K) is also shown to correspond to the location of the macular cross-section abnormality and the peripapillary wedge defect.

Comment

This case demonstrates the importance of reviewing sectoral RNFL measurements and macular measurements in addition to average RNFL measurements in order to fully appreciate the structural involvement of the disease.

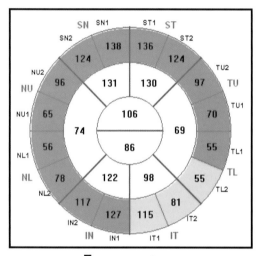

F. RNFL analysis.

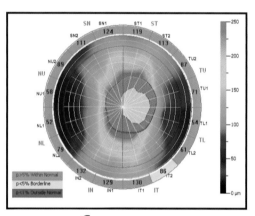

G. ONH analysis.

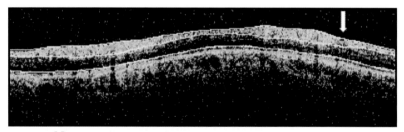

H. Circumpapillary RNFL cross-section image from the ONH scanning pattern.

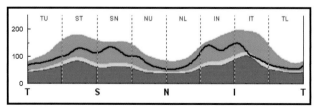

I. Circumpapillary RNFL thickness analysis from ONH scan.

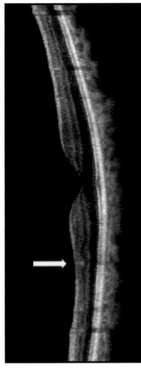

J. Macular cross-line
image.

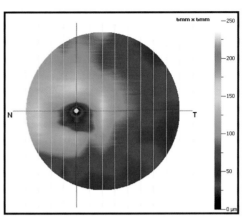

K. Macular ganglion cell complex
thickness map.

Case 12-5. Local Structural Damage Shown in SD-OCT Optic Disc and Macular Analysis With Corresponding Functional Loss

Clinical Summary

This case presents the right eye of a 65-year-old female with normal tension glaucoma treated with latanoprost. Best-corrected visual acuity is 20/20, IOP is 8 mm Hg, and central corneal thickness is 528 μm. The anterior segment examination shows open angles and a mild nuclear sclerotic cataract.

The dilated fundus exam reveals an ONH with a cup-to-disc ratio of 0.8 and a thin neuroretinal rim at 7:00 with a corresponding RNFL wedge defect (A). Humphrey visual field shows a superior nasal step and central scotoma (B). HRT MRA shows abnormalities of the inferior and nasal regions (C).

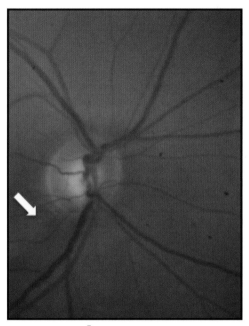

A. Disc photo.

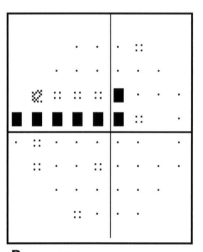

B. Visual field pattern deviation, mean deviation = -3.70 dB.

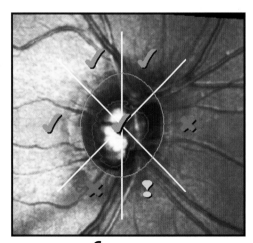

C. HRT MRA.

Cirrus HD-OCT

Cirrus HD-OCT imaging reveals a focal defect in the inferior temporal region (D-F). The arrow in D (part A) points to the location of the focal RNFL thinning. Parts B and C (of D) show that the only region in which the RNFL thickness is outside normal limits is the inferotemporal region. E shows an inferotemporal wedge defect clearly demarcated in the region shown in red in F. A thin rim also appears in the inferotemporal region, where the disc margin nearly meets the cup margin (F). Note the eye movement appearing in the en face image as discontinuity of the blood vessels at the inferior nasal region. The motion occurred below the plane where the circumpapillary RNFL measurements were recorded, and therefore these measurements can be reliably used.

The macular cube scan (G) shows the continuation of the RNFL defect throughout the inferior macula and along the vertical cross section, especially when compared to the superior macula (H, arrow). The macular cube ganglion cell analysis shows the defect in the thickness map (I), deviation map (J), and sector analysis (K).

Comment

This case demonstrates a locally thin RNFL along with macular thinning shown with SD-OCT that corresponds to the visual field abnormality.

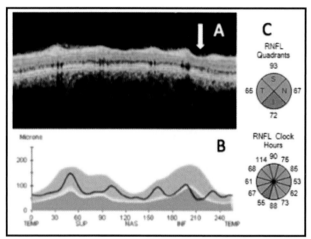

D. Optic Disc Cube scan. (A) Circumpapillary RNFL cross section. (B) RNFL thickness compared to a normative database. (C) RNFL sectoral analysis.

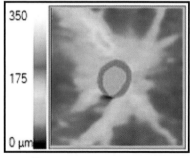

E. RNFL thickness map.

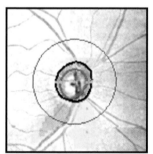

F. RNFL deviation map on en face image with ONH disc and cup margins.

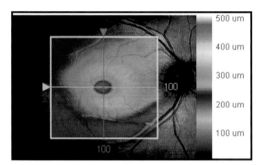

G. Macular cube thickness analysis on LSO image.

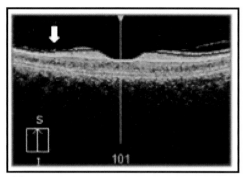

H. Macular vertical cross-section image.

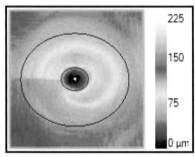

I. Macular cube ganglion cell analysis thickness map.

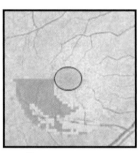

J. Macular cube ganglion cell analysis deviation map.

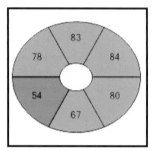

K. Macular cube ganglion cell analysis sectors.

Case 12-6. Inferotemporal Damage Evident by Clinical Exam and Imaging With Fluctuating Visual Field Defects

Clinical Summary

This case presents the left eye of an 86-year-old female with primary open-angle glaucoma treated with bimatoprost. Best-corrected visual acuity is 20/30, IOP is 15 mm Hg, and central corneal thickness is 532 μm. The anterior segment examination shows open angles, a moderate nuclear sclerotic cataract, and cortical opacities. The dilated fundus exam reveals an ONH with a cup-to-disc ratio of 0.8 and an inferotemporal notch. Humphrey visual field shows superior central and nasal step defects with nonspecific changes in the inferior hemifield (A, B).

The Table indicates the mean RNFL thickness measurement for Cirrus HD-OCT (borderline) and RTVue-100 (within normal limits).

C and D provide 3D OCT-1000 cross-sectional images on the ONH and macula for comparison with the following images acquired with Cirrus HD-OCT and RTVue-100.

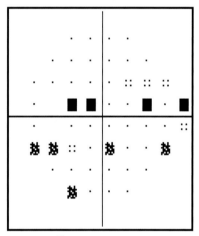

A. Visual field 1
pattern deviation,
mean deviation = -3.36 dB.

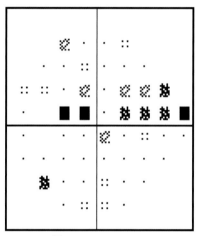

B. Visual field 2
pattern deviation,
mean deviation = -3.37 dB.

RNFL Thickness Measurements

Device	RNFL Thickness (μm)
Cirrus HD-OCT	65
RTVue-100	83

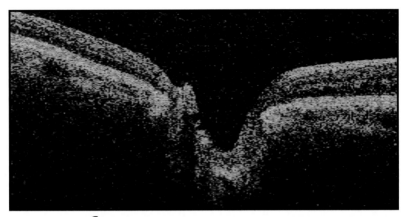

C. 3D OCT-1000 ONH cross-section image.

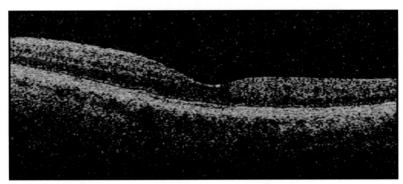

D. 3D OCT-1000 macular cross-section image.

Cirrus HD-OCT

Cirrus HD-OCT shows a thin RNFL in the entire inferior region but most pronounced in the inferotemporal region as indicated by the cross-section image (E, part A, arrow). The RNFL thickness profile demonstrates a clear localized RNFL defect within a thin inferior sector (E, part B). The sector analysis (E, part C) shows an abnormal thickness in the inferior quadrant, but more specifically at the 5:00 location. F and G show the extension of the thin RNFL, in the inferotemporal region, along with a superonasal wedge defect that is more clearly detected on the deviation map. Note that the circumpapillary RNFL analysis did not detect the superior defect. This can be explained by the close proximity of the defect to the disc margin while the sampling location of the circular scan is mostly outside the involved region. The macular cube scan and cross section (H, I) show a slight abnormal thickness inferiorly. This is indicated by the deep blue hues in the pseudocolor thickness map. The glaucomatous damage is mostly pronounced in the macular cube ganglion cell analysis thickness map (J), deviation map (K), and sectors (L) where the macula was thin over a broad area. A superonasal defect is also apparent corresponding to the early superior peripapillary thinning.

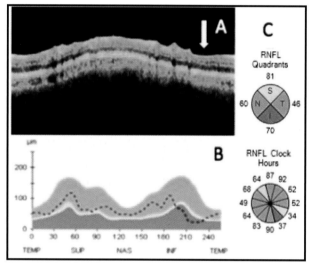

E. Optic Disc Cube scan. (A) Circumpapillary RNFL cross section. (B) RNFL thickness compared to a normative database. (C) RNFL sectoral analysis.

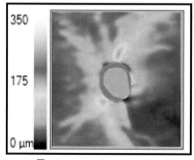

F. RNFL thickness map.

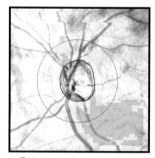

G. RNFL deviation map on en face image with ONH disc and cup margins.

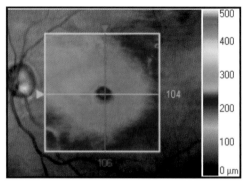

H. Macular cube thickness analysis on LSO image.

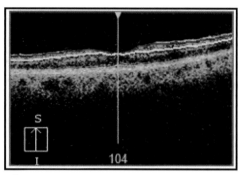

I. Macular vertical cross-section image.

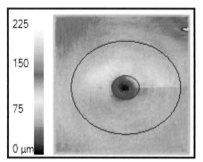

J. Macular cube ganglion cell analysis thickness map.

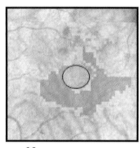

K. Macular cube ganglion cell analysis deviation map.

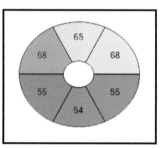

L. Macular cube ganglion cell analysis sectors.

RTVue-100

RTVue-100 ONH scan shows the same infero-temporal focal damage (M, arrow) best shown in N and O, where the measured thickness of the damaged region is categorized outside normal limits. The macular ganglion cell complex scan (P) shows a severely thin inner retinal complex, especially in the entire inferior macula where the green level of thickness is reduced to blue. Q also shows that thinning is most abnormal in the inferior region with an additional area of abnormality in the superior region. This might correspond with the nonspecific changes observed in the inferior visual field.

Comment

This case demonstrates the importance of reviewing the RNFL thickness deviation map or the ONH analysis map along with the macular ganglion cell complex map to identify the full extent of the retinal involvement. This case also illustrates situations where structural findings substantially exceed the functional deficit.

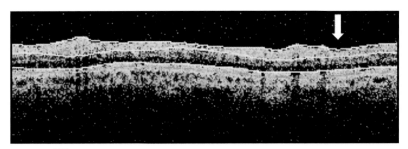

M. Circumpapillary RNFL cross-section image from the ONH scanning pattern.

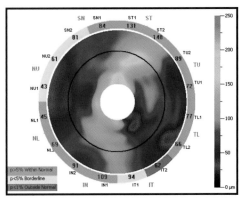

N. ONH analysis.

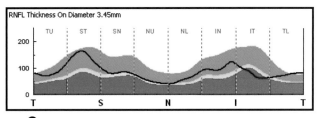

O. Circumpapillary RNFL thickness analysis from ONH scan.

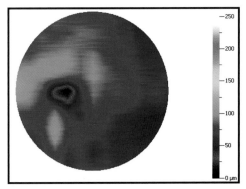

P. Macular ganglion cell complex thickness map.

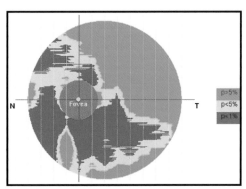

Q. Macular ganglion cell complex significance map.

Case 12-7. Structural Changes Confirm Early Visual Field Scotoma

Clinical Summary

This case presents the right eye of a 65-year-old female with primary open-angle glaucoma treated surgically with trabeculectomy with mitomycin C and medically with memantine only. Ocular examination reveals a best-corrected visual acuity of 20/25, IOP of 7 mm Hg, and central corneal thickness of 547 μm. The anterior segment examination shows an elevated superior bleb without leaks and a mild nuclear sclerotic cataract. ONH evaluation (A) shows the cup-to-disc ratio to be 0.9. Visual field testing shows a prominent inferior arcuate and nasal scotoma along with a questionable early superior nasal step (B). HRT MRA shows a local defect in the superotemporal region only (C), while GDx shows a profound decrease in reflectivity in the superior quadrant with substantial inferior RNFL loss (D).

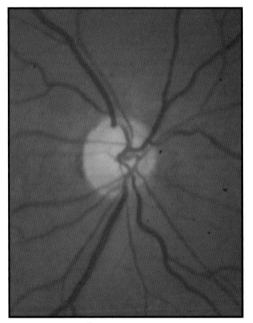

A. Disc photo.

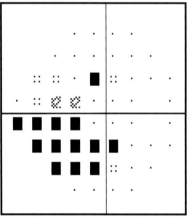

B. Visual field pattern deviation, mean deviation = -10.51 dB.

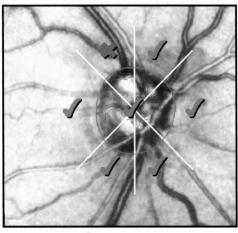

C. HRT MRA.

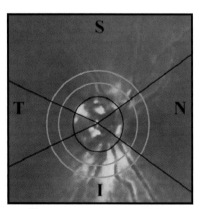

D. GDx enhanced corneal compensation nerve fiber thickness map.

Stratus TD-OCT

The TD-OCT RNFL scan reveals a thin RNFL across most of the circumpapillary region (E). The RNFL thickness profile shows a thin layer throughout the scan, most pronounced in the superior region with less damage in the inferior region (F).

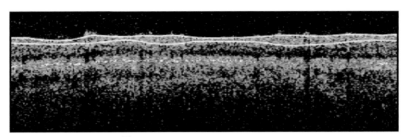

E. RNFL cross-section image.

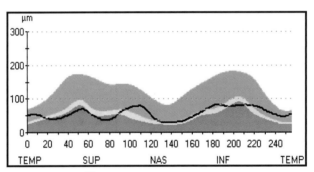

F. RNFL thickness profile.

Cirrus HD-OCT

The Cirrus Optic Disc Cube scan also reveals a globally thin RNFL, with an average RNFL thickness of 60 μm (G, part C). Superior and inferior quadrants were reported as abnormal while the corresponding clock hours in the inferior region were only within the borderline range. G (part B) shows an RNFL thickness profile similar to the TD-OCT profile, with slightly less damage in the inferior region. H shows the RNFL thickness map, where the small remaining yellow coloring indicates a large area of thin RNFL. A large area of significantly thin RNFL is noticeable in the deviation map in the superior hemifield, with less damage in the inferior region (I).

Comment

This case demonstrates the importance of the imaging devices in ensuring a precise diagnosis. While the inferior visual field defect was evident, the finding in the superior hemifield was questionable. The imaging results enforce the findings in both the superior and inferior hemifields.

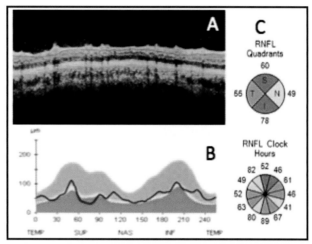

G. Optic Disc Cube scan. (A) Circumpapillary RNFL cross section. (B) RNFL thickness compared to a normative database. (C) RNFL sectoral analysis.

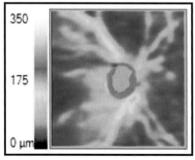

H. RNFL thickness map.

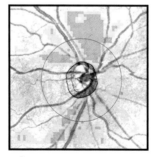

I. RNFL deviation map on en face image with ONH disc and cup margins.

Case 12-8. TD-OCT Imaging Correlated Better With the Visual Field Than SD-OCT

Clinical Summary

This case presents the right eye of a 72-year-old female with pseudoexfoliative glaucoma treated with argon laser trabeculoplasty, trabeculectomy, and topically with dorzolamide/timolol. Best-corrected visual acuity is 20/200, and IOP is 10 mm Hg. The anterior segment examination shows open angles, with a well-centered posterior chamber intraocular lens. The dilated fundus exam reveals an ONH with a cup-to-disc ratio of 0.9 (A). Humphrey visual field shows a dense superior and inferior nasal step and an arcuate scotoma with early superior and inferior central scotoma (B). HRT MRA (C) shows all sectors to be outside normal limits.

The Table shows both TD- and SD-OCT indicated that the mean RNFL thickness is outside normal limits.

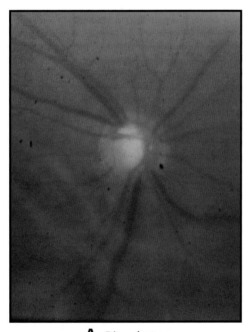

A. Disc photo.

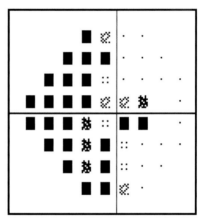

B. Visual field pattern deviation, mean deviation = -13.94 dB.

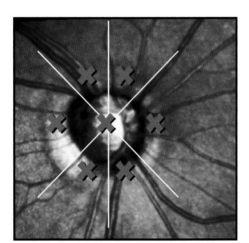

C. HRT MRA.

RNFL Thickness Measurements

Device	RNFL Thickness (µm)
Stratus TD-OCT	51
Cirrus HD-OCT	56

Stratus TD-OCT

TD-OCT imaging shows the RNFL thickness to be outside the normal range inferiorly, superiorly, and temporally, sparing the nasal region (D-F). This structural imaging corresponds well with the visual field findings. Note that the structural involvement in the temporal region corresponds with the central scotoma.

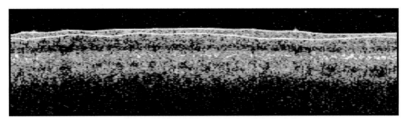

D. RNFL cross-section image.

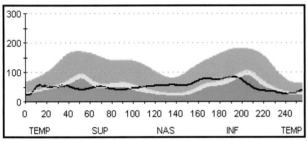

E. RNFL thickness profile.

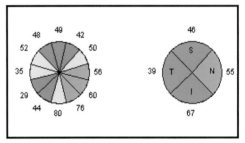

F. RNFL sectoral thickness analysis.

Cirrus HD-OCT

Differing from the TD-OCT findings, SD-OCT (G-I) shows RNFL thickness to be outside the normal range only in the superior and inferior regions. This is shown best in the sector analysis of G (part C), where the temporal and nasal sectors are within the normal range. The thickness (H) and deviation maps (I) show extensive damage mostly in the superior and inferior regions.

Comment

This case demonstrates a visual field defect that best correlates with the RNFL thickness assessment presented in TD-OCT image analysis.

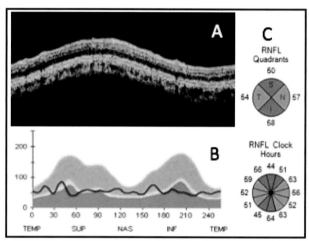

G. Optic Disc Cube scan. (A) Circumpapillary RNFL cross section. (B) RNFL thickness compared to a normative database. (C) RNFL sectoral analysis.

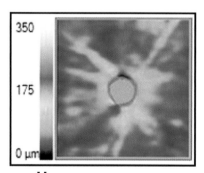

H. RNFL thickness map.

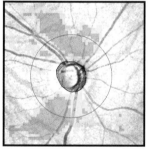

I. RNFL deviation map on en face image with ONH disc and cup margins.

Case 12-9. Strong Agreement Between SD-OCT and TD-OCT in Advanced Primary Open-Angle Glaucoma

Clinical Summary

This case presents the right eye of a 73-year-old female with primary open-angle glaucoma treated with a trabeculectomy with mitomycin C with no further use of ocular medications. Best-corrected visual acuity is 20/30, and IOP is 8 mm Hg. The anterior segment examination shows a cystic bleb without leaks, wide-open angles, and a centered posterior chamber intraocular lens. The dilated fundus exam reveals an ONH with a cup-to-disc ratio of 0.9 (A). Humphrey visual field displays dense superior and inferior arcuate scotomas (B). GDx enhanced corneal compensation imaging shows reduced birefringence in both the superotemporal and inferonasal regions (C).

The Table shows both TD- and SD-OCT measured the mean RNFL thickness to be outside normal limits.

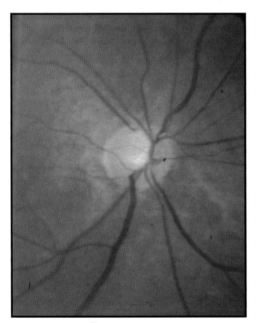

A. Disc photo.

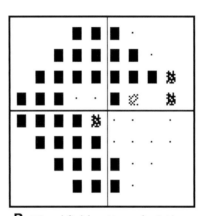

B. Visual field pattern deviation, mean deviation = -17.92 dB.

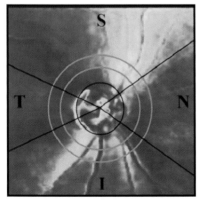

C. GDx enhanced corneal compensation nerve fiber thickness map.

RNFL Thickness Measurements

Device	RNFL Thickness (μm)
Stratus TD-OCT	52
Cirrus HD-OCT	53

Stratus TD-OCT

Imaging with Stratus TD-OCT displays obliteration of the RNFL double-hump pattern with a thin RNFL in the superior and inferior poles (D [white arrows], E) that were marked as outside normal limits at 6:00, 7:00, 10:00, 11:00, and 12:00. A borderline RNFL thickness is determined at 4:00 and 5:00 (F).

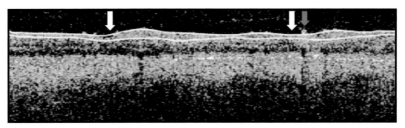

D. RNFL cross-section image.

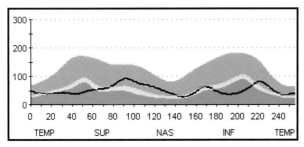

E. RNFL thickness profile.

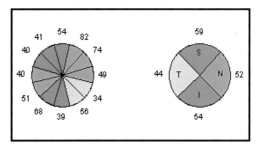

F. RNFL sectoral thickness analysis.

Cirrus HD-OCT

Imaging with Cirrus HD-OCT demonstrates overall findings similar to those provided by TD-OCT, judging by the color codes for the comparison with normative values (G). However, closer attention on the sectoral measurements shows a lesser degree of localized damage recorded by SD-OCT in clock hours 6 and 11 compared to those recorded by TD-OCT. However, this did not affect the overall RNFL thickness provided by the 2 devices (52 and 53 μm). The main reason for the localized discrepancy between the devices is due to the segmentation software that delineates the boundaries of the RNFL. This can be seen in the focal thickness RNFL in the center of the thin inferior region (D, G, part A [red arrow]). In TD-OCT the RNFL segmentation crosses through the localized thickening while in SD-OCT the delineation follows the tissue more closely. The marked structural damage is clearly visible in the RNFL thickness map and the deviation map corresponding to the perimetric damage (H, I).

Comment

This case demonstrates a strong agreement between Stratus TD-OCT and Cirrus HD-OCT that corresponds well with the visual field defect.

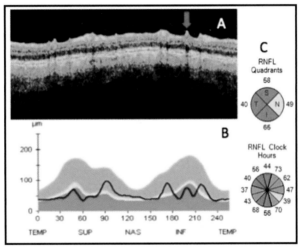

G. Optic Disc Cube scan. (A) Circumpapillary RNFL cross section. (B) RNFL thickness compared to a normative database. (C) RNFL sectoral analysis.

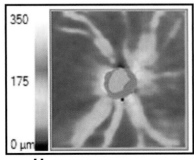

H. RNFL thickness map.

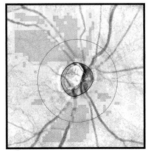

I. RNFL deviation map on en face image with ONH disc and cup margins.

Case 12-10. Global Structural Damage Sparing the Fovea Corresponded to Advanced Visual Field Loss With Remaining Central Vision

Clinical Summary

This case presents the right eye of a 61-year-old female with primary open-angle glaucoma treated with brinzolamide, brimonidine/timolol, and travoprost. She has an extensive ocular surgical history including selective laser trabeculoplasty, a failed trabeculectomy, and placement of both a Baerveldt tube shunt and an Ahmed glaucoma valve implant. Best-corrected visual acuity is 20/30, IOP is 14 mm Hg, and central corneal thickness is 523 μm. The anterior segment examination shows a vascularized superior bleb, 2 patent peripheral iridotomies, the Ahmed tube in proper position within the anterior chamber, and a centered posterior chamber intraocular lens. The dilated fundus exam reveals near total disc cupping.

Visual field shows a severely depressed field sparing only central vision (A). Imaging with HRT (B) displays an MRA outside normal limits, with the exception of the temporal quadrant, and imaging with GDx reveals widespread reduced birefringence throughout the entire peripapillary region (C).

The Table shows both TD- and SD-OCT mean RNFL thickness measurements are outside normal limits.

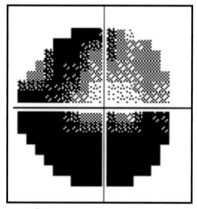

A. Visual field grayscale, mean deviation = -24.16 dB.

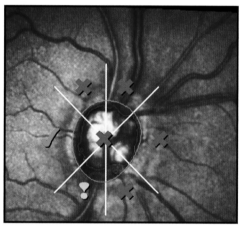

B. HRT MRA.

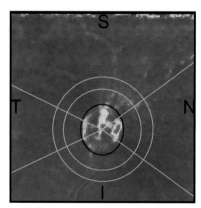

C. GDx enhanced corneal compensation nerve fiber thickness map.

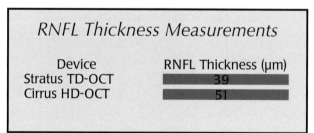

RNFL Thickness Measurements

Device	RNFL Thickness (μm)
Stratus TD-OCT	39
Cirrus HD-OCT	51

Stratus TD-OCT

Imaging from TD-OCT shows marked damage with a flat thickness profile and relative sparing nasally (D-F). It is notable that even with very advanced glaucomatous damage, the global OCT RNFL thickness measurements are rarely reported beneath 35 μm. In this case, clock hour 10 reports values as low as 20 μm. This is likely marking the "floor effect" of OCT measurements, representing remaining supportive glial tissue.

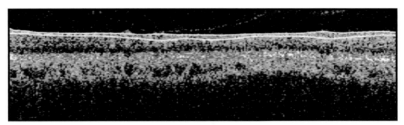

D. RNFL cross-section image.

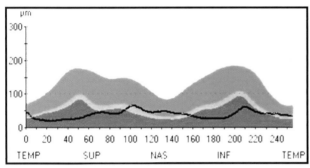

E. RNFL thickness profile.

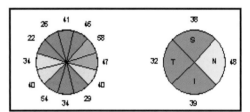

F. RNFL sectoral thickness analysis.

Cirrus HD-OCT

Cirrus HD-OCT imaging of the RNFL shows a severely thin RNFL in all areas sparing the nasal region (G-I). G (part B) shows the circumpapillary RNFL thickness to be outside normal limits in most regions of the scan. H shows a marked reduction in thickness globally, and I shows the significant thickness deviation in comparison to a normative database, indicated by the red coloring.

Cirrus HD-OCT imaging of the macula indicates a thin retina in the macular region (J, K). The nasal region and the fovea remain at a normal thickness level while all other sectors are thinner than normal (L). The green center of L correlates well with the central vision remaining in this advanced glaucoma case, with the maculopapillar bundle conveying the axons that originate in the fovea and approach the nasal sector creating a near-normal thickness. The macular cube ganglion cell analysis illustrates similar results with thinning in all regions except the inferonasal sector (M-O).

Comment

This case demonstrates OCT's ability to quantify severe damage to the structure of the retina in advanced glaucoma.

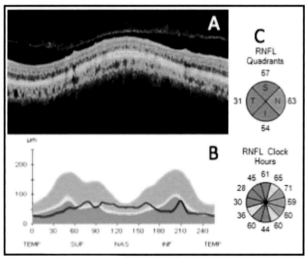

G. Optic Disc Cube scan. (A) Circumpapillary RNFL cross section. (B) RNFL thickness compared to a normative database. (C) RNFL sectoral analysis.

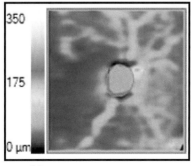

H. RNFL thickness map.

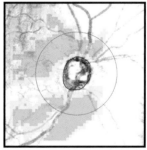

I. RNFL deviation map on en face image with ONH disc and cup margins.

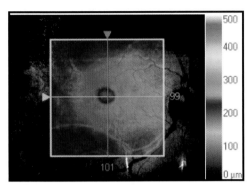

J. Macular cube thickness analysis on LSO image.

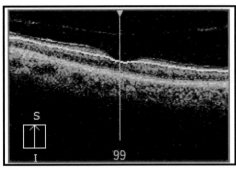

K. Macular vertical cross-section image.

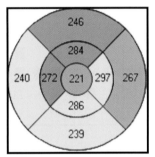

L. Macular sectoral thickness analysis.

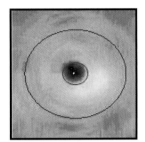

M. Macular cube ganglion cell analysis thickness map.

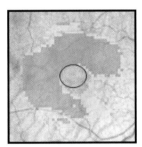

N. Macular cube ganglion cell analysis deviation map.

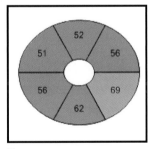

O. Macular cube ganglion cell analysis sectors.

Case 12-11. Functional Abnormalities in Visual Field Not Found by SD-OCT Structural Imaging

Clinical Summary

This case presents the right eye of a 51-year-old female with primary open-angle glaucoma and a positive family history of glaucoma in both parents. Best-corrected visual acuity is 20/20, IOP is 18 mm Hg, and there is a notably thick cornea with a central corneal thickness of 631 μm. The anterior segment examination shows wide-open angles and a mild nuclear sclerotic cataract. The dilated fundus exam reveals an ONH with a cup-to-disc ratio of 0.7 (A). Humphrey visual field shows a superior arcuate scotoma (B). HRT MRA analysis shows the ONH to be within normal limits in each sector and borderline globally (C).

As shown in the Table, all global OCT mean RNFL thickness measurements remained in the normal range.

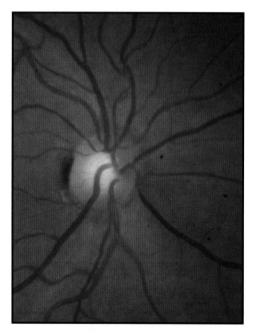

A. Disc photo.

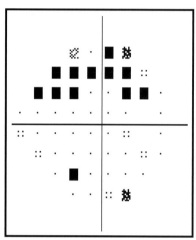

B. Visual field pattern deviation, mean deviation = -4.82 dB.

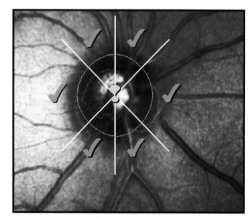

C. HRT MRA.

RNFL Thickness Measurements

Device	RNFL Thickness (μm)
Cirrus HD-OCT	91
RTVue-100	102
Spectralis HRA+OCT	114

Cirrus HD-OCT

The Optic Disc Cube scan shows a normal thickness profile with global and sectoral thickness measurements all within the normal range (D).

Normal macular configuration and thickness is demonstrated in the thickness map (E) and the cross-section image (F).

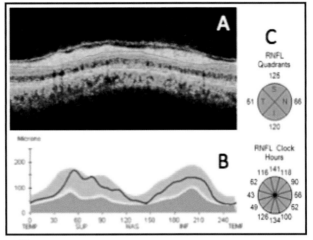

D. Optic Disc Cube scan. (A) Circumpapillary RNFL cross section. (B) RNFL thickness compared to a normative database. (C) RNFL sectoral analysis.

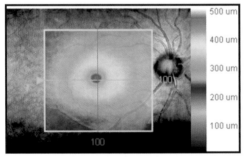

E. Macular cube thickness analysis on LSO image.

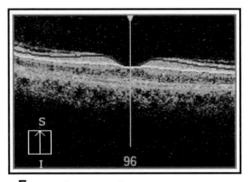

F. Macular vertical cross-section image.

Spectralis HRA+OCT

Spectralis HRA+OCT imaging indicates a normal circumpapillary RNFL thickness (G) and normal macular scan (H). The delineation of the RNFL boundaries failed in the temporal aspects of G as shown by the thickness profile in that region, which exceeds the upper limit of the normal thickness range.

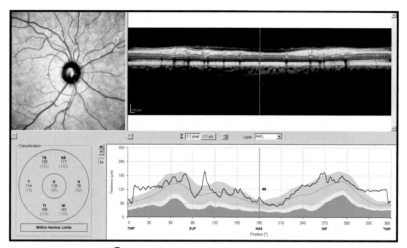

G. Circumpapillary RNFL analysis.

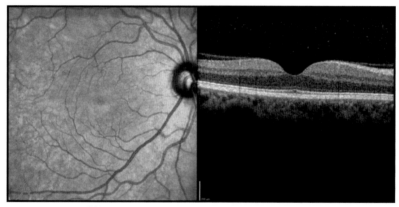

H. (Left) Infrared CSLO image of macula.
(Right) SD-OCT line scan across macula.

RTVue-100

RTVue-100 imaging shows a slight, very localized thin RNFL in a section of the temporal circumpapillary RNFL (I-K). This thin RNFL would be expected to cause a central scotoma and, therefore, does not match the visual field finding. The macular area shows a normal thickness on the ganglion cell complex analysis and the vertical cross-sectional image (L, M).

Comment

This case demonstrates agreement among the imaging modalities, which show normal structural findings that do not correspond with the visual field findings.

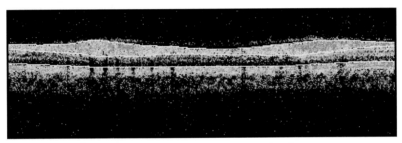

I. Circumpapillary RNFL cross-section image.

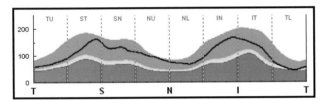

J. Circumpapillary RNFL thickness analysis.

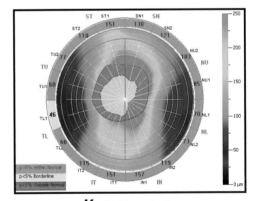

K. ONH analysis.

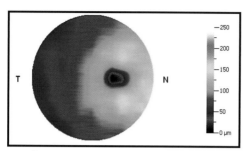

L. Macular ganglion cell complex thickness map.

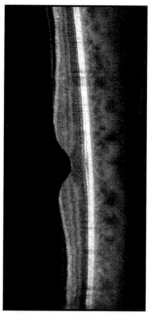

M. Macular cross-line image.

Case 12-12. Normal Visual Field With Contradicting SD-OCT and HRT Imaging

Clinical Summary

This case presents a 67-year-old female with increased IOP in the low 30s prior to starting medical therapy and currently being treated with latanoprost. Best-corrected visual acuity is 20/25, and IOP is 12 mm Hg. The anterior segment examination shows wide-open angles, a trace nuclear sclerotic cataract, and pseudoexfoliative peripheral capsular changes.

The dilated fundus exam reveals an ONH with a cup-to-disc ratio of 0.7 (A). Consecutive visual fields are full (B); however, HRT analysis (C) indicates abnormalities throughout the disc area sparing temporally.

The Table shows that all OCT devices indicated an RNFL thickness within normal limits compared to a normative database.

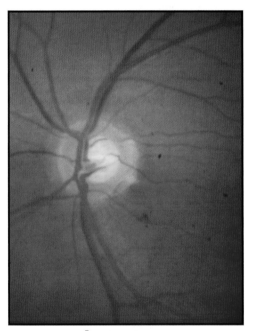

A. Disc photo.

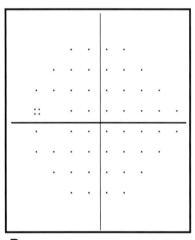

B. Visual field pattern deviation, mean deviation = 0.15 dB.

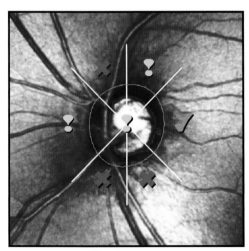

C. HRT MRA.

RNFL Thickness Measurements

Device	RNFL Thickness (μm)
Stratus TD-OCT	79
Cirrus HD-OCT	77
RTVue-100	92
Spectralis HRA+OCT	87

Cirrus HD-OCT

Cirrus HD-OCT imaging reveals a normal Optic Disc Cube scan (D) where the circumpapillary RNFL thickness is within the normal range, except for borderline abnormalities of the superior and 2:00 region (D, part C). The thickness and deviation maps (E, F) show some superotemporal abnormalities. Note that the RNFL wedge defects are detected in the superior, superotemporal, and inferior regions on the cube scan, but only crossed the sampling ring at the tip of the defects thus showing minimal effect on the RNFL thickness measurements.

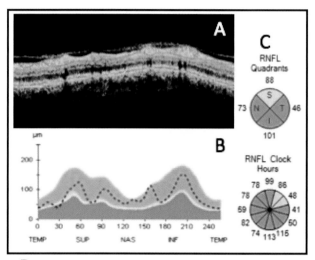

D. Optic Disc Cube scan. (A) Circumpapillary RNFL cross section. (B) RNFL thickness compared to a normative database. (C) RNFL sectoral analysis.

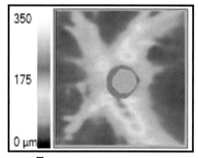

E. RNFL thickness map.

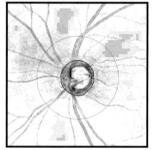

F. RNFL deviation map on en face image with ONH disc and cup margins.

Spectralis HRA+OCT

Spectralis HRA+OCT imaging also reveals a normal circumpapillary RNFL thickness (G) with a global mean RNFL thickness of 87 μm. Spectralis macular imaging, along a horizontal line crossing the foveal region, also appears normal (H).

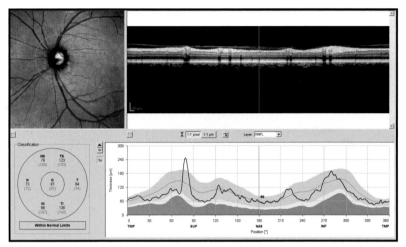

G. Circumpapillary RNFL analysis.

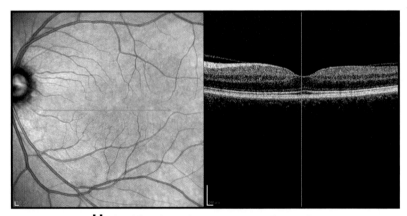

H. (Left) Infrared CSLO image of macula.
(Right) SD-OCT line scan across macula.

RTVue-100

The ONH analysis (I-K) shows a normal RNFL thickness in the region surrounding the ONH. The vertical ONH cross scan reveals a large cup. The macular thickness is normal in both the ganglion cell complex (L) and the cross-line image (M).

Comment

This case illustrates the importance of obtaining data within the entire peripapillary scanning window, as the glaucomatous RNFL effect was noticeable only outside the conventional sampling ring location.

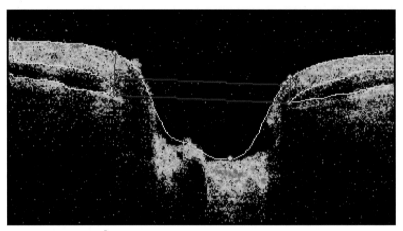

I. ONH vertical cross-section image.

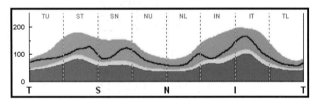

J. Circumpapillary RNFL thickness analysis obtained from ONH scan.

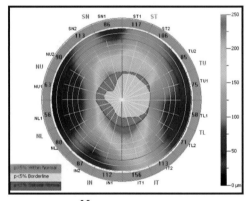

K. ONH analysis.

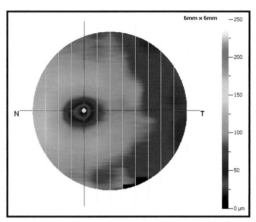

L. Macular ganglion cell complex thickness map.

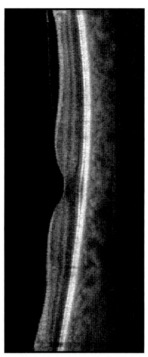

M. Macular cross-line image.

Case 12-13. Imaging Displayed Abnormal Structure With Normal Functional Testing

Clinical Summary

This case presents the left eye of a 47-year-old female with a history of systemic steroid use referred for increased cupping and given the diagnosis of glaucoma suspect. Best-corrected visual acuity is 20/20, and IOP is 10 mm Hg. The anterior segment examination shows wide-open angles. The dilated fundus exam reveals an ONH with a cup-to-disc ratio of 0.9, with a locally thin inferior neuroretinal rim and peripapillary atrophy (A). Repetitive Humphrey visual fields are full (B). Imaging with HRT (C) displays an MRA outside normal limits globally, inferiorly, and nasally.

The Table shows that Cirrus HD-OCT mean RNFL thickness is measured within normal limits.

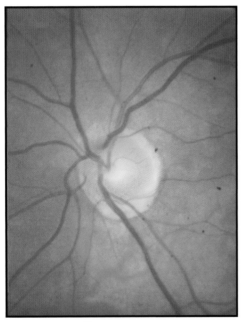

A. Disc photo.

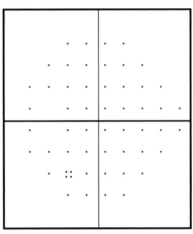

B. Visual field pattern deviation, mean deviation = 0.1 dB.

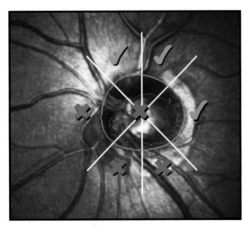

C. HRT MRA.

RNFL Thickness Measurements

Device	RNFL Thickness (µm)
Cirrus HD-OCT	85
Stratus TD-OCT	96

Stratus TD-OCT

Imaging with Stratus TD-OCT displays RNFL thickness to be in the borderline range in the inferior quadrant and at 6:00, 7:00, and 9:00 (D-F). This agrees with the HRT MRA analysis shown in C.

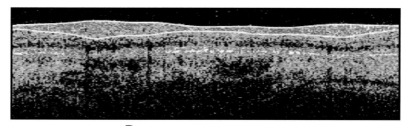

D. RNFL cross-section image.

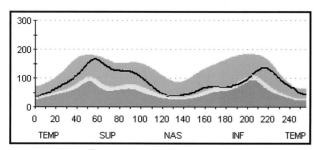

E. RNFL thickness profile.

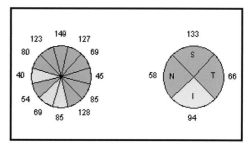

F. RNFL sectoral thickness analysis.

Cirrus HD-OCT

Imaging with Cirrus HD-OCT demonstrates RNFL thickness to be in the borderline range at 6:00 with global and quadrant parameters within normal limits (G, part C). However, the Optic Disc Cube scan thickness and deviation maps (H, I) show a clear thin RNFL in the inferior aspect of the disc and another wedge defect in the temporal aspect of the disc.

Comment

This case demonstrates the use of quantitative objective measures for early indication of structural damage in glaucoma suspects. The agreement among all imaging devices on the appearance of structural damage in the absence of functional evidence at that time strongly suggests a preperimetric status of glaucomatous damage. The importance in assessing the deviation map for Cirrus for regions outside the circular sampling location is illustrated in this case as the damage was minimally evident in the circular profile, while clearly detectable in the map.

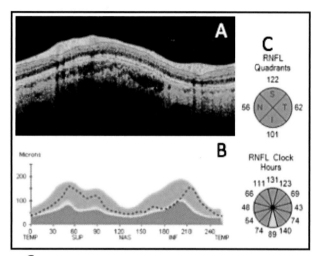

G. Optic Disc Cube scan. (A) Circumpapillary RNFL cross section. (B) RNFL thickness compared to a normative database. (C) RNFL sectoral analysis.

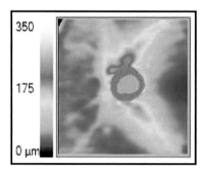

H. RNFL thickness map.

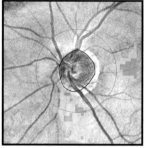

I. RNFL deviation map on en face image with ONH disc and cup margins.

Case 12-14. Imaging Displayed Abnormal Structure While Function Remained Normal

Clinical Summary

This case presents the left eye of a 59-year-old healthy female with suspected glaucoma. Best-corrected visual acuity is 20/20, and IOP is 12 mm Hg. The anterior segment exam shows open angles. Disc photographs reveal large cupping and peripapillary atrophy (A). The visual field is full (B), and HRT MRA (C) shows no disc abnormalities.

The Table shows that the mean global RNFL thickness measurements from both TD- and SD-OCT remain within the normal range, despite local abnormal RNFL thickness measurements.

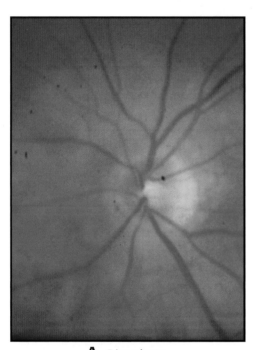

A. Disc photo.

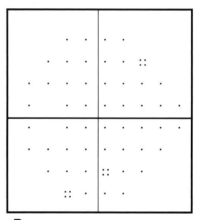

B. Visual field pattern deviation, mean deviation = -0.56 dB.

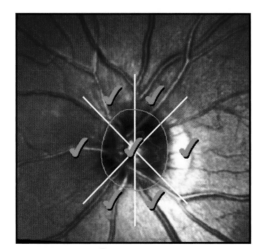

C. HRT MRA.

RNFL Thickness Measurements

Device	RNFL Thickness (μm)
Stratus TD-OCT	98
Cirrus HD-OCT	85
RTVue-100	92

Cirrus HD-OCT

Cirrus HD-OCT imaging reveals a thin RNFL in the inferior region (D). It should be noted that the RNFL defect is very focal, confined to 6:00, but when the RNFL thickness is summarized for the inferior quadrant where it includes the normal thickness measurements for 5:00 and 7:00, the sector is only labeled as borderline. The thickness and deviation maps (E, F) demonstrate a clear inferior wedge defect. The macular cube, however, reveals no apparent abnormalities in G through I.

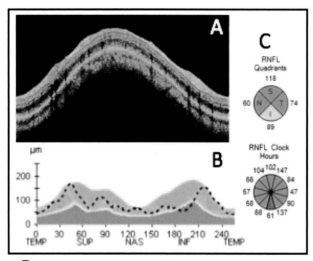

D. Optic Disc Cube scan. (A) Circumpapillary RNFL cross section. (B) RNFL thickness compared to a normative database. (C) RNFL sectoral analysis.

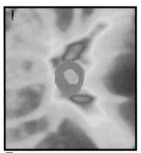

E. RNFL thickness map.

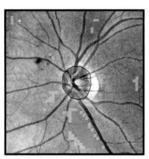

F. RNFL deviation map on en face image with ONH disc and cup margins.

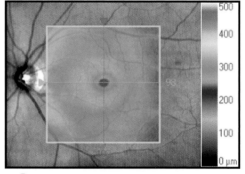

G. Macular cube thickness analysis on LSO image.

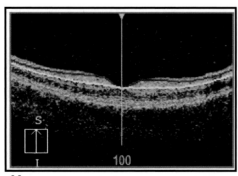

H. Macular vertical cross-section image.

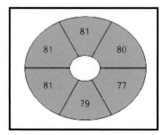

I. Macular cube ganglion cell analysis sectors.

RTVue-100

RTVue-100 imaging indicates a thin RNFL inferiorly, in both the RNFL (J) and ONH (K-M) scans. Similar to the Cirrus analysis of the macula, the cross-line image (N) and the ganglion cell complex analysis (O) show no abnormalities.

Comment

This case demonstrates a local abnormality detected with all imaging devices that is not apparent in the functional testing, creating a shift in the diagnosis from suspect to preperimetric glaucoma.

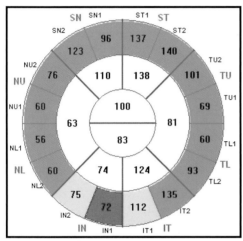

J. RNFL analysis.

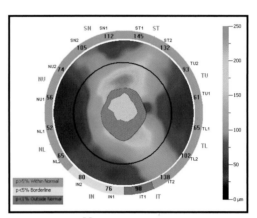

K. ONH analysis.

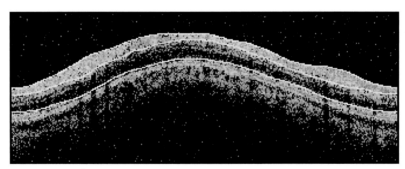

L. Circumpapillary RNFL cross-section image.

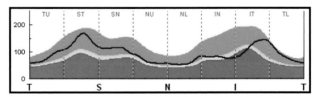

M. Circumpapillary RNFL thickness analysis.

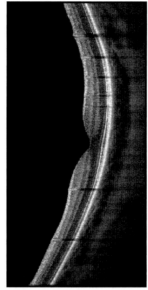

N. Macular cross-line image.

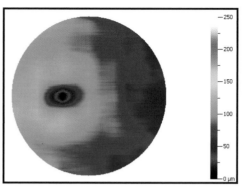

O. Macular ganglion cell complex thickness map.

Case 12-15. SD-OCT Clock Hour Retinal Nerve Fiber Layer Thicknesses Corresponded to Visual Field Abnormalities But Disagreed With HRT

Clinical Summary

This case presents the right eye of a 51-year-old female diagnosed with early primary open-angle glaucoma. Best-corrected visual acuity is 20/25, IOP is 17 mm Hg, and central corneal thickness is 576 μm. The anterior segment examination shows wide-open angles and a mild nuclear sclerotic cataract. The dilated fundus exam reveals an ONH with a cup-to-disc ratio of 0.8 (A). Visual field displays an early superior arcuate scotoma reproducible in 2 visits (B, C). HRT (D) shows MRA parameters outside normal limits superiorly, nasally, and globally. GDx enhanced corneal compensation nerve fiber thickness map shows a normal thickness, as shown in E.

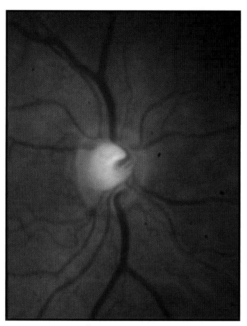

A. Disc photo.

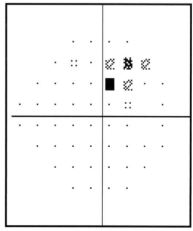

B. Visit 1. Visual field pattern deviation, mean deviation = 1.52 dB.

C. Visit 2. Visual field pattern deviation, mean deviation = 0.98 dB.

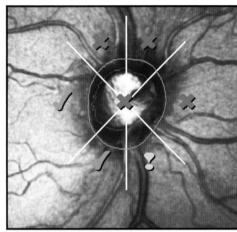

D. HRT MRA.

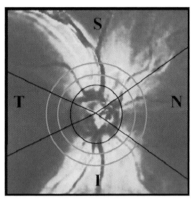

E. GDx enhanced corneal compensation nerve fiber thickness map.

Stratus TD-OCT

Stratus fast RNFL scan shows the RNFL thickness in the circumpapillary region to be in the normal range (F-H), shown by the black thickness line remaining in the green region, except for a focal temporal region where the RNFL thickness is approaching the borderline range.

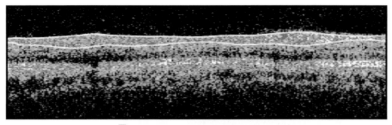

F. RNFL cross-section image.

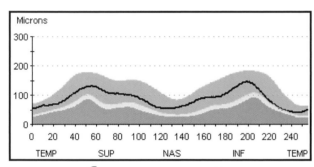

G. RNFL thickness profile.

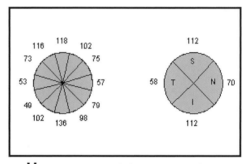

H. RNFL sectoral thickness analysis.

Cirrus HD-OCT

Cirrus Optic Disc Cube scan reveals the mean and sector circumpapillary RNFL thicknesses to be in the normal range (I). The clock hour thickness analysis (I, part C), however, shows 8:00 as a borderline thickness, as reflected in the RNFL thickness profile where a localized temporal region goes deep into the borderline zone (I, part B), similar to Stratus TD-OCT findings. J and K show normal thickness and deviation maps.

Comment

This case demonstrates an early abnormality shown with SD-OCT that coincides with early visual field scotoma and disagrees with the HRT MRA.

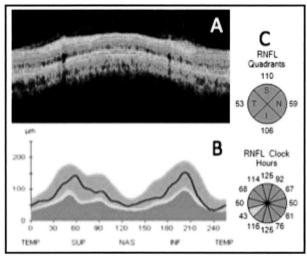

I. Optic Disc Cube scan. (A) Circumpapillary RNFL cross section. (B) RNFL thickness compared to a normative database. (C) RNFL sectoral analysis.

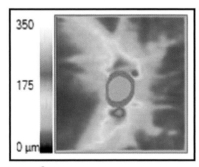

J. RNFL thickness map.

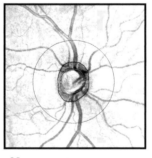

K. RNFL deviation map on en face image with ONH disc and cup margins.

Case 12-16. Ganglion Cell Complex Analysis Showed Structural Damage More Severe Than Would Be Expected Based Upon Visual Field

Clinical Summary

This case presents the right eye of a 77-year-old female with primary open-angle glaucoma treated with travoprost. Best-corrected visual acuity is 20/25, and IOP is 13 mm Hg. The anterior segment examination shows wide-open angles, a mild nuclear sclerotic cataract, and cortical opacities. Humphrey visual field shows an early inferior arcuate scotoma (A). The dilated fundus exam reveals an ONH with a cup-to-disc ratio of 0.8 and peripapillary atrophy (B). The mean RNFL thickness measurement for Cirrus HD-OCT was marked in the borderline region, whereas the RTVue-100 mean RNFL measurement was within normal limits, as shown in the Table.

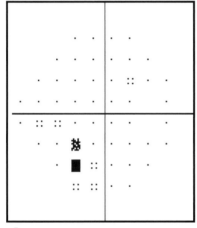

A. Visual field pattern deviation, mean deviation = 0.36 dB.

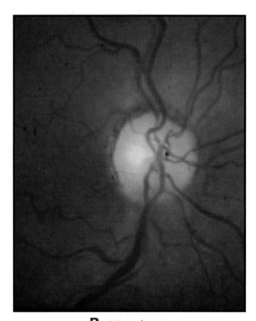

B. Disc photo.

RNFL Thickness Measurements

Device	RNFL Thickness (µm)
Cirrus HD-OCT	71
RTVue-100	98

Cirrus HD-OCT

Cirrus HD-OCT shows RNFL abnormalities superotemporally, superonasally, and inferotemporal (C-E). The most prominently thin RNFL appears superiorly, which correlates with the visual field abnormality. A thin superotemporal rim was also shown in E that correlates with the RNFL damage. The images acquired of the macula (F-I) are within normal limits; however, the macular ganglion cell deviation map and sector analysis (J) indicate prominent damage mainly superiorly.

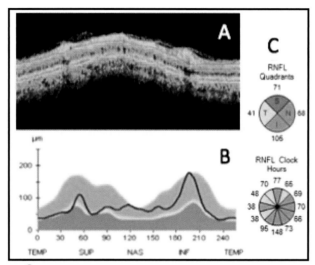

C. Optic Disc Cube scan. (A) Circumpapillary RNFL cross section. (B) RNFL thickness compared to a normative database. (C) RNFL sectoral analysis.

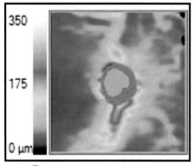

D. RNFL thickness map.

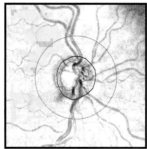

E. RNFL deviation map on en face image with ONH disc and cup margins.

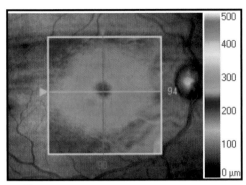

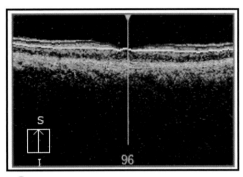

F. Macular cube thickness analysis on LSO image.

G. Macular vertical cross-section image.

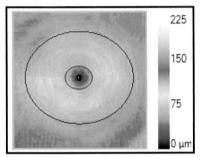

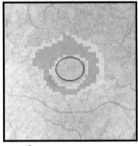

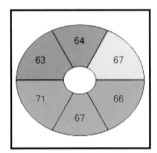

H. Macular cube ganglion cell analysis thickness map.

I. Macular cube ganglion cell analysis deviation map.

J. Macular cube ganglion cell analysis sectors.

RTVue-100

RTVue-100 ONH imaging (K, L) indicates a borderline RNFL thickness in the inferotemporal region. RTVue, however, failed to report abnormalities in the superotemporal region (M), where Cirrus shows the most advanced damage. The RTVue-100 ganglion cell complex thickness map (N, O), however, shows a thin superotemporal inner retinal complex of the macula, which corresponds to visual field and Cirrus analysis of damage.

Comment

This case illustrates a situation where Cirrus HD-OCT better highlights the ONH damage and both Cirrus HD-OCT and RTVue-100 ganglion cell complex analysis show macular abnormalities that correspond with the early visual field findings.

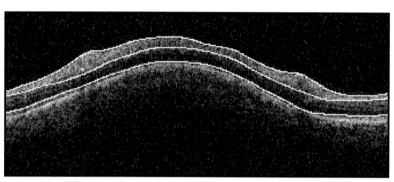

K. Circumpapillary RNFL cross-section image.

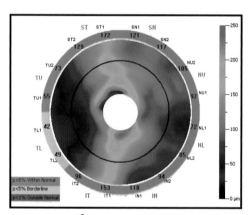

L. ONH analysis.

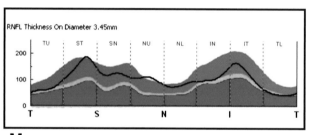

M. Circumpapillary RNFL thickness analysis obtained from ONH scan.

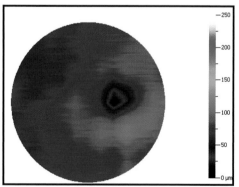

N. Macular ganglion cell complex thickness map.

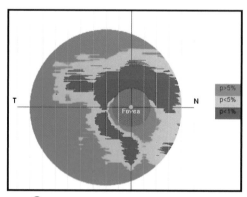

O. Macular ganglion cell complex significance map.

Case 12-17. Early Structural Damage Both Superiorly and Inferiorly Only Reflected in One Visual Field Hemifield

Clinical Summary

This case presents the left eye of a 61-year-old female with primary open-angle glaucoma treated with latanoprost. Best-corrected visual acuity is 20/20, IOP is 16 mm Hg, and there is a notably thick cornea with a central corneal thickness of 677 µm. The anterior segment examination shows wide-open angles and a mild nuclear sclerotic cataract. The dilated fundus exam reveals an ONH with a cup-to-disc ratio of 0.8 and thin neuroretinal rim inferiorly and nasally (A). Visual field shows a reproducible early superior defect (B). HRT (C) shows MRA parameters outside normal limits in the superonasal region and borderline globally and in the superotemporal, temporal, and temporal inferior regions. GDx enhanced corneal compensation nerve fiber thickness map shows an atypical birefringence pattern superiorly with possible reduction in RNFL superotemporally (D).

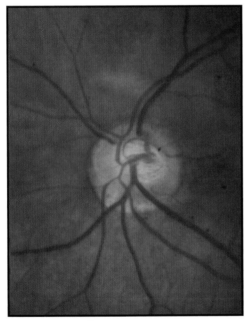

A. Disc photo.

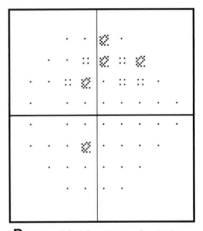

B. Visual field pattern deviation, mean deviation = -0.13 dB.

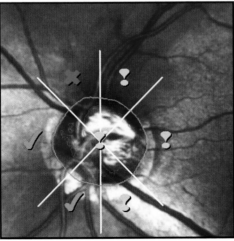

C. HRT MRA.

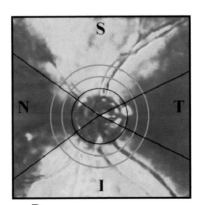

D. GDx enhanced corneal compensation nerve fiber thickness map.

Stratus TD-OCT

Stratus fast RNFL scan shows a thin superior and inferior region (E-G). Inferior RNFL appears to be more damaged than the superior RNFL, as indicated by both F and G.

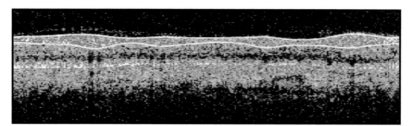

E. RNFL cross-section image.

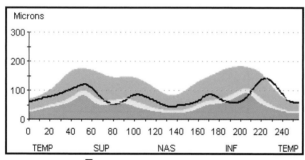

F. RNFL thickness profile.

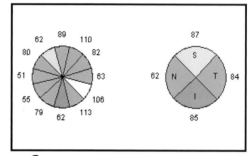

G. RNFL sectoral thickness analysis.

Cirrus HD-OCT

Cirrus Optic Disc Cube scan reveals a thin RNFL in the superior and inferior regions (H, I) with prominent wedge defects adjacent to both poles (J). Like the Stratus fast RNFL scan, the Cirrus Optic Disc Cube scan indicates the damage to be more advanced inferiorly.

Comment

This case demonstrates agreement between TD-OCT and SD-OCT, where the more severe structural damage correlates well with the visual field defect. The additional structural damage identified with both iterations is not shown in the visual field.

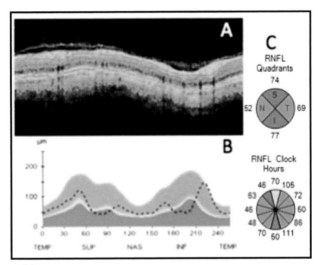

H. Optic Disc Cube scan. (A) Circumpapillary RNFL cross section. (B) RNFL thickness compared to a normative database. (C) RNFL sectoral analysis.

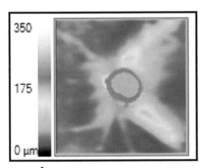

I. RNFL thickness map.

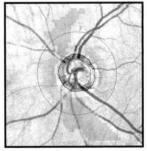

J. RNFL deviation map on en face image with ONH disc and cup margins.

Case 12-18. Advanced Structural Damage Both Superiorly and Inferiorly Only Reflected in One Visual Field Hemifield

Clinical Summary

This case presents the left eye of a 62-year-old female with normal tension glaucoma treated with bimatoprost and timolol. Best-corrected visual acuity is 20/20, and IOP is 10 mm Hg. The anterior segment examination shows wide-open angles and a mild nuclear sclerotic cataract. The dilated fundus exam reveals an ONH with a cup-to-disc ratio of 0.8 and large temporal peripapillary atrophy (A). Humphrey visual field shows a dense superior arcuate scotoma (B). Imaging with HRT shows MRA (C) to be outside normal limits superonasally and borderline inferiorly and globally. D and E, obtained with 3D OCT-1000, show a large cup and a thin inferior macula.

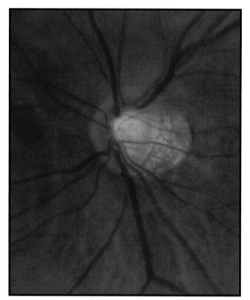

A. Disc photo.

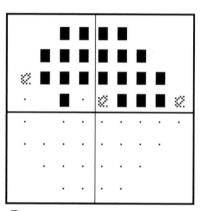

B. Visual field pattern deviation, mean deviation = -11.37 dB.

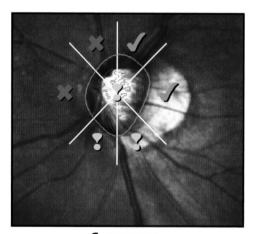

C. HRT MRA.

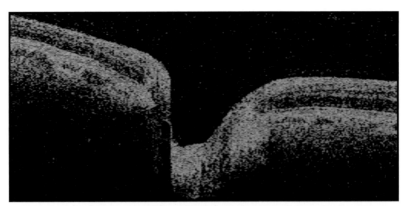

D. 3D OCT-1000 ONH cross-section image.

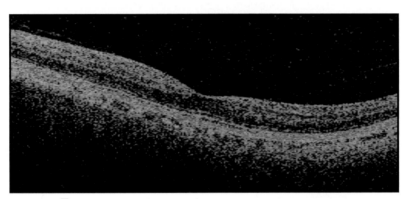

E. 3D OCT-1000 vertical macular cross-section image.

RTVue-100

The RTVue-100 ONH scan shows a severely thin RNFL inferotemporally and to a lesser degree superonasally (F-H). The ganglion cell complex analysis (I, J) displays severe widespread damage, which appears to be more widespread than the damage to the RNFL circumpapillary area.

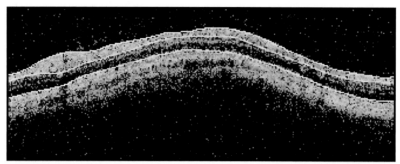

F. Circumpapillary RNFL cross-section image from ONH scan pattern.

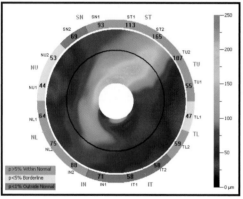

G. ONH analysis.

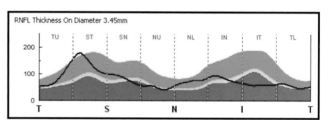

H. Circumpapillary RNFL thickness analysis from ONH scan pattern.

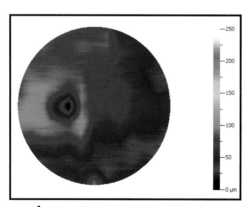

I. Macular ganglion cell complex thickness map.

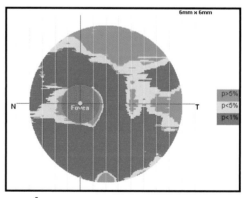

J. Macular ganglion cell complex significance map.

Cirrus HD-OCT

Cirrus HD-OCT shows a severely thin RNFL in the inferior and superior regions with global RNFL thickness outside normal limits at 56 μm (K-M). There is strong agreement with the RNFL thickness analyses between abnormal RTVue sections (G) and Cirrus clock hours (K, part C). M shows a thin rim in the inferotemporal region, which corresponds to the wide inferotemporal RNFL damage. The macular cube scan analysis shows a thin retina inferiorly, shown as the increased blue shading in N and outside normal range in the macular sectoral thickness analysis map (O). However, the ganglion cell analysis (P-R) demonstrates marked damage throughout the macula similar to the findings of the RTVue-100 ganglion cell complex analysis.

Comment

This case demonstrates that RNFL structural damage might show more severe damage than reflected in the visual field. The more significant structural damage inferiorly in this case corresponds well with the dense superior functional deficit.

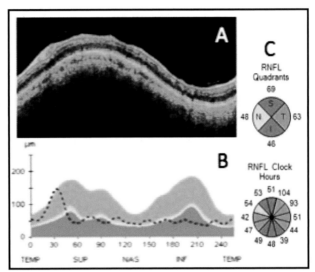

K. Optic Disc Cube scan. (A) Circumpapillary RNFL cross section. (B) RNFL thickness compared to a normative database. (C) RNFL sectoral analysis.

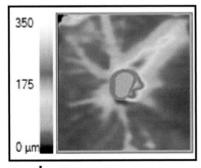

L. RNFL thickness map.

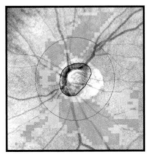

M. RNFL deviation map on en face image with ONH disc and cup margins.

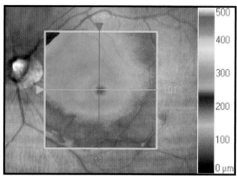

N. Macular cube thickness analysis on LSO image.

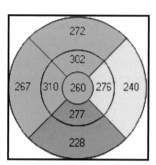

O. Macular sectoral thickness analysis.

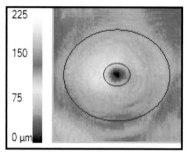

P. Macular cube ganglion cell analysis thickness map.

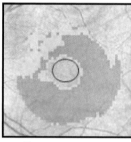

Q. Macular cube ganglion cell analysis deviation map.

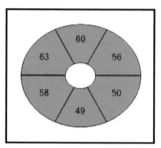

R. Macular cube ganglion cell analysis sectors.

Case 12-19. Imaging Revealed Structural Damage to Be Greater Than Would Be Expected Based Upon the Visual Field

Clinical Summary

This case presents the left eye of a 53-year-old female with primary open-angle glaucoma treated with bimatoprost. Best-corrected visual acuity is 20/20, IOP is 14 mm Hg, and central corneal thickness is 548 μm. The anterior segment examination shows wide-open angles and a mild nuclear sclerotic cata-ract. The dilated fundus exam reveals an ONH with a cup-to-disc ratio of 0.9, with the neuroretinal rim thin-nest superotemporally (A). Visual field pattern devia-tion shows a reproducible minimal defect in the infe-rior region (B), and HRT MRA shows abnormalities in the inferior, temporal, and superotemporal regions (C). GDx enhanced corneal compensation indicates widespread reduced birefringence (D).

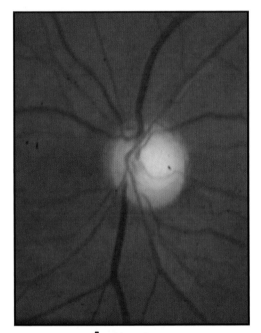

A. Disc photo.

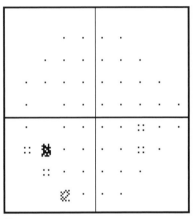

B. Visual field pattern deviation, mean deviation = -0.55 dB.

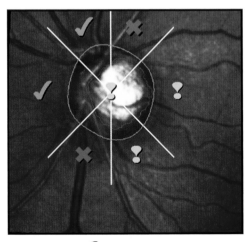

C. HRT MRA.

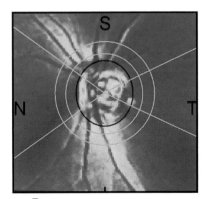

D. GDx enhanced corneal compensation nerve fiber thickness map.

Stratus TD-OCT

TD-OCT imaging reveals a thin RNFL throughout the circumpapillary RNFL (E) and most noticeable in the superotemporal region (F, G). The global mean RNFL thickness is 59 µm and outside normal limits when compared to the normative distribution.

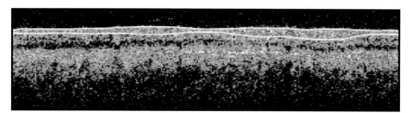

E. RNFL cross-section image.

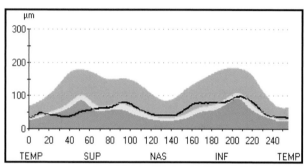

F. RNFL thickness profile.

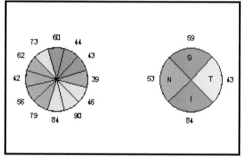

G. RNFL sectoral thickness analysis.

Cirrus HD-OCT

Cirrus HD-OCT agrees with TD-OCT in reporting a mean RNFL thickness outside normal limits (H). The RNFL thickness profile (H, part B) is similar to that of TD-OCT. Like TD-OCT, SD-OCT shows severe abnormalities exist in all regions except nasally (I, J).

Comment

This case demonstrates a situation where both iterations of OCT show advanced structural involvement, yet the functional assessment only shows an early deficit.

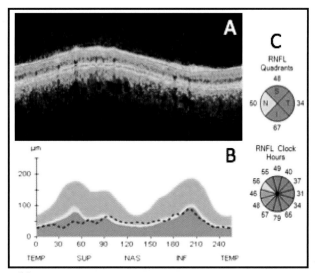

H. Optic Disc Cube scan. (A) Circumpapillary RNFL cross section. (B) RNFL thickness compared to a normative database. (C) RNFL sectoral analysis.

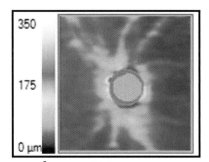

I. RNFL thickness map.

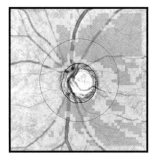

J. RNFL deviation map on en face image with ONH disc and cup margins.

Case 12-20. Glaucomatous Progression Shown With Visual Field, HRT, and OCT

Clinical Summary

This case presents the right eye of an 80-year-old male with pigmentary glaucoma and narrow angles treated with laser peripheral iridotomy, dorzolamide/timolol, brimonidine, and travoprost. Best-corrected visual acuity is 20/25, IOP is 13 mm Hg, and central corneal thickness is 580 µm. The anterior segment examination shows patent peripheral iridotomy and a mild nuclear sclerotic cataract. The dilated fundus exam reveals a cup-to-disc ratio of 0.8. The visual field shows a superior arcuate scotoma (A), along with a Guided Progression Analysis indicating possible progression (B) and a decrease in visual field index over the span of 2 years (C).

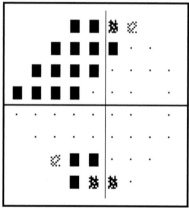

A. Visit 4. Visual field pattern deviation, mean deviation = -8.24 dB.

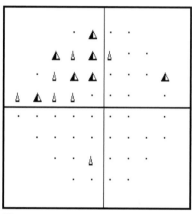

B. Visual field Guided Progression Analysis for Visit 4, possible progression.

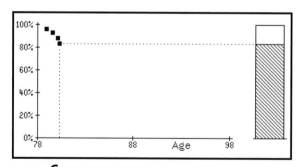

C. Visual field index slope for 2 years.

Cirrus HD-OCT

The mean RNFL thickness for SD-OCT decreased from 85 to 72 µm over the follow-up period covered with Cirrus HD-OCT imaging. The RNFL thickness profile demonstrates a deepening into the outside normal limit (red) zone in the inferotemporal and superotemporal sections when comparing Visit 1 with Visit 4 (D and G, parts B). This is also shown in the clock hour analysis where these sectors switched from borderline to outside normal limits. Thinning of the RNFL can be also observed in the RNFL thickness map (E, H) but is more evident when comparing the RNFL deviation maps (F, I) with substantial expansion of thin (red) regions.

The Guided Progression Analysis highlights the inferior region as the site of structural progression. The location of likely progression is marked in the change map (J, upper panel) and the inferior thickness plot (J, left lower panel). The rate of inferior RNFL thickness change was found to be -15.7 µm/ year.

Comment

This case demonstrates perfectly coinciding longitudinal functional and structural changes.

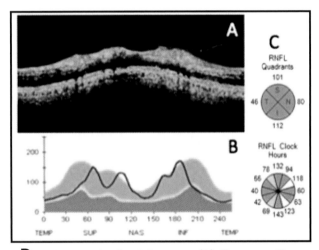

D. Visit 1. Optic Disc Cube scan. (A) Circumpapillary RNFL cross section. (B) RNFL thickness compared to a normative database. (C) RNFL sectoral analysis.

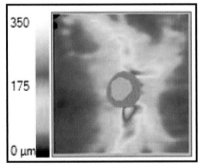

E. Visit 1. RNFL thickness map.

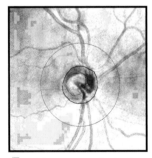

F. Visit 1. RNFL deviation map on en face image with ONH disc and cup margins.

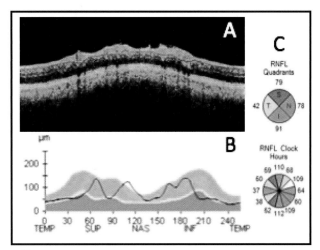

G. Visit 4. Optic Disc Cube scan. (A) Circumpapillary RNFL cross section. (B) RNFL thickness compared to a normative database. (C) RNFL sectoral analysis.

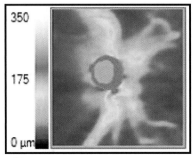

H. Visit 4. RNFL thickness map.

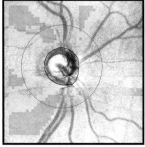

I. Visit 4. RNFL deviation map on en face image with ONH disc and cup margins.

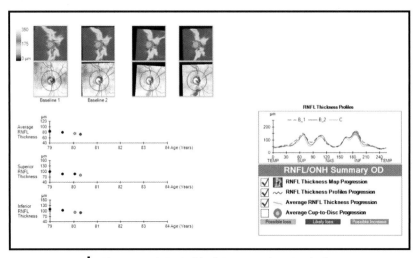

J. Cirrus HD-OCT Guided Progression Analysis.

Case 12-21. OCT Structural Imaging Confirms Stable Glaucomatous Damage

Clinical Summary

This case presents the left eye of a 69-year-old female with primary open-angle glaucoma treated with selective laser trabeculoplasty, brimonidine/timolol, and bimatoprost. Best-corrected visual acuity is 20/30, and IOP is 12 mm Hg. The anterior segment examination shows open angles and a trace nuclear sclerotic cataract. The dilated fundus exam reveals a tilted disc with cup-to-disc ratio of 0.9 and considerable peripapillary atrophy (A). Baseline visual field shows a superior nasal scotoma (B) and visual field index analysis over the period of follow-up indicates a downward trend that does not reach the statistically significant level (C). Guided Progression Analysis indicates possible progression; however, no defect characteristic of glaucoma is shown to be progressing (D).

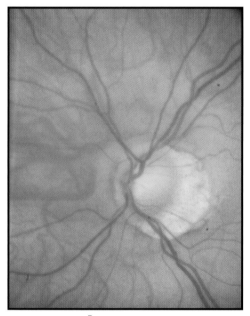

A. Disc photo.

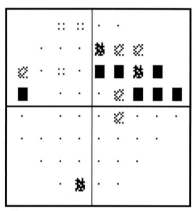

B. Visual field pattern deviation, mean deviation = -2.74 dB.

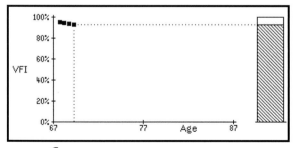

C. Visual field index slope for Visit 4 follow-up period.

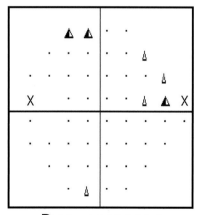

D. Visual field Guided Progression Analysis for Visit 4, possible progression.

Stratus TD-OCT

Imaging from Stratus TD-OCT shows damage both superiorly and inferiorly (E-G) with no clear evidence of progression during the follow-up period (H).

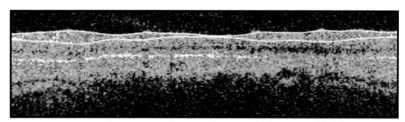

E. Visit 4. RNFL cross-section image.

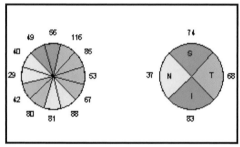

F. Visit 4. RNFL sectoral thickness analysis.

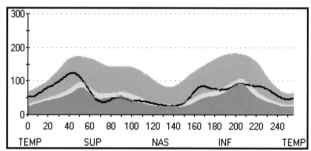

G. Visit 4. RNFL thickness profile.

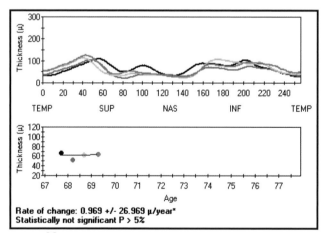

H. TD-OCT Guided Progression Analysis for Visits 1 through 4.

Cirrus HD-OCT

Imaging of the RNFL with Cirrus HD-OCT, demonstrates agreement with Stratus with both superior and inferior damage (I-K) and no progression detected during the follow-up period (L).

Comment

This case demonstrates SD-OCT's ability to determine the glaucomatous damage is stable when visual field presents with unclear results.

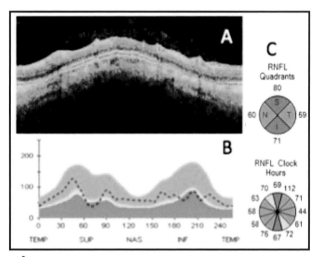

I. Visit 4. Optic Disc Cube scan. (A) Circumpapillary RNFL cross section. (B) RNFL thickness compared to a normative database. (C) RNFL sectoral analysis.

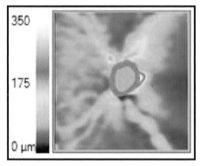

J. Visit 4. RNFL thickness map.

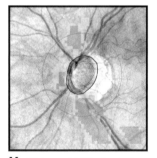

K. Visit 4. RNFL deviation map on en face image with ONH disc and cup margins.

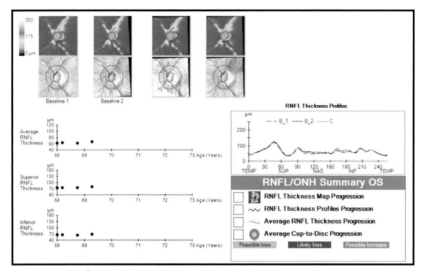

L. Cirrus HD-OCT Guided Progression Analysis.

Case 12-22. OCT Confirms Stable Damage While Visual Field Damage Too Severe to Report Change

Clinical Summary

This case presents the left eye of a 62-year-old male with pigmentary glaucoma treated with dorzolamide/timolol and travoprost. Best-corrected visual acuity is 20/20, IOP is 13 mm Hg, and central corneal thickness is 564 µm. The anterior segment examination shows a centered posterior chamber intraocular lens and open angles with pigmentary deposition. The dilated fundus exam reveals a cup-to-disc ratio of 0.9 (A, B). Visual field shows a superior arcuate scotoma where damage was too severe to report further change on the Guided Progression Analysis and a fluctuating visual field index over the follow-up period (C-E).

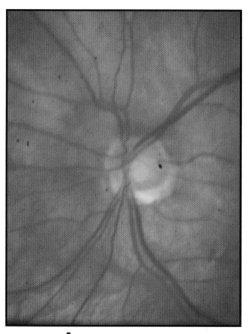 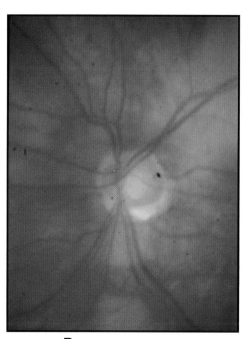

A. Visit 2. Disc photo. **B.** Visit 4. Disc photo.

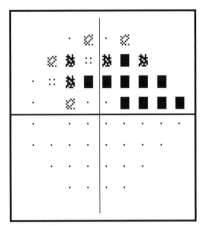

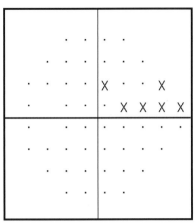

C. Visit 4. Visual field pattern deviation, mean deviation = -7.73 dB.

D. Visual field Guided Progression Analysis for Visit 4.

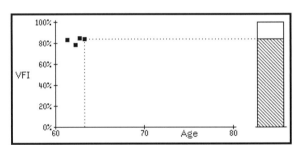

E. Visual field index slope for Visit 4 follow-up period.

Stratus TD-OCT

Imaging from Stratus TD-OCT shows marked damage both superiorly and inferiorly (F, G) and no progression over the follow-up period (H).

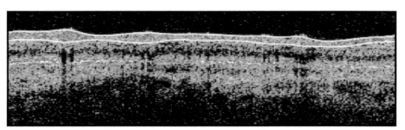

F. Visit 4. RNFL cross-section image.

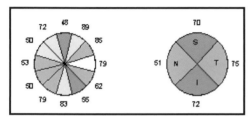

G. Visit 4. RNFL sectoral thickness analysis.

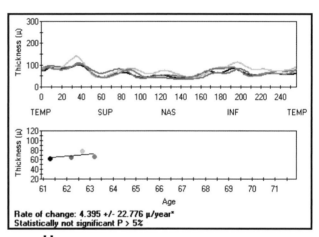

H. TD-OCT Guided Progression Analysis for Visits 1 through 4.

Cirrus HD-OCT

Imaging of the RNFL with Cirrus HD-OCT demonstrates agreement with TD-OCT with both superior and inferior damage (I, part C). The wider RNFL thinning in the inferior sector (J, K) corresponds with the marked superior arcuate scotoma in the visual field, while the narrower superior RNFL wedge defect is not accompanied with a corresponding visual field deficit. Cirrus Guided Progression Analysis (L), for the identical visits shown with both visual field and TD-OCT, shows stable RNFL measurements. Note that the variability in RNFL measurements obtained with SD-OCT in the consecutive visits is substantially lower than with TD-OCT. It should be noted that even in the most advanced RNFL damage, OCT reports a value in the range of 30 to 40 µm (floor effect) reflecting the residual supporting tissue. This should be considered when assessing change over time in the area of advanced damage.

Comment

This case demonstrates an inconclusive fluctuating visual field index and an out-of-range visual field Guided Progression Analysis that does not allow assessment of further progression, with corresponding RNFL defects that are nonprogressing by TD-OCT and Cirrus HD-OCT.

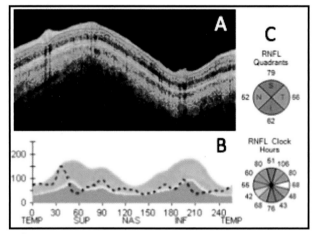

I. Visit 4. Optic Disc Cube scan. (A) Circumpapillary RNFL cross section. (B) RNFL thickness compared to a normative database. (C) RNFL sectoral analysis.

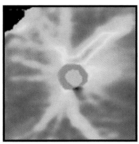

J. Visit 4.
RNFL thickness map.

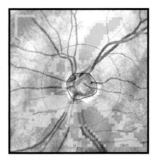

K. Visit 4. RNFL deviation
map on en face image
with ONH disc and cup
margins.

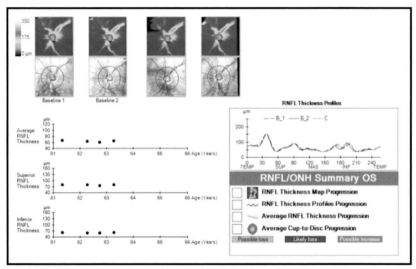

L. Cirrus HD-OCT Guided Progression Analysis.

Case 12-23. Focal Structural Progression With Fluctuating Visual Field Defect

Clinical Summary

This case presents the left eye of a 75-year-old male with primary open-angle glaucoma treated with brimonidine/timolol and latanoprost. Best-corrected visual acuity is 20/25, and IOP ranged from 12 to 25 mm Hg. The anterior segment examination shows open angles, a moderate nuclear sclerotic cataract, and pigment on the anterior capsule. The dilated fundus exam reveals an ONH with a cup-to-disc ratio of 0.8 throughout the follow-up period (A-C). During the interim of follow-up, a splinter hemorrhage was noted at 6:00 on the disc margin (A, arrow), which was resolved at follow-up visits. No visual field progression is noted by comparing printouts from each time point (D-F), visual field index (G), or Guided Progression Analysis (H) during this period. HRT topographic change analysis (TCA) shows an increase in the size of the thinning in the temporal inferior region of the optic disc (I-M).

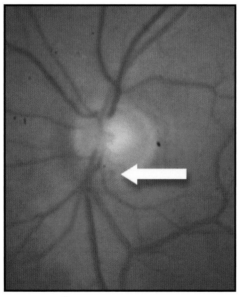

A. Visit 2. Disc photo.

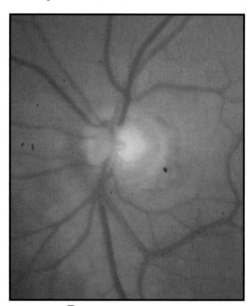

B. Visit 3. Disc photo.

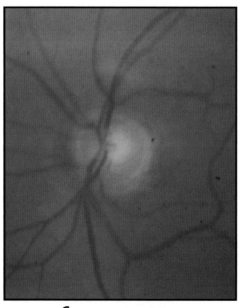

C. Visit 5. Disc photo.

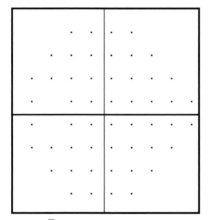

D. Visit 1. Visual field
pattern deviation,
mean deviation = 0.33 dB.

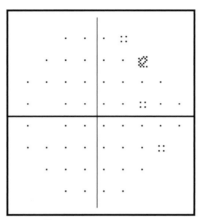

E. Visit 2. Visual field
pattern deviation,
mean deviation = 1.08 dB.

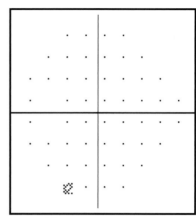

F. Visit 5. Visual field
pattern deviation,
mean deviation = -2.34 dB.

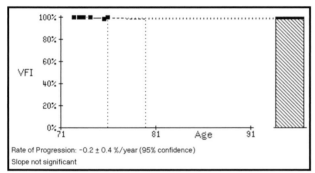

G. Visual field index slope for Visit 5
follow-up period.

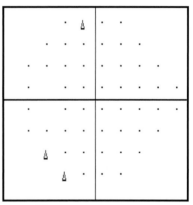

H. Visual field Guided
Progression Analysis for Visit 5.

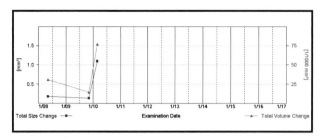

I. HRT topographic change analysis.

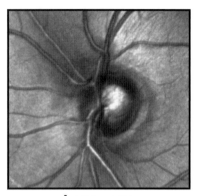

J. Visit 1. TCA.

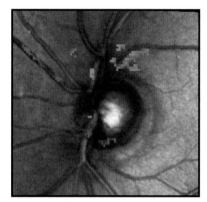

K. Visit 3. TCA.

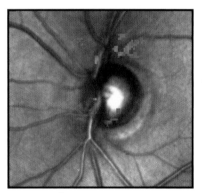

L. Visit 4. TCA.

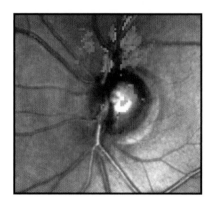

M. Visit 5. TCA.

Stratus TD-OCT

Stratus TD-OCT at the last visit shows a localized focal thinning in the RNFL cross section (N) that progressed during the period of follow-up as indicated by the clock hour analysis (O) and the Guided Progression Analysis (P).

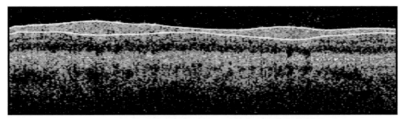

N. RNFL cross-section image from Visit 4.

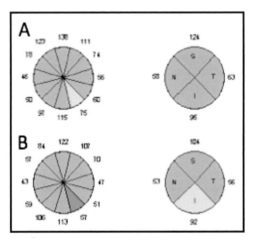

O. RNFL sectoral thickness analysis.
(A) Visit 2. (B) Visit 4.

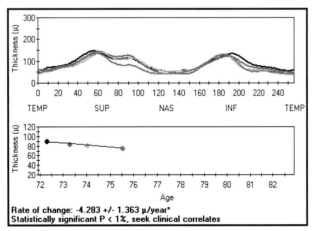

P. TD-OCT Guided Progression Analysis for
Visits 1 through 4.

Cirrus HD-OCT

Cirrus Optic Disc Cube scan shows a thin RNFL in the inferotemporal region on the cross section (Q, part A, arrow), thickness profile, and in the clock hour analysis at 5:00 (Q). The thickness map (R) and deviation map (S) also show an RNFL wedge defect in the temporal inferior region.

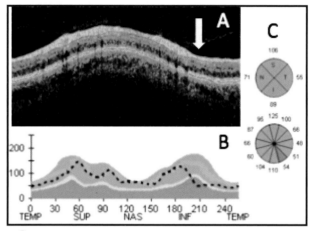

Q. Visit 5. Optic Disc Cube scan. (A) Circumpapillary RNFL cross section with arrow pointing to region of thinning. (B) RNFL thickness compared to a normative database. (C) RNFL sectoral analysis.

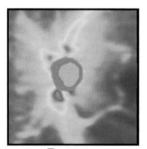

R. Visit 5. RNFL thickness map.

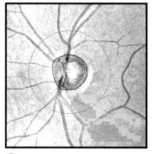

S. Visit 5. RNFL deviation map on en face image with ONH disc and cup margins.

RTVue-100

RTVue-100 RNFL progression analysis is shown in T where gradual thinning is shown in the infero-temporal region. The RNFL thickness in this sector decreases from 103 to 74 μm over the follow-up period. RNFL thinning is also apparent on the RNFL thickness profile (U), where the defect in the infero-temporal region dives deeper into the red region. RTVue-100 macular retinal thickness progression shows no thinning to the macula (V).

RTVue-100 ganglion cell complex progression analysis (W) shows progressive changes to the inner retinal complex occur over the follow-up period. The thinning occurs in the inferior macula, though the average ganglion cell thickness also reports thinning (lower left plot). The global quantification (average ganglion cell complex, lower right table), however, is misleading by showing a gradual thinning but within the normal limit. Because the actual thinning is localized, the thinning is less pronounced when averaged across the entire macula. This emphasizes the importance of assessment using the map rather than relying on the global quantification analysis.

Comment

This case demonstrates a focal structural defect at the site of a disc hemorrhage, with progressive damage, noted both in the RNFL and ganglion cell complex analysis.

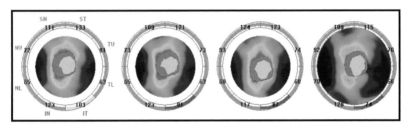

T. RNFL progression analysis for ONH scan during follow-up period.

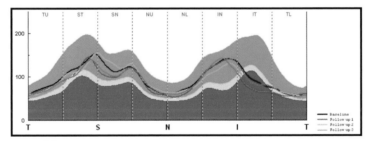

U. RNFL thickness distribution progression analysis during follow-up period.

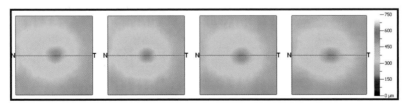

V. Macular retinal thickness progression analysis during follow-up period.

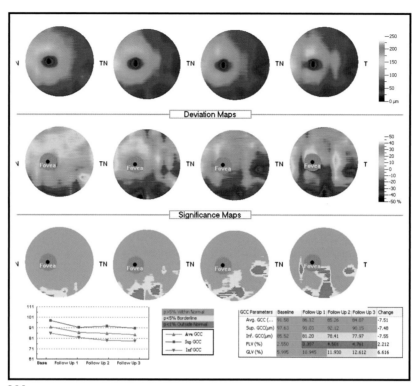

W. Ganglion cell complex thickness progression during follow-up period.

Case 12-24. Rapid Progression Structurally and Functionally

Clinical Summary

This case presents the left eye of a 74-year-old female with secondary open-angle glaucoma following 2 Descemet's stripping automated endothelial keratoplasties (DSAEK) and steroid response, treated with selective laser trabeculoplasty, bimatoprost, brimonidine, timolol, and rimexolone. Best-corrected visual acuity is 20/80, IOP is 18 mm Hg, and central corneal thickness is 625 μm. The anterior segment examination shows DSAEK attached, open angles, and a well-centered posterior chamber intraocular lens. The dilated fundus exam reveals a cup-to-disc ratio of 0.8 with a neuroretinal rim thinnest inferiorly (A). Visual field shows an initial small superior nasal step that rapidly progresses to extensive defect in both hemifields (B-D). The visual field grayscale is shown for this case because Visit 3 involved a severely depressed field, for which the pattern deviation plot could not be generated.

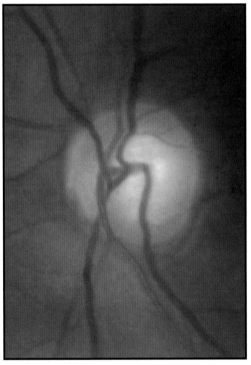

A. Visit 2. Disc photo.

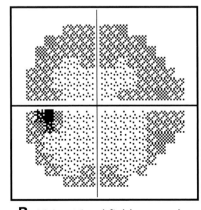

B. Visit 1. Visual field grayscale.

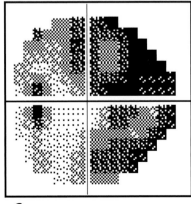

C. Visit 2. Visual field grayscale.

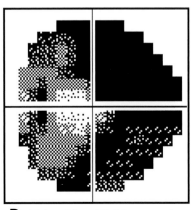

D. Visit 3. Visual field grayscale.

HRT TCA shows progression over the follow-up
period both superiorly and inferiorly (E, F).

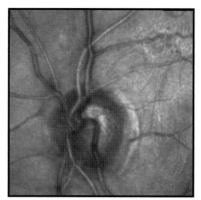

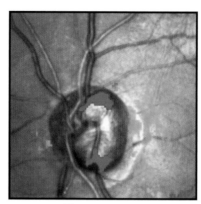

E. Visit 1. TCA.   **F.** Visit 3. TCA.

Stratus TD-OCT

Stratus TD-OCT shows an abnormally thin RNFL thickness globally in the cross-section image (G) and an RNFL thickness outside the normal range for all quadrants other than nasal (H). TD-OCT Guided Progression Analysis shows substantial thinning across the RNFL thickness profiles and a steep downward trend for the average RNFL thickness measurements during the follow-up period (I). Due to the poor signal in the inferior region, at Visit 3, the segmentation analysis failed to detect the boundaries of the RNFL and reported an erroneous thickness.

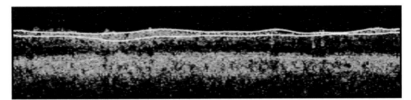

G. RNFL cross-section image from Visit 3.

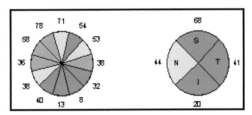

H. Visit 3. RNFL sectoral analysis.

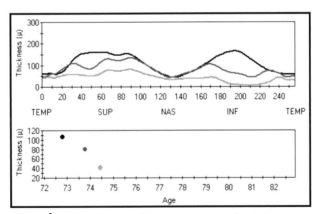

I. TD-OCT Guided Progression Analysis for Visits 1 through 3.

Cirrus HD-OCT

The RNFL thickness and deviation map for Visit 3's Optic Disc Cube scan shows marked thinning superotemporally and inferotemporally (J, K). This was also verified in the cross-section image and RNFL thickness profile (L, parts A and B). The quadrant analysis shows RNFL thickness outside the normal range superiorly and inferiorly. This differs from the TD-OCT analysis due to the higher signal quality obtained by the SD-OCT scan, as shown by the cross-section images (G, L, part A).

Cirrus Guided Progression Analysis shows progressive thinning on the RNFL thickness and deviation maps superiorly and inferiorly (M, top left). The average RNFL thickness plots show possible progression for the overall, superior, and inferior thickness (M, bottom left). The RNFL thickness profile also shows possible progression over the follow-up period. Over this period of follow-up, mean RNFL thickness decreased by 42 μm. Guided Progression Analysis defines "possible" progression when a significant rate of change appears once and "likely" when a significant slope is confirmed in an additional test. Because this patient only had 3 tests, the steep change is labeled as "possible" progression.

Comment

This case demonstrates a situation where structure and function coincide in showing a very rapid rate of progression.

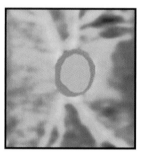

J. Visit 3.
RNFL thickness map.

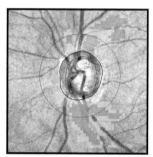

K. Visit 3. RNFL deviation map on en face image with ONH disc and cup margins.

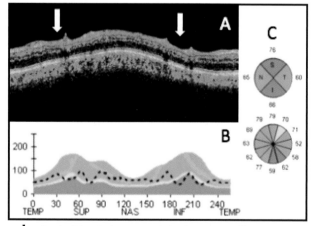

L. Optic Disc Cube scan. (A) Circumpapillary RNFL cross section. (B) RNFL thickness compared to a normative database. (C) RNFL sectoral analysis.

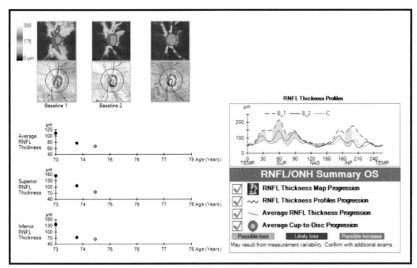

M. Cirrus HD-OCT Guided Progression Analysis.

Case 12-25. Structure and Function Coincide in Glaucoma Progression Diagnosis

Clinical Summary

This case presents the right eye of a 71-year-old female with primary open-angle glaucoma treated with selective laser trabeculoplasty and brimonidine/timolol. Best-corrected visual acuity is 20/20, IOP is 13 mm Hg, and central corneal thickness is 578 µm. The anterior segment examination shows open angles and a moderate nuclear sclerotic cataract. The dilated fundus exam reveals an ONH with a cup-to-disc ratio of 0.9 with a neuroretinal rim thinnest inferiorly (A-C). During the follow-up period, there was a clear worsening of the visual field scotoma (D-G) that was identified as significant progression by the visual field index analysis (H) and likely progression by the Guided Progression Analysis (I). HRT TCA (J-M) shows consistent thinning that was most notable in the inferotemporal and superior regions.

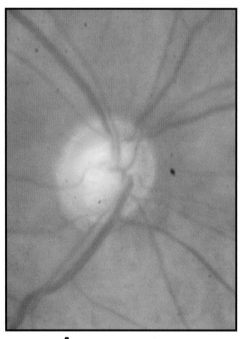

A. Year 2. Disc photo.

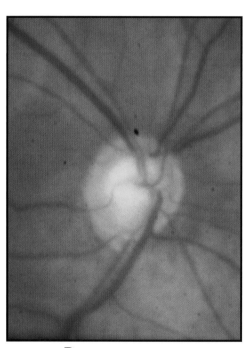

B. Year 3. Disc photo.

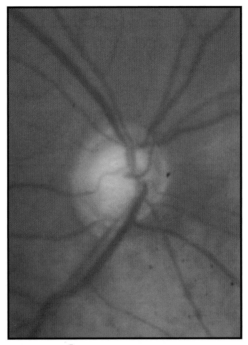

C. Year 4. Disc photo.

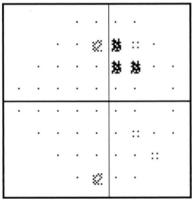

D. Year 1. Visual field
pattern deviation,
mean deviation = -0.41 dB.

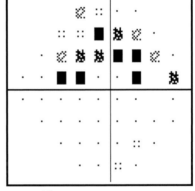

E. Year 2. Visual field
pattern deviation,
mean deviation = -1.40 dB.

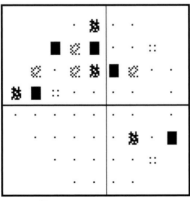

F. Year 3. Visual field
pattern deviation,
mean deviation = -3.23 dB.

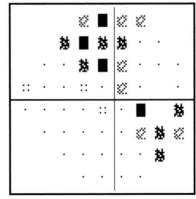

G. Year 4. Visual field
pattern deviation,
mean deviation = -3.29 dB.

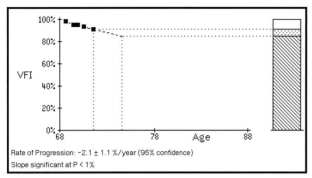

H. Visual field index slope for 4-year follow-up period.

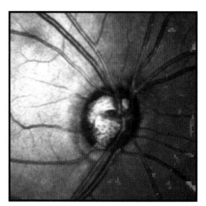

I. Visual field Guided Progression Analysis for Year 4.

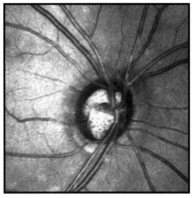

J. Year 1. TCA.

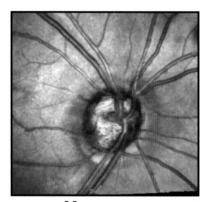

K. Year 2. TCA.

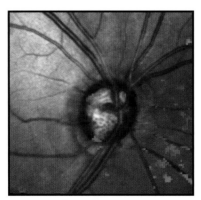

L. Year 3. TCA.

M. Year 4. TCA.

Stratus TD-OCT

The TD-OCT cross-section image shows a thin superior and inferior region (N) with total obliteration of the inferior RNFL hump. RNFL sectoral analysis shows some degree of abnormal thickness in all regions except for the temporal quadrant (O). TD-OCT Guided Progression Analysis indicates significant progression over the follow-up period (P). Average RNFL thickness decreased from 63 to 47 μm during the follow-up span.

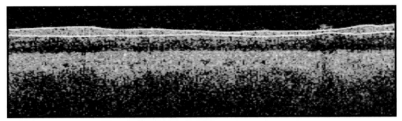

N. Year 4. RNFL cross-section image.

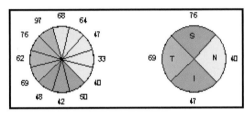

O. Year 4. RNFL sectoral analysis.

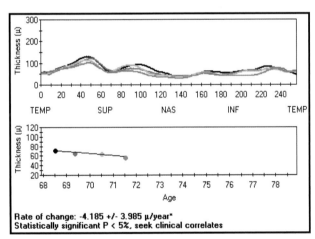

P. TD-OCT Guided Progression Analysis for Visits 1 through 4.

Cirrus HD-OCT

Cirrus HD-OCT shows a severely thin RNFL in the inferior region with a focal abnormality in the superior region (Q, part A, arrows). The RNFL thickness profile and sectoral analysis show the inferior region thickness reaches the outside normal range (Q, parts B and C), though the overall damage is somewhat less pronounced than reported by TD-OCT. The inferior abnormality is also apparent on the RNFL thickness and deviation maps (R, S).

The macular cube thickness analysis shows the inferior retinal thickness is also outside the normal range when compared to a normative distribution of age-matched patients (T, U) as a direct continuation of the inferior peripapillary involvement. Ganglion cell analysis (V-X) shows similar inferior damage with early superior damage corresponding to the early peripapillary RNFL thinning.

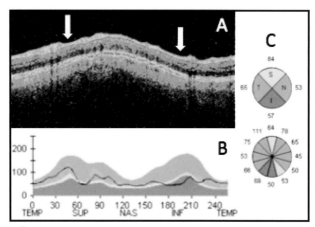

Q. Year 4. Optic Disc Cube scan. (A) Circumpapillary RNFL cross section with arrow pointing to region of thinning. (B) RNFL thickness compared to a normative database. (C) RNFL sectoral analysis.

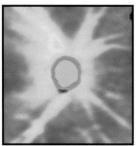

R. Year 4. RNFL thickness map.

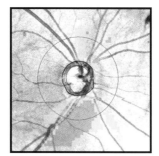

S. Year 4. RNFL deviation map on en face image with ONH disc and cup margins.

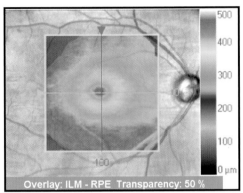

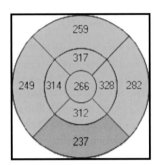

T. Year 4. Macular cube thickness analysis on LSO image.

U. Year 4. Macular sectoral thickness analysis.

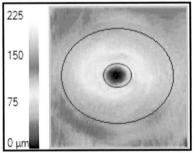

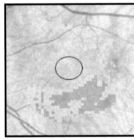

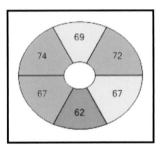

V. Year 4. Macular cube ganglion cell analysis thickness map.

W. Year 4. Macular cube ganglion cell analysis deviation map.

X. Year 4. Macular cube ganglion cell analysis sectors.

RTVue-100

RTVue-100 ONH scan progression analysis shows thinning to the peripapillary RNFL as shown by a reduction in the yellow and red color immediately surrounding the superior portion of the disk (Y). The circumpapillary RNFL thickness obtained on a 3.4-mm diameter circle shows a stable thickness inferiorly and progressive thinning superiorly (Z). At Year 4, the superior region RNFL thickness is in the borderline range, whereas the inferior thickness is outside the normal range. This analysis suggests that while the inferior RNFL thickness is outside the normal range, it is nonprogressing. The superior region, however, appears to progress over this period of follow-up (Z).

RTVue-100 ganglion cell complex progression analysis (AA) indicates both superior and inferior progression over the period of follow-up. The average ganglion cell complex thickness is in the normal range for the first 2 visits and progressed to borderline by Visit 3 (Follow-up 2). The inferior ganglion cell complex thickness at baseline was also within the normal range, but then progressed to the outside normal range by Visit 3. The lower left plot shows the downward trend for the average, superior, and inferior ganglion cell complex thickness (AA).

The Table displays the OCT mean RNFL thickness measurements that were outside normal limits for the follow-up period. TD-OCT measurements are much smaller than SD-OCT measurements and experienced a greater loss of thickness. RTVue-100 decreased from 78 to 74 μm over the follow-up period.

Comment

This case demonstrates glaucoma progression where function and structural analysis from both peripapillary and macular regions correspond.

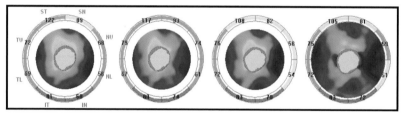

Y. RNFL progression analysis for ONH scan during follow-up period.

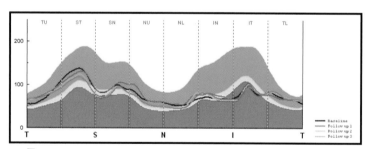

Z. RNFL thickness distribution progression analysis during follow-up period.

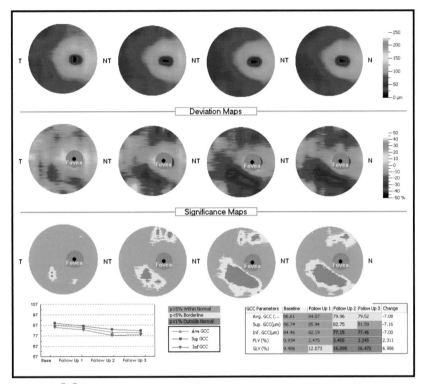

AA. Ganglion cell complex thickness progression during follow-up period.

Mean RNFL Thicknesses				
Device	RNFL Thickness (μm)			
	Year 1	Year 2	Year 3	Year 4
Stratus TD-OCT	63	57	56	47
Cirrus HD-OCT	NA	NA	NA	65
RTVue-100	78	81	76	74

Case 12-26. Progression Shown by Structural Imaging While Visual Field Damage Remained Stable

Clinical Summary

This case presents the left eye of a 67-year-old female with primary open-angle glaucoma treated with travoprost and brimonidine. Best-corrected visual acuity is 20/20, IOP is 14 mm Hg, and central corneal thickness is 533 μm. Anterior segment examination shows open angles and a moderate nuclear sclerotic cataract. The dilated fundus exam reveals an ONH with a cup-to-disc ratio of 0.8 (A-C). The visual field shows a dense inferior nasal step and a fluctuating superior nasal step (D-G). Neither of these defects shows progression by Guided Progression Analysis (H), nor did the visual field index show significant progression (I). HRT TCA (J-M) did not report any significant change within the ONH.

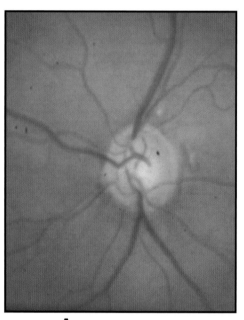

A. Year 2. Disc photo.

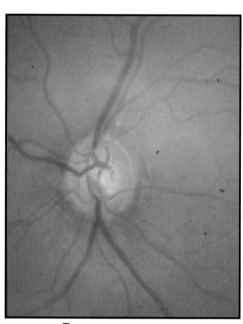

B. Year 3. Disc photo.

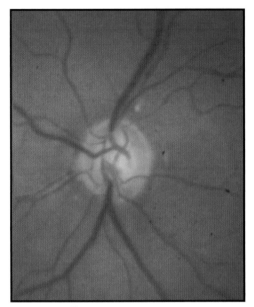

C. Year 4. Disc photo.

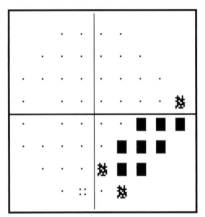

D. Year 1. Visual field
pattern deviation,
mean deviation = -4.64 dB.

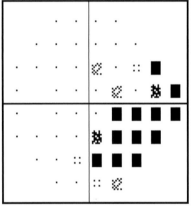

E. Year 2. Visual field
pattern deviation,
mean deviation = -5.89 dB.

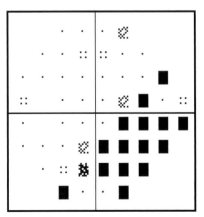

F. Year 3. Visual field
pattern deviation,
mean deviation = -7.62 dB.

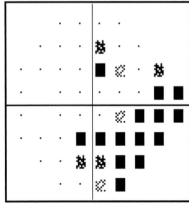

G. Year 4. Visual field
pattern deviation,
mean deviation = -6.04 dB.

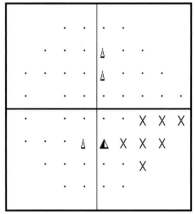

H. Visual field Guided
Progression Analysis for Year 4.

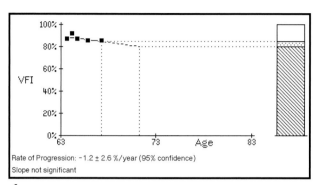

Rate of Progression: −1.2 ± 2.6 %/year (95% confidence)
Slope not significant

I. Visual field index slope for 4-year follow-up period.

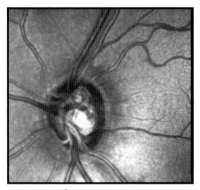

J. Year 1. TCA.

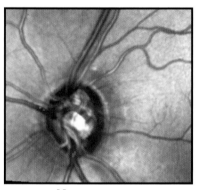

K. Year 2. TCA.

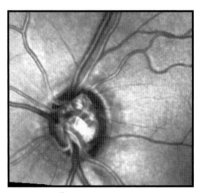

L. Year 3. TCA.

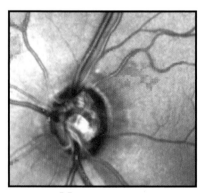

M. Year 4. TCA.

Stratus TD-OCT

Stratus TD-OCT RNFL cross section at the end of the follow-up period shows thinning in both poles of the optic disc (N, O). Guided Progression Analysis of the RNFL scan (P) shows a downward trend in average RNFL thickness but does not reach statistical significance.

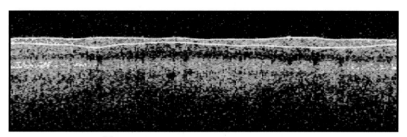

N. Year 4. RNFL cross-section image.

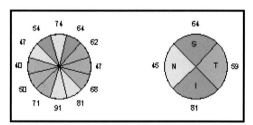

O. Year 4. RNFL sectoral analysis.

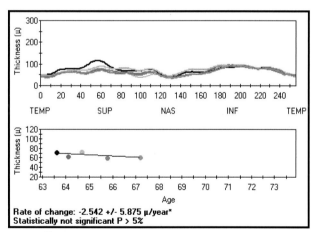

P. TD-OCT Guided Progression Analysis for Years 1 through 4.

3D OCT-1000

Topcon 3D OCT-1000 imaging of the circumpapillary RNFL shows a focally thin RNFL in the superotemporal area (Q, arrow). The ONH image shows large cupping (R) and the horizontal macular cross section appears normal (S).

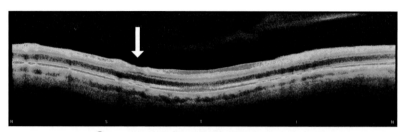

Q. Year 4. Circumpapillary RNFL image.

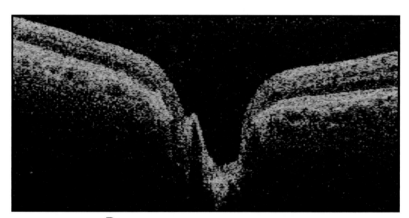

R. Year 4. ONH cross-section image.

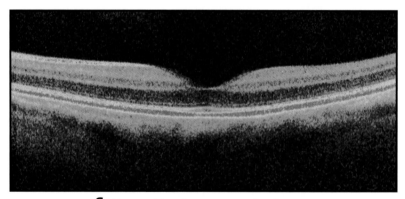

S. Year 4. Macular cross-section image.

Cirrus HD-OCT

Cirrus HD-OCT imaging of the circumpapillary RNFL shows RNFL thickness outside normal limits superiorly and inferiorly (T). RNFL wedge defects are evident in the superotemporal and inferior regions (U, V). The macular scans (W, X) show no damage and a normal thickness throughout all of the sectors. However, the ganglion cell analysis shows inferotemporal abnormality and, to a lesser extent, a superotemporal abnormality (Y-AA) corresponding to both RNFL wedge defects.

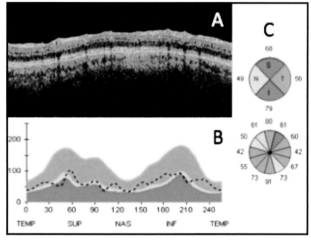

T. Year 4. Optic Disc Cube scan. (A) Circumpapillary RNFL cross section. (B) RNFL thickness compared to a normative database. (C) RNFL sectoral analysis.

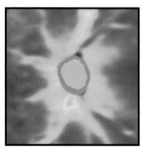

U. Year 4. RNFL thickness map.

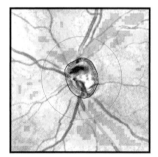

V. Year 4. RNFL deviation map on en face image with ONH disc and cup margins.

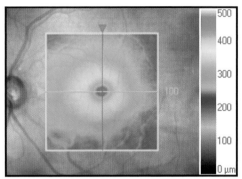

W. Year 4. Macular cube thickness
analysis on LSO image.

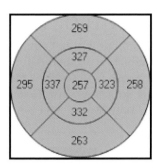

X. Year 4. Macular cube
sectoral thickness
analysis.

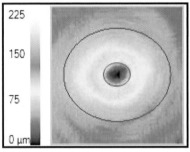

Y. Year 4. Macular cube ganglion
cell analysis thickness map.

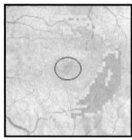

Z. Year 4. Macular
cube ganglion cell
analysis deviation map.

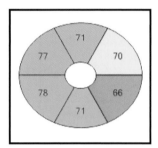

AA. Year 4.
Macular cube ganglion
cell analysis sectors.

RTVue-100

RTVue-100 RNFL scan progression (BB, CC) shows inconsistencies in the severity of the damage. The ONH scan progression analysis (DD, EE) is equally inconsistent with the most severe damage consistently appearing in the superior and inferior regions.

RTVue-100 ganglion cell complex progression analysis (FF) indicates superior progression that corresponds to the visual field defect. The average ganglion cell complex thickness remains in the normal region across all visits; however, the focal loss volume remains outside normal limits. This parameter has been shown to be an early indicator of glaucomatous damage.

The Table shows that all mean RNFL thickness measurements from the imaging devices were either borderline or outside normal limits compared to a normative database. TD-OCT initially reports the measurement as borderline; however, it progressed over the period of follow-up. RTVue-100 found the RNFL thickness to be abnormal throughout the entirety of the follow-up.

Comment

This case demonstrates a patient with substantial functional loss, where no functional progression can be detected, while the structural assessment shows gradual loss. Fluctuating damage in the superior visual field was associated with stable structural loss.

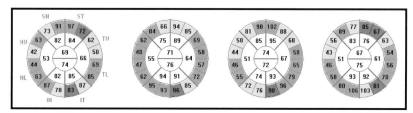

BB. RNFL progression analysis during follow-up period.

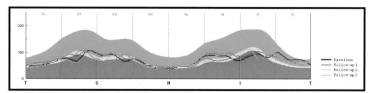

CC. RNFL thickness progression analysis during follow-up period.

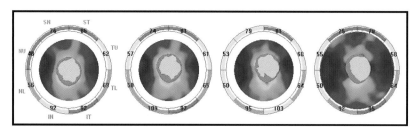

DD. RNFL progression analysis for ONH scan during follow-up period.

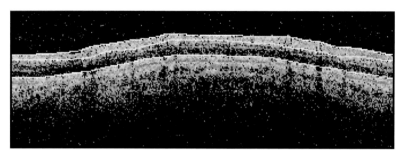

EE. RNFL cross-section image from ONH scan.

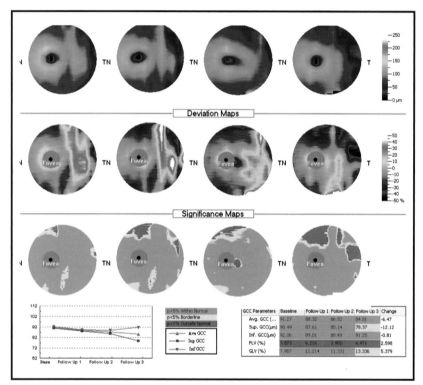

FF. Ganglion cell complex thickness progression during follow-up period.

Mean RNFL Thicknesses

Device	RNFL Thickness (µm)			
	Year 1	Year 2	Year 3	Year 4
Stratus TD-OCT	75	73	61	62
Cirrus HD-OCT	NA	NA	NA	63
RTVue-100	71	73	72	70

Chapter 13

Optical Coherence Tomography for Neuro-Ophthalmology

Carlos Mendoza-Santiesteban, MD; Matthew D. Lazzara, MD; and
Thomas R. Hedges III, MD

- Proving Maculopathy That May Mimic Optic Neuropathy
- Optic Neuropathy in the Presence of Retinopathy
- Functional Loss of Vision
- Optic Nerve Swelling
- Vitreopapillary Traction
- Compressive Optic Neuropathy
- Optic Neuritis
- Toxic, Hereditary, and Nutritional Optic Neuropathy
- Conclusion

In neuro-ophthalmic practice, optical coherence tomography (OCT) is very useful in identifying maculopathy that mimics optic neuropathy. Most of these conditions are illustrated in the section dealing with retinal disorders. OCT provides structural evidence of normality when there may be functional or fictitious loss of vision and may be relied upon when there has been long-standing functional loss of vision. OCT has been useful in our experience in dealing with a variety of conditions associated with optic disc swelling, including papilledema, pseudopapilledema, and anterior ischemic optic neuropathy (AION). OCT can be useful in many cases of optic atrophy, including optic neuritis and optic nerve compression.

Proving Maculopathy That May Mimic Optic Neuropathy

Previously, the diagnosis of occult maculopathy mimicking optic neuropathy depended on subtle and often indirect findings. Frequently, this also required ruling out optic neuropathy, sometimes at significant expense. It was not unusual for neuro-ophthalmologists to become engaged in a dialogue with a retina specialist who insisted that a patient with unexplained visual loss had optic neuropathy, when the neuro-ophthalmologist was sure that the problem was indeed macular but had no clear way of proving this. Central serous retinopathy was a common maculopathy that could mimic optic neuropathy yet could easily be identified with fundus fluorescein angiography. However, now, with more refined OCT techniques,[1,2] other retinal conditions mimicking optic neuropathy are more easily proven.

OCT reliably and consistently demonstrates macular holes and epiretinal membranes.[3] Another group of conditions, now more easily identified using OCT, the occult outer retinopathies, includes multiple evanescent white-dot syndrome, acute zonal occult outer retinopathy, and acute idiopathic blind spot enlargement syndrome. These conditions are especially easy to identify with high-resolution OCT whereby the inner/outer segment (IS/OS) junction is usually affected in the retinal areas corresponding

Schuman JS, Puliafito CA, Fujimoto JG, Duker JS, eds.
Optical Coherence Tomography of Ocular Diseases,
Third Edition (pp 469-548).
© 2013 SLACK Incorporated.

to the clinical findings.[4-8] These diagnoses are also made with more assurance using multifocal electroretinography. However, OCT is much easier and quicker for the patient and usually suffices.

OCT helps in localizing the cause of microscotomas to the outer retina. However, we still do not have a good understanding of the pathophysiology of this condition. Hopefully, with more detailed OCT, the mechanism by which these microscotomas occur will become apparent. The structural findings in some patients with microscotoma that we see with OCT do resemble those that are seen with phototoxic maculopathy,[9-11] which can result in a very discrete area of IS/OS loss in such individuals. It also resembles what is occasionally seen in patients with epiretinal membrane.[12]

Bilateral central visual loss in young people with apparently normal-appearing retinas and optic nerves has been a diagnostic dilemma until recently. Frequently, these children have required a variety of rather expensive investigations. Although multifocal electroretinography can identify juvenile retinal degeneration or Stargardt's disease when it does occur, OCT does show distinctive macular outer retinal changes early on, and OCT may become the standard way of making this diagnosis in the future.[13] Multifocal electroretinography may be difficult in young children, although we have been able to use this approach in some individuals as young as 6 years of age. We have also found that OCT is as sensitive in identifying hydroxychloroquine retinopathy as multifocal electroretinography.[14] OCT allows neuro-ophthalmologists to make a diagnosis of occult maculopathy much more efficiently; this has saved time and has saved patients considerable expense.

Optic Neuropathy in the Presence of Retinopathy

OCT can identify optic neuropathy when there is nerve fiber layer (NFL) loss, and this may be the first clue that there is an insidious optic neuropathy occurring such as with optic nerve sheath meningiomas. In individuals with a mild decrease in visual acuity, mild color vision loss, and subtle visual field constriction, finding NFL thinning provides more objective evidence that there is an optic neuropathy that requires further investigation. We have been impressed with how optic nerve head (ONH) analysis by OCT will identify optic neuropathy in the presence of a known maculopathy. Even though

such individuals may have visual field characteristics that are more typical of optic neuropathy, such as bitemporal hemianopia, frequently a concomitant maculopathy makes the interpretation of subjective psychophysical tests difficult. Finding characteristic NFL changes on OCT does help motivate us at least to obtain magnetic resonance imaging (MRI) scans when a retinal surgeon sends a patient in whom the possibility of an optic neuropathy coexisting with maculopathy arises.

Functional Loss of Vision

OCT can provide further objective evidence of normal structure in patients suspected of having functional visual loss. However, one must remember that retinal nerve fiber layer (RNFL) degeneration does take time to develop, and a normal RNFL thickness does not always rule out a compressive optic neuropathy. However, in patients who have had functional visual loss for many months or years, a normal RNFL thickness, along with a normal macular scan, is strong, objective evidence that there is no structural pathology accounting for visual loss that is likely functional in nature.

Optic Nerve Swelling

We have attempted to use OCT to differentiate mild papilledema from pseudopapilledema. OCT can show ONH drusen, and, when there are significant drusen, one would expect the RNFL to be thin.[15] However, in those individuals with congenitally crowded ONHs and without significant drusen, we have found that OCT shows thickening of the NFL, similar to that which occurs in mild papilledema.[16] Therefore, we now use OCT to observe such individuals with suspected pseudopapilledema over time, just the way we used to use photographs for this purpose. If OCT does not show any change in the NFL thickness over time, then we can assume that such individuals were born with crowded nerves and thicker NFL. The finding of thickened NFL on circumferential OCTs in patients with pseudopapilledema is not surprising, considering that there is axoplasmic flow stasis in these individuals, just as there is in those with true papilledema. Of course, one must remember that patients with pseudopapilledema can develop increased intracranial pressure and these 2 conditions may occur simultaneously. Recently, one report showed evidence that peripapillary subretinal fluid may be seen exclusively in patients with pathologic optic nerve swelling either from increased intracranial pressure or from ischemic optic neuropathy. Perhaps this may be the best way to distinguish mild papilledema from pseudopapilledema in the future.[17]

We also have been using OCT to follow up patients with papilledema. The main problem with this has been in interpreting what appears to be normalization of the RNFL thickness when there is concomitant optic atrophy, which also leads to reduction in the thickness of the NFL over time. However, we have some indication that there may be a pattern of NFL change, which may indicate that there is optic atrophy superimposed upon papilledema. When the thickness of the superior NFL diminishes while the thickness of the inferior NFL remains elevated, the likelihood of visual field loss appears to rise, indicating the onset of atrophic papilledema, rather than improvement in the papilledema.

One observation that OCT has allowed is the visualization of subretinal fluid in patients with papilledema.[18] This may correlate with loss of visual acuity, which is a reversible phenomenon. The degree of subretinal fluid in the foveal region seems to correlate with the degree of visual acuity loss, and, just as in patients with central serous retinopathy, the prognosis for recovery of visual acuity remains good. In our practice, when there is loss of visual acuity and this can be demonstrated to be due to subretinal fluid by OCT, we do not feel that this is definitely an indication for urgent intervention surgically. The source of the fluid is not entirely clear. Because there is frequently a communication between the subfoveal fluid and the peripapillary subretinal fluid that we also described, the possibility that the fluid could be coming from the choroid remains the best possibility. There may be disruption of the connections between Bruch's membrane and the optic nerve that are disturbed because of the swelling of the nerve, allowing for serous fluid to leak under the retina in the peripapillary space and then, in some individuals, track into the subfoveal region.

Subretinal fluid has also been observed in patients with AION.[19] When there is loss of visual acuity in patients with AION associated with subfoveal fluid, this may have significant implications with regard to treatment. Patients with subretinal fluid from AION, like patients with subretinal fluid from papilledema, also have a good prognosis for spontaneous recovery of visual acuity as the subretinal fluid resorbs.

Vitreopapillary Traction

OCT has also been very useful in our practice in patients with suspected optic disc swelling due to vitreopapillary traction.[20] Vitreopapillary traction may be difficult to prove by ophthalmoscopy alone. However, OCT clearly shows vitreous adhesions to the ONH, and in some of these individuals, there may be simultaneous, vitreomacular traction. When the latter occurs, the resolution of the pseudopapilledema caused by vitreopapillary traction can be relieved surgically.

Compressive Optic Neuropathy

There have been some interesting OCT findings in patients with compressive optic neuropathy.[21,22] However, from a practical point of view, we have not found OCT to be all that useful in managing patients with compressive optic neuropathy. We do not feel that OCT aids in the prognosis any more than ophthalmoscopic observation of the RNFL does. Our main goal in managing patients with compressive optic neuropathy is to prevent any RNFL loss, and visual field testing remains the main tool in identifying compressive optic neuropathy before optic atrophy develops. As opposed to patients with ONH disease, glaucoma being the main example, visual field changes usually precede NFL changes, and we continue to follow all of our patients with compressive optic neuropathy primarily monitoring their visual fields.

Optic Neuritis

From a practical point of view, OCT is occasionally useful in managing patients with optic neuritis.[23-29] Although OCT can serve as a biomarker for the progression of demyelinating disease, it may not always reflect the overall degree of demyelination occurring in such individuals. Certainly OCT will be useful in studies of the effectiveness of various drugs in the treatment of demyelinating disease from an investigational point of view, but for the day-to-day management of patients with multiple sclerosis, OCT is probably only going to be as useful as MRI scanning to monitor the overall condition of the patient. Although there have been reports of OCT helping to distinguish patients with neuromyelitis optica from those with multiple sclerosis, the degree of NFL dropout is reflected by the degree of visual loss demonstrated by visual acuity testing or visual field testing, so OCT in and of itself is not all that useful in that regard.

Toxic, Hereditary, and Nutritional Optic Neuropathy

Toxic, hereditary, and nutritional optic neuropathy have in common selective loss of retinal nerve fibers in the maculopapillary bundle. OCT demonstrates this pattern very well in most cases. A variety of interesting observations have been made in these patients, particularly in Leber's hereditary optic neuropathy.[30-34] Whether OCT will provide prognostic information regarding these conditions remains to be seen.

Conclusion

Although OCT has become very useful in our practice over the past several years, we try to remain aware of some of the limitations of OCT. OCT can be normal in patients with compressive optic neuropathy, and visual field testing remains the most important diagnostic tool in the diagnosis and follow-up of patients with compressive optic neuropathy. OCT can be normal in patients with some occult maculopathies, and multifocal electroretinography may be needed to identify maculopathy in these patients and to prevent extensive evaluations, searching for other diagnoses.

A bad OCT is like a bad MRI or a bad computed tomography scan. There may be errors in RNFL analysis. Sometimes the algorithm used by the OCT machine will fail and false measurements of the RNFL or the macula may occur. It is important to check the alignment of the circular scans when analyzing RNFL measurements. If the scan is not properly placed with respect to the ONH, inaccurate measurements may follow. This is especially problematic in patients with swollen optic nerves where the presence of subretinal fluid and marked elevation of the NFL may provide measurements that are inaccurate because they are out of the range of the normal algorithm. Perhaps in patients with ONH swelling, a larger diameter scanning circle should be used for RNFL analysis.

Also, there may be errors in macular analysis. To avoid this, because most macular diagnoses rely on a more qualitative evaluation of the OCT, we always obtain line scans, which incorporate the ONH and the macula. This allows for a better view of the anatomic details of the macula, which are not always clear on the typical macular scans. OCT may identify concurrent optic nerve and macular disease. Therefore, we image the macula as well as the RNFL in every patient in whom we obtain OCT.

References

1. Huang D, Swanson EA, Lin CP, et al. Optical coherence tomography. *Science*. 1991;254(5035):1178-1181.
2. Fujimoto JG, Brezinski ME, Tearney GJ, et al. Optical biopsy and imaging using optical coherence tomography. *Nat Med*. 1995;1(9):970-972.
3. Ko TH, Witkin AJ, Fujimoto JG, et al. Ultrahigh-resolution optical coherence tomography of surgically closed macular hole. *Arch Ophthamol*. 2006;124:827-836.
4. Witkin AJ, Ko TH, Fujimoto JG, et al. Ultra-high resolution optical coherence tomography assessment of photoreceptors in retinitis pigmentosa and related diseases. *Am J Ophthlamol*. 2006;142:945-952.
5. Pieroni CG, Witkin AJ, Ko TH, et al. Ultrahigh resolution optical coherence tomography in non-exudative age related macular degeneration. *Br J Ophthalmol*. 2006;90(2):191-197.
6. Ko TH, Fujimoto JG, Duker JS, et al. Comparison of ultrahigh and standard resolution optical coherence tomography for imaging of macular pathology and repair. *Ophthalmology*. 2004;111:2033-2043.
7. Drexler W, Sattmann H, Hermann B, et al. Enhanced visualization of macular pathology with the use of ultrahigh-resolution optical coherence tomography. *Arch Ophthalmol*. 2003;121(5):695-705.
8. Srinivasan VJ, Wojtkowski M, Witkin AJ, et al. High-definition and 3-dimensional imaging of macular pathologies with high-speed ultrahigh-resolution optical coherence tomography. *Ophthalmology*. 2006;113:2054-2065.
9. Garg SJ, Martidis A, Nelson ML, et al. Optical coherence tomography chronic solar retinopathy. *Am J Ophthalmol*. 2004;137:351-354.
10. Chen RW, Gorczynska I, Srinivasan VJ, et al. High-speed ultrahigh resolution optical coherence tomography findings in chronic solar retinopathy. *Retin Cases Brief Rep*. 2008;2(2):101-102.
11. Kaushik S, Gupta V, Gupta A. Optical coherence tomography findings in solar retinopathy. *Ophthlamic Surg Lasers Imaging*. 2004;35(1):52-55.
12. Witkin AJ, Wojtkowski M, Reichel E, et al. Photoreceptor disruption secondary to posterior vitreous detachment as visualized using high-speed ultrahigh resolution optical coherence tomography. *Arch Ophthalmol*. 2007;125(11):1579-1580.
13. Ergun E, Hermann B, Wirtitsch M, et al. Assessment of central visual function in Stargardt's disease/fundus flavimaculatus with ultrahigh-resolution optical coherence tomography. *Invest Ophthalmol Vis Sci*. 2005;46:310-316.
14. Rodriguez-Padilla JA, Hedges TR, Monson B, et al. High-speed ultra–high-resolution optical coherence tomography findings in hydroxychloroquine retinopathy. *Arch Ophthalmol*. 2007;125:775-780.
15. Roh S, Noecker RJ, Schuman, JS, Hedges TR, Weiter JJ, Mattox C. Effect of optic nerve head drusen on nerve fiber layer thickness. *Ophthalmology*. 1998;105:878-885.
16. Karam EZ, Hedges TR. Optical coherence tomography of the retinal nerve fibre layer in mild papilloedema and pseudopapilloedema. *Br J Ophthalmol*. 2005;89:294-298.

17. Johnson LN, Diehl ML, Hamm CW, et al. Differentiating optic disc edema from optic nerve head drusen on optical coherence tomography. *Arch Ophthalmol.* 2009;127(1):45-49.

18. Hoye VJ, Berrocal AM, Hedges TR, Amaro-Quireza ML. Optical coherence tomography demonstrates subretinal macular edema from papilledema. *Arch Ophthalmol.* 2001;119:1287-1290.

19. Hedges TR, Vuong, LN, Gonzalez-Garcia AO, Mendoza-Santiesteban CE, Amaro-Quiereza AL. Subretinal fluid from anterior ischemic optic neuropathy demonstrated by optical coherence tomography. *Arch Ophthalmol.* 2008;126:812-815.

20. Hedges TR, Flattem NL, Bagga A. Vitreopapillary traction confirmed by optical coherence tomography. *Arch Ophthalmol.* 2006;124:279-281.

21. Kanamori A, Nakamura M, Matsui N, et al. Optical coherence tomography detects characteristic retinal nerve fiber layer thickness corresponding to band atrophy of the optic discs. *Ophthalmology.* 2004;111:2278-2283.

22. Monteiro MLR, Leal BC, Rosa AAM, Bronstein MD. Optical coherence tomography analysis of axonal loss in band atrophy of the optic nerve. *Br J Ophthalmol.* 2004;88:896-899.

23. Zaveri MS, Conger A, Salter A, et al. Retinal imaging by laser polarimetry and optical coherence tomography evidence of axonal degeneration in multiple sclerosis. *Arch Neurol.* 2008;65(7):924-928.

24. Frohman EM, Dwyer MG, Frohman T, et al. Relationship of optic nerve and brain conventional and non-conventional MRI measures and retinal nerve fiber layer thickness, as assessed by OCT and GDx: a pilot study. *J Neurol Sci.* 2009;282(1-2):96-105.

25. Costello F, Hodge W, Pan YI, et al. Tracking retinal nerve fiber layer loss after optic neuritis: a prospective study using optical coherence tomography. *Mult Scler.* 2008;14(7):893-905.

26. Henderson AP, Trip SA, Schlottmann PG, et al. An investigation of the retinal nerve fibre layer in progressive multiple sclerosis using optical coherence tomography. *Brain.* 2008;131(Pt 1):277-287.

27. Pulicken M, Gordon-Lipkin E, Balcer LJ, et al. Optical coherence tomography and disease subtype in multiple sclerosis. *Neurology.* 2007;69(22):2085-2092.

28. Gordon-Lipkin E, Chodkowski B, Reich DS, et al. Retinal nerve fiber layer is associated with brain atrophy in multiple sclerosis. *Neurology.* 2007;69(16):1603-1609.

29. Ratchford JN, Quigg ME, Conger A, et al. Optical coherence tomography helps differentiate neuromyelitis optica and MS optic neuropathies. *Neurology.* 2009;73(4):302-308.

30. Barboni P, Savini G, Valentino ML, et al. Retinal nerve fiber layer evaluation by optical coherence tomography in Leber's hereditary optic neuropathy. *Ophthalmology.* 2005;112(1):120-126.

31. Barboni P, Carbonelli M, Sadun A, et al. Natural history of Leber's hereditary optic neuropathy: longitudinal analysis of the retinal nerve fiber layer by optical coherence tomography. *Ophthalmology.* 2010;113(3):623-627.

32. Savini G, Barboni P, Valentino ML, et al. Retinal nerve fiber layer evaluation by optical coherence tomography in unaffected carriers with Leber hereditary optic neuropathy mutations. *Ophthalmology.* 2005;112(1):127-131.

33. Chicani CM, Carelli V, Berezovsky A, et al. Leber's hereditary optic neuropathy: Project Brazil/LHON—8 year summary. *Vision Panamericana.* 2009;170-177.

34. Chai SJ, Foroozan R. Decreased retinal nerve fibre layer thickness detected by optical coherence tomography in patients with ethambutol induced optic neuropathy. *Br J Ophthalmol.* 2007;91:895-897.

Index to Cases

Case 13-1. Nutritional Optic Neuropathy

Clinical Summary

A 35-year-old female is noted to have optic disc pallor on routine examination. Visual acuities are 20/25 on the right and 20/20 on the left. Visual fields (Humphrey 30-2) show central depression on pattern deviation on both sides (A).

Fundus examination shows temporal pallor and dropout of the NFL in the maculopapillary bundles on both sides (B, C).

Optical Coherence Tomography

On SD-OCT, RNFL thickness analysis shows thin NFL in the maculopapillary regions on thickness deviation and thin NFL measurements temporally on quadrantic analysis as well as on normative data histograms in both eyes (D).

Macular thickness maps (E, F) show thinning nasal, superior, and inferior to the foveas bilaterally reflecting maculopapillary bundle NFL loss, which was seen in the line scans.

Central macular thickness in the 9-zone map shows normal values reflecting the normal retinal thickness indicating the absence of nerve fibers in the foveolar region. Line high-resolution B-scans show almost complete absence of nerve fibers in the papillomacular bundle (G, H).

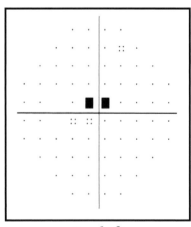

A—left

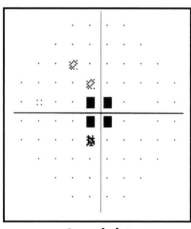

A—right

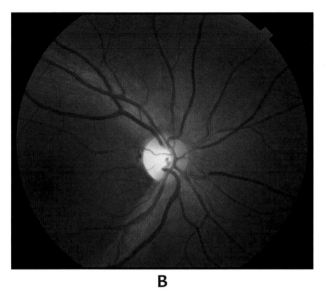

B

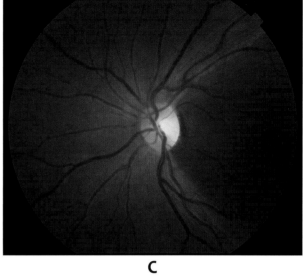

C

D

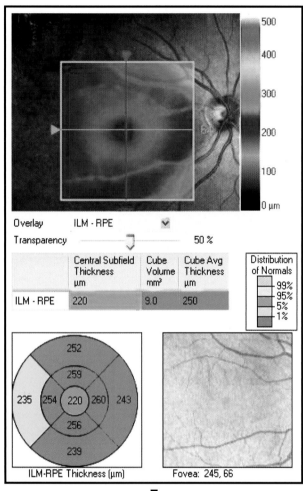

E

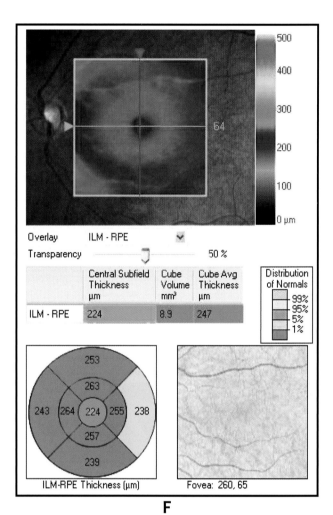

F

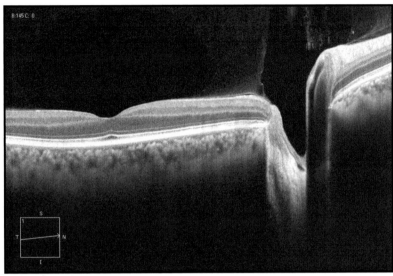

G

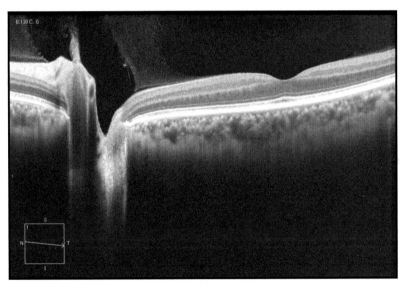

H

Case 13-2. Leber's Hereditary Optic Neuropathy

Clinical Summary

A 27-year-old otherwise healthy male has trouble reading print and road signs. He smokes cigarettes. Visual acuities are 20/200 on the right and 20/80 on the left. Color vision is minimally depressed. Visual fields show central scotomas on both sides (A).

Red-free fundus imaging shows mild optic disc swelling with telangiectatic vessels within the RNFL (B, C).

Optical Coherence Tomography

TD-OCT shows thickening of the NFL superiorly and inferiorly in both eyes (D, E).

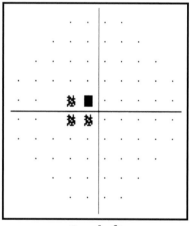

A—left

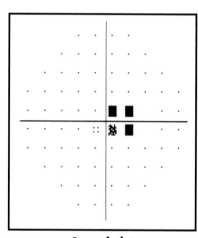

A—right

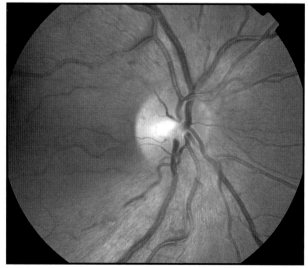

B

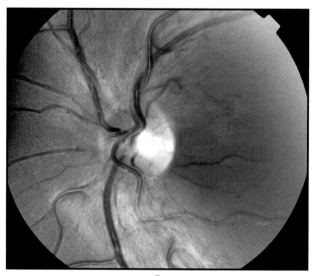

C

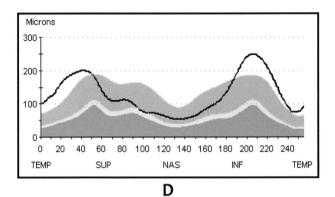

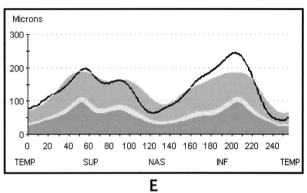

D   **E**

Follow-Up

Mitochondrial DNA analysis shows the 11778 deletion. Months later, visual acuities had declined to 6/200 on the right and 2/200 on the left. The central visual field defects had worsened (F).

On fundus examination, both ONHs had developed significant temporal pallor and loss of the normal RNFL appearance (G, H).

TD-OCT shows RNFL thinning, most prominent temporally (I, J).

Serial analysis of the RNFL over time shows progressive thinning, especially in the maculopapillary regions (K).

Comment

This particular case demonstrates the early NFL swelling and the highly selective, progressive maculopapillary RNFL dropout that has been described in the literature both clinically and by OCT in patients with Leber's hereditary optic neuropathy.

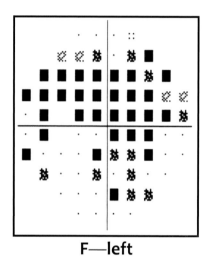

F—left

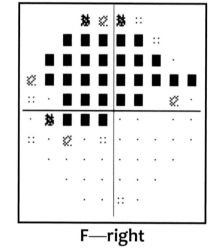

F—right

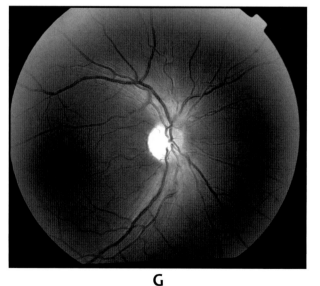

G

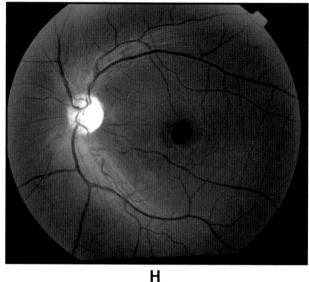

H

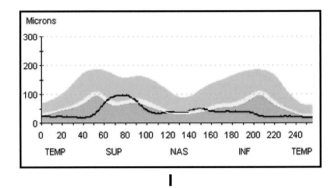

I

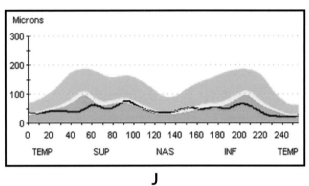

J

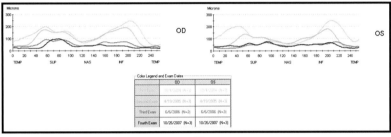

K

Case 13-3. Mild Optic Neuritis

Clinical Summary

A 30-year-old otherwise healthy male notes trouble focusing with his right eye more than the left eye over a period of days. Visual acuities are 20/25 on the right and 20/25 on the left. The right visual field shows a paracentral scotoma, and the left visual field shows mild, patchy, paracentral depression (A).

The fundi appear normal (B, C).

MRI scan shows evidence of demyelinating disease (D).

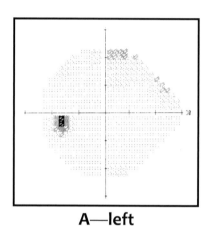

A—left

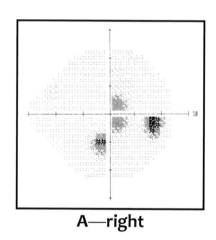

A—right

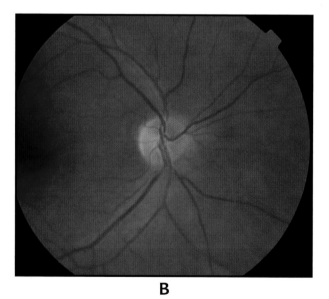

B

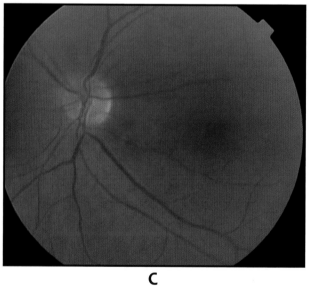

C

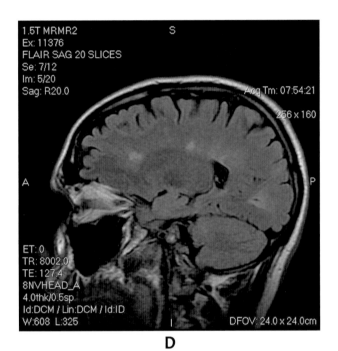

D

Follow-Up

Four years later, he notes blurred vision in the left eye, especially when he is overheated. Visual acuities are 20/15 on the right and 20/30 on the left. Visual fields (Humphrey program 30-2) now show minimal changes on the right and a nasal paracentral scotoma on the left (E).

Optical Coherence Tomography

TD-OCT showed superior and temporal thinning of the NFL bilaterally (F).

His vision improved, and he remained neurologically stable on interferon. Although he had no new visual symptoms, his RNFL became thinner, and then stabilized as seen on serial analysis of the RNFL (G).

On his last visit, TD- and SD-OCTs of the RNFL could be compared (H, I).

Comment

In this case, OCT shows RNFL dropout after episodes of optic neuritis and during a period when the patient with multiple sclerosis is asymptomatic. The loss of nerve fibers during the asymptomatic period is not readily evident ophthalmoscopically.

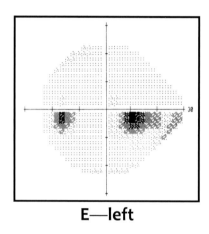

E—left

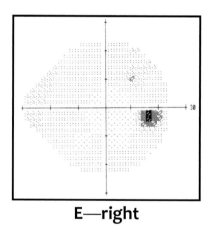

E—right

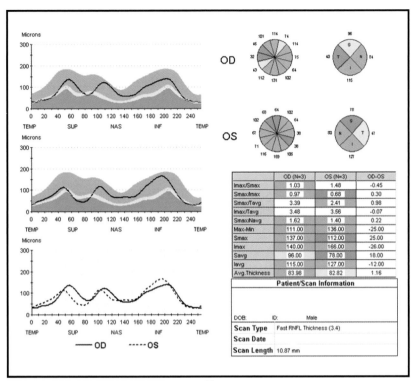

F

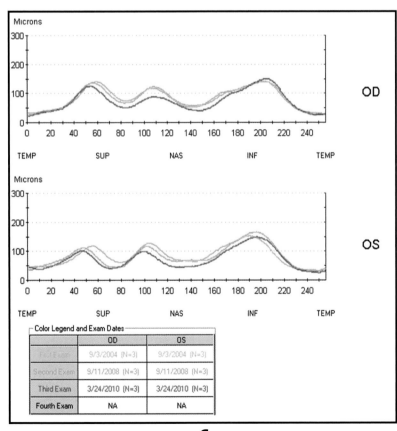

G

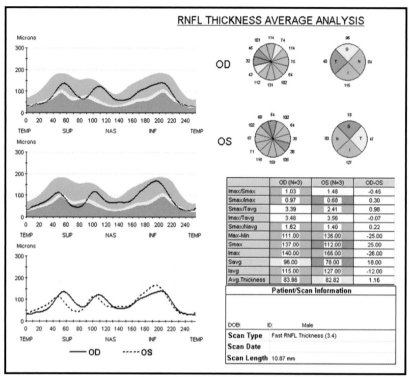

H

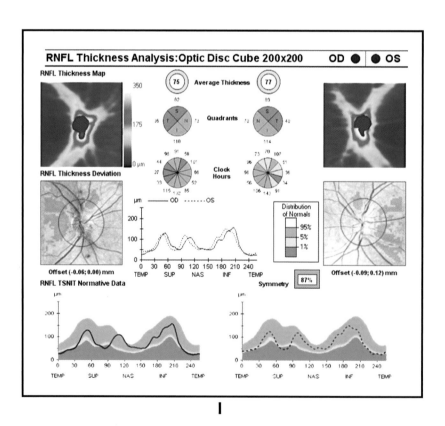

I

Case 13-4. Severe Optic Neuritis

Clinical Summary

A 43-year-old female developed the onset of blurred vision in the right eye progressing over a period of days. MRI is unremarkable. Her vision improved spontaneously and then worsened over a period of weeks. Examination shows visual acuities of 20/50 on the right and 20/15 on the left. There is a relative afferent pupillary defect on the right. Visual field testing shows central loss on the right (A).

Fundus examination shows mild swelling of the right optic disc (B) and a normal optic nerve on the left (C).

Optical Coherence Tomography

TD-OCT line scans show thickening of the RNFL on the right but a normal NFL on the left (D).

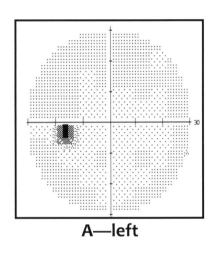

A—left

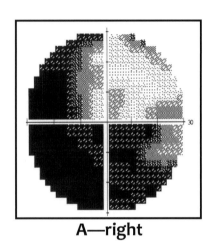

A—right

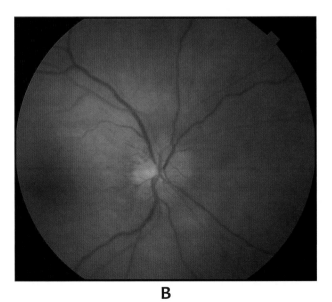

B

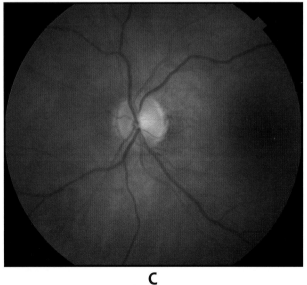

C

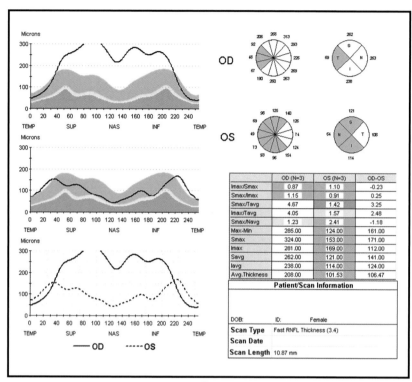

D

Follow-Up

Vision improved after a course of intravenous high-dose corticosteroids followed by oral cortico-steroid. Follow-up shows visual acuities of 20/20 on the right and 20/15 on the left. The visual field improved. The optic disc swelling resolved (E, F).

The subsequent development of optic atrophy can be seen on the SD-OCT of the NFL in the right eye, and this can be compared to the TD-OCT done at the same time (G, H).

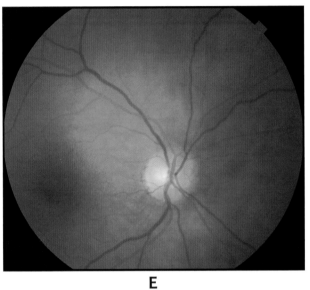

E

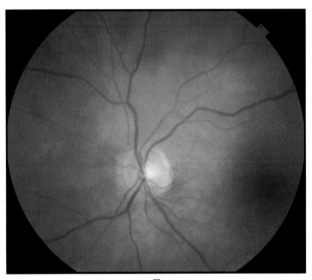

F

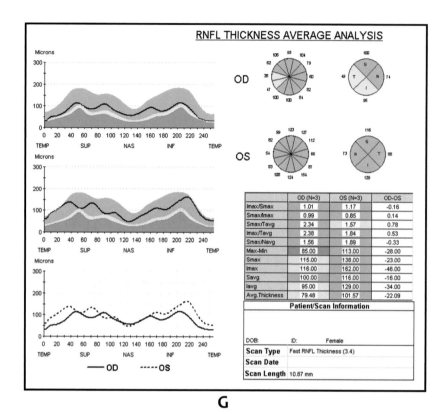

G

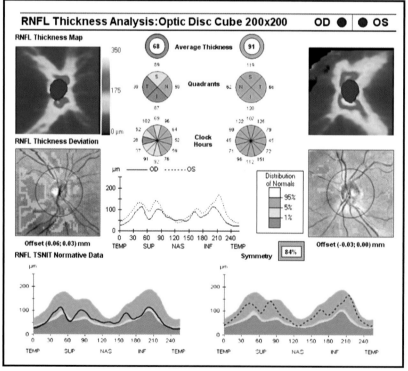

H

Case 13-5. Unilateral Compressive Optic Neuropathy

Clinical Summary

A 75-year-old female was unhappy with the results of cataract surgery in her right eye. An orbital tumor was found on MRI (A). Attempted orbital decompression at another institution was not successful.

Her vision progressively declined in the right eye. On her last examination, visual acuities are hand motions on the right and 20/30 on the left. There is a relative afferent pupillary defect. Visual fields show severe generalized loss on the right (B).

Optic atrophy is present on fundus examination (C).

Optical Coherence Tomography

OCT shows NFL thinning on the right, but still with average thicknesses of 64 μm indicating the possibility of visual recovery if the tumor could be decompressed; however, the patient continues to refuse surgery (D).

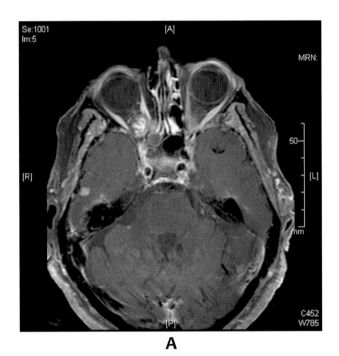

A

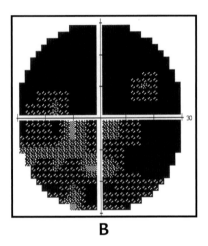

B

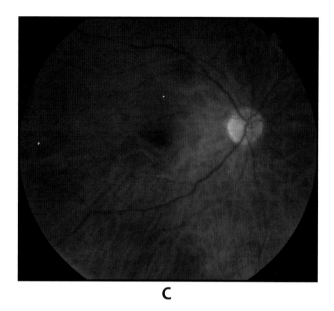

C

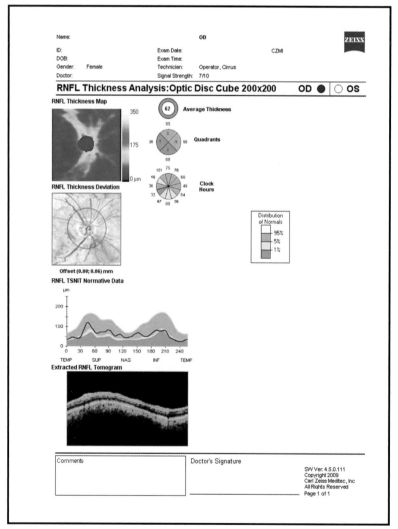

D

Case 13-6. Chiasmal Compressive Optic Neuropathy (Band Atrophy)

Clinical Summary

A 50-year-old male notes decreased vision in his right eye. Examination shows bitemporal hemianopia. MRI scan shows a large pituitary adenoma (A).

The tumor was debulked, and he remained stable for 13 years. On last examination, visual acuities are 20/25 on the right and 20/20 on the left. Visual field examination (Humphrey program 30-2) shows mild nasal loss on the right and mild temporal loss on the left (B).

Fundus examination shows mild optic atrophy (C, D).

Optical Coherence Tomography

SD-OCT shows a pattern atrophy characterized by predominant loss of nerve fibers in the nasal and temporal zones seen best in the deviation map (E).

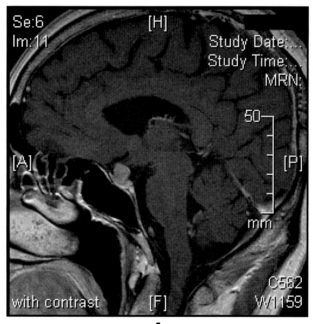

A

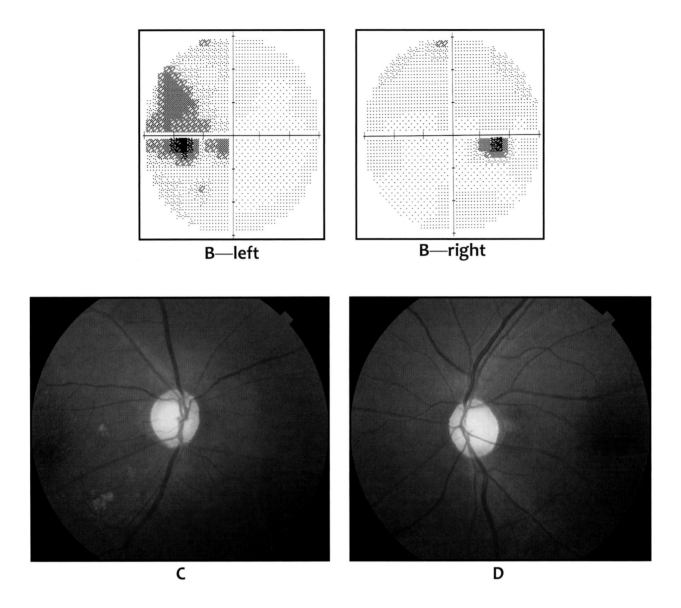

B—left   **B—right**

C   **D**

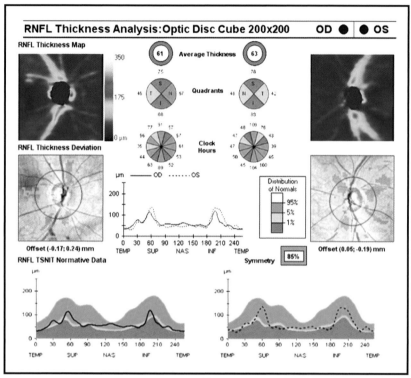

E

Case 13-7. Compressive Optic Neuropathy With Optic Swelling

Clinical Summary

A 65-year-old female notes slowly progressive loss of vision in her right eye. Her cataract surgeon suspects that she might have an optic nerve problem. Visual acuities are 20/60 on the right and 20/20 on the left. There is a relative afferent pupillary defect. Visual field testing (Humphrey program 30-2) shows peripheral loss (A).

Funduscopic examination shows swelling in the ONH with optociliary shunt vessels (B).

Optical Coherence Tomography

OCT shows thickening of the NFL on the right side (C).

Contrast computed tomography scan shows an intrinsic optic nerve tumor, apparently an optic nerve sheath meningioma (D).

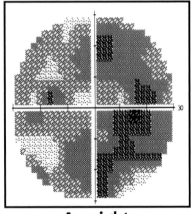

A—right

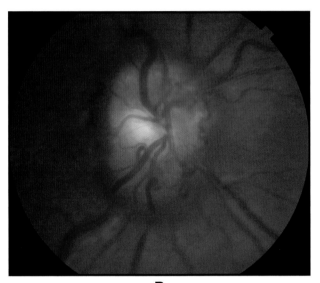

B

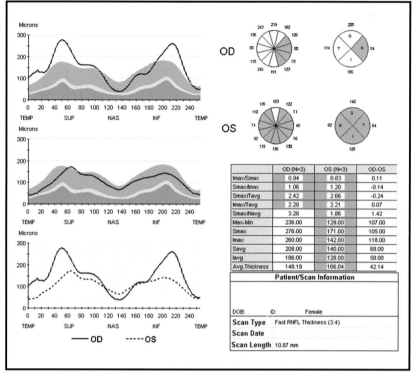

	OD (N=3)	OS (N=3)	OD-OS
Imax/Smax	0.94	0.83	0.11
Smax/Imax	1.06	1.20	-0.14
Smax/Tavg	2.42	2.66	-0.24
Imax/Tavg	2.28	2.21	0.07
Smax/Navg	3.28	1.86	1.42
Max-Min	236.00	129.00	107.00
Smax	276.00	171.00	105.00
Imax	260.00	142.00	118.00
Savg	208.00	140.00	68.00
Iavg	186.00	128.00	58.00
Avg.Thickness	148.19	106.04	42.14

Patient/Scan Information

DOB:	ID: Female
Scan Type	Fast RNFL Thickness (3.4)
Scan Date	
Scan Length	10.87 mm

C

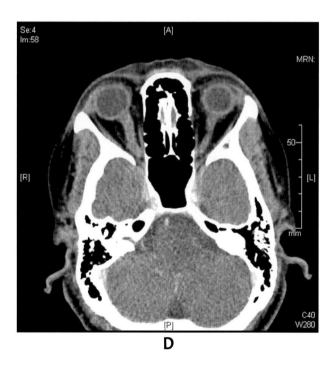

D

Case 13-8. Mild Congenital Optic Nerve Head Crowding

Clinical Summary

A 19-year-old female is evaluated by an optometrist for contact lens intolerance. She also complains of headaches. Visual acuities are 20/20 on the right and 20/20 on the left. Automated visual fields are normal on both sides.

Fundus examination shows crowded ONHs without drusen (A, B).

Optical Coherence Tomography

High-density line scans in the SD-OCT show elevation of both ONHs but no evidence of drusen (C, D).

NFL thickness analysis of both TD- (E) and SD-OCTs (F) show increased average thicknesses of the superonasal portion of the optic disc in both eyes.

Comment

The TD- and SD-OCTs are very similar, but the SD-OCT may be more accurate because of reduced acquisition time and the larger amount of data used to calculate RNFL thickness.

OCT cannot distinguish congenital crowding from mild papilledema except by following patients over time, whereas OCT measurements will not change with crowding but will change if there is pathological optic disc swelling.

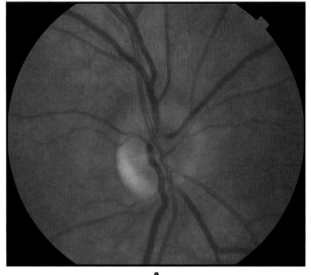

A

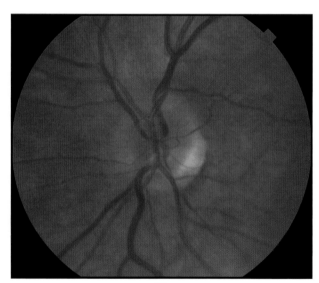

B

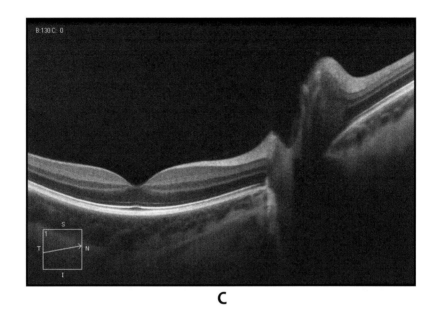

C

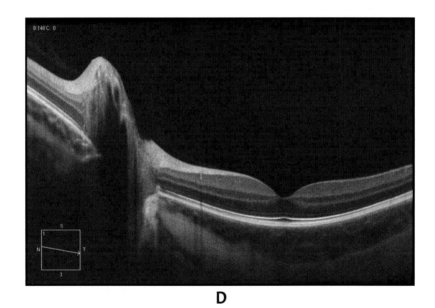

D

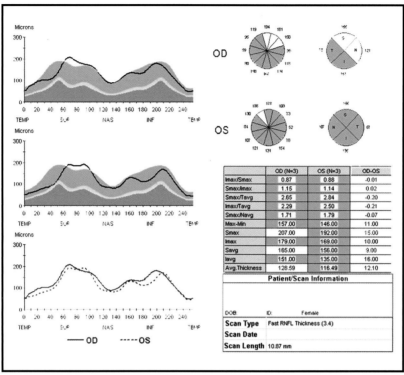

E

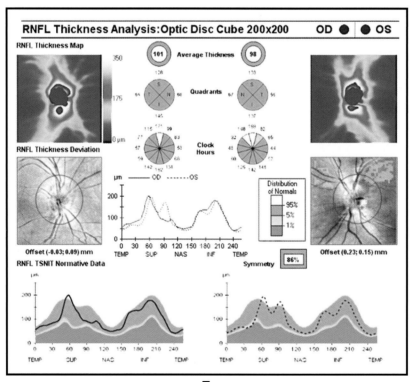

F

Case 13-9. Mild Optic Nerve Head Drusen

Clinical Summary

A 17-year-old healthy, asymptomatic male is found on routine examination to have elevated ONHs bilaterally. MRI scan is normal, and a lumbar puncture shows a normal opening pressure. Visual acuities are 20/20 on the right and 20/20 on the left. Automated visual field testing (Humphrey program 30-2) shows an inferior nasal visual field defect on the right and a nonspecific superior visual field defect on the left (A).

Fundus examination shows elevation of the right optic nerve without hemorrhage or obscuration of the blood vessels (B). The left ONH appears similar with some anomalous and tortuous blood vessels emanating from the optic disc (C).

Optical Coherence Tomography

TD-OCT line scans show ONH elevation and shadows suggesting buried drusen (D, E).

TD-OCT RNFL thickness analysis shows superior thinning of the NFL on the right on quadrantic analysis and RNFL profile plot (F).

A B-scan ultrasound of the right eye shows high reflectivity at the level of the ONH consistent with calcified optic disc drusen (G, H).

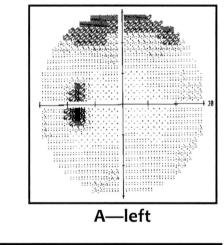

A—left

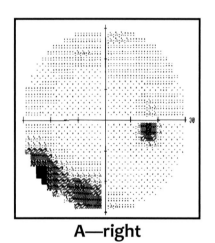

A—right

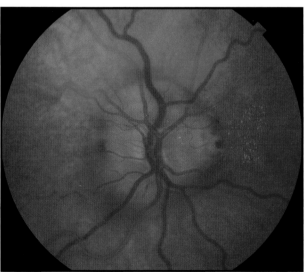

B

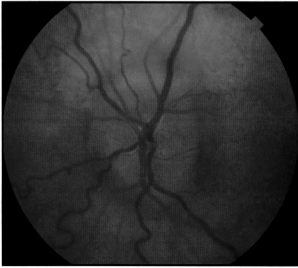

C

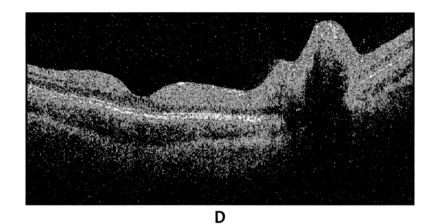

D

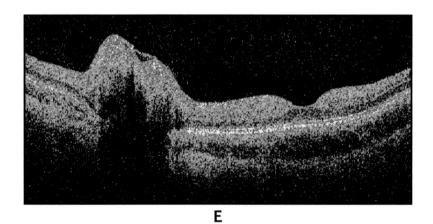

E

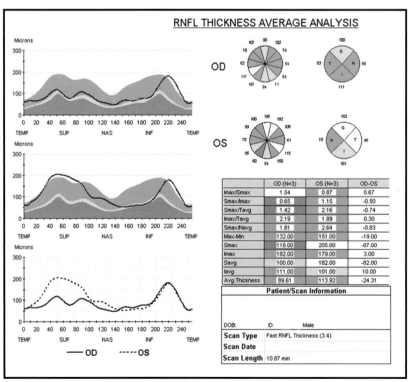

F

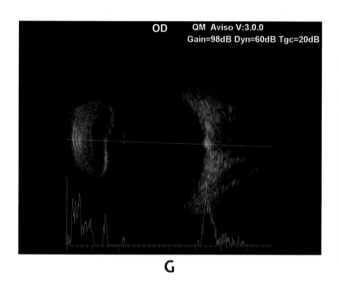

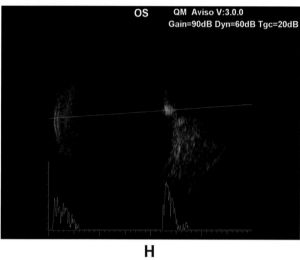

G

H

Case 13-10. Severe Optic Disc Drusen

Clinical Summary

A 52-year-old male is found to have elevated ONHs in both eyes with extensive readily visible drusen. Visual acuities are 20/20 on the right and 20/20 on the left. Automated visual field testing shows dense inferior altitudinal field loss on the right side and patchy peripheral defects and a mild inferior arcuate scotoma on the left (A).

Fundus examination of the right ONH shows elevation with multiple optic disc drusen, and similar findings are seen on the left (B, C).

Optical Coherence Tomography

SD-OCT line scans through the ONHs highlight numerous drusen along with the elevated ONHs (D, E).

SD-OCT RNFL thickness analysis shows diffuse RNFL thinning in the right eye greater than the left eye with some temporal sparing evident in the quadrantic analysis and compared to the normative RNFL data (F).

Comment

OCT is a useful objective method to monitor retinal nerve fiber loss in patients with optic disc drusen.

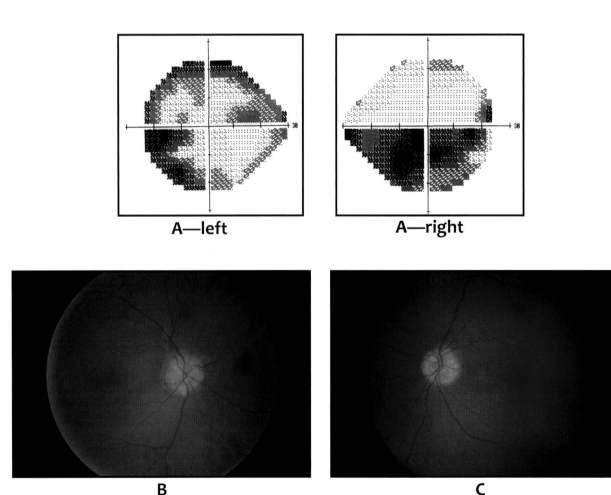

A—left   A—right

B   C

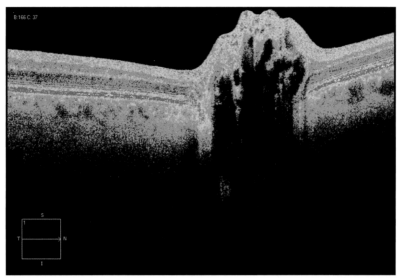

D

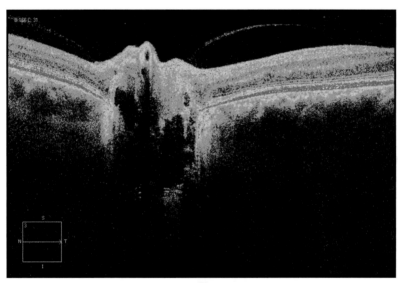

E

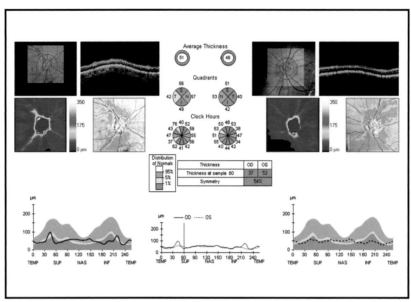

F

Case 13-11. Mild Papilledema

Clinical Summary

A 20-year-old obese female developed headaches and nausea. A computed tomographic scan of the head is unremarkable and opening pressure on lumbar puncture is greater than 500 mm of water. Visual acuities are 20/20 on the right and 20/25 on the left. Automated visual fields (Humphrey 30-2) show no abnormalities on the left side. The right visual field shows some minimal central defects probably secondary to artifact (A).

Fundus examination shows mild elevation of the ONH with some blurring of the disc margins sparing the temporal regions suggestive of mild papilledema (B). The left ONH shows similar findings (C).

Optical Coherence Tomography

SD-OCT line scan shows elevation of the ONHs (D, E).

SD-OCT RNFL thickness analysis shows NFL swelling in both eyes, especially superiorly and inferiorly seen on the quadrantic thickness map, quadrantic analysis, and RNFL thickness profile plot (F).

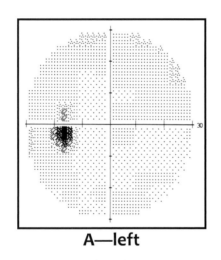

A—left

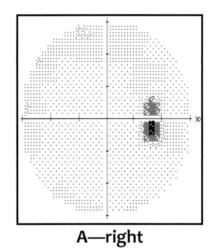

A—right

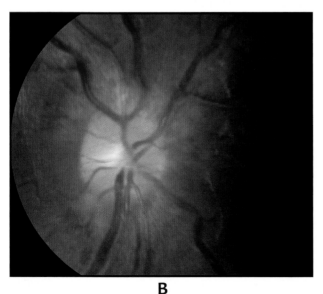

B

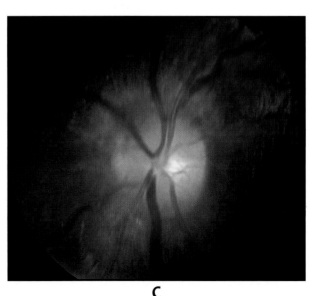

C

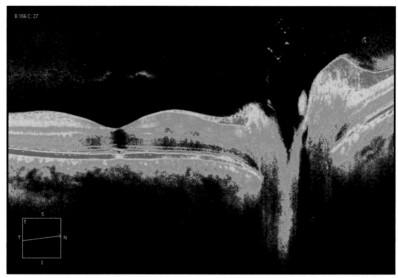

D

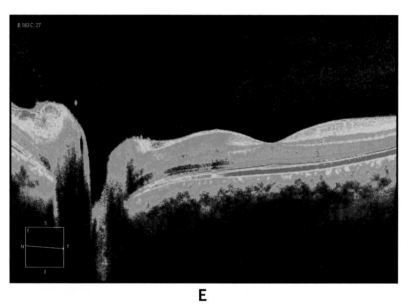

E

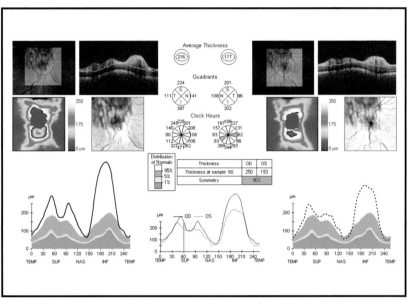

F

Case 13-12. Moderate Papilledema

Clinical Summary

A 25-year-old overweight female developed headaches and "strained" vision. In the emergency room, a physician notes papilledema. MRI scan is normal. Opening pressure on lumbar puncture is 380 mm of water. Visual acuities are 20/20 on the right and 20/20 on the left. The visual fields are normal. Fundus examination shows mild to moderate papilledema with disc hemorrhages (A, B).

Optical Coherence Tomography

SD-OCT line scans show elevation of both ONHs with normal retinas (C, D).

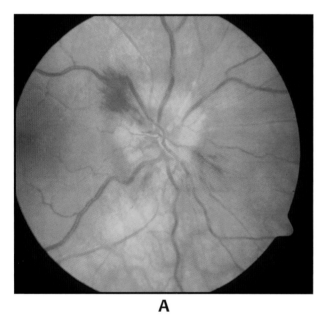

A

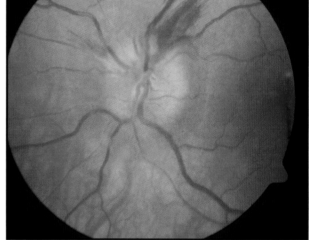

B

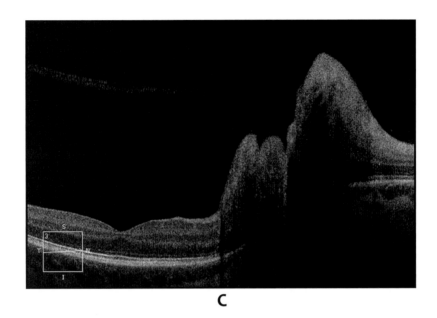

C

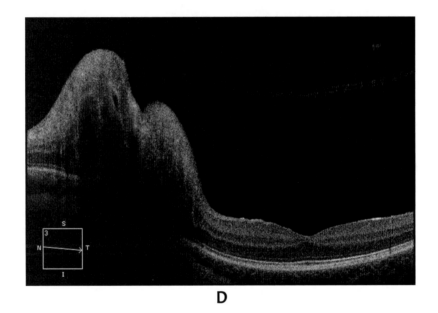

D

Follow-Up

She is treated with weight loss alone. SD-OCT glaucoma progression analysis shows improvement in the RNFL swelling over the next 5 months, followed by slight worsening as she regains weight (E, F).

When her NFL appears normal at the third visit, the ONHs also appear normal (G, H).

When OCT shows more NFL thickening, the fundus examination shows mild recurrence of the optic disc swelling, which subsequently resolved (I, J).

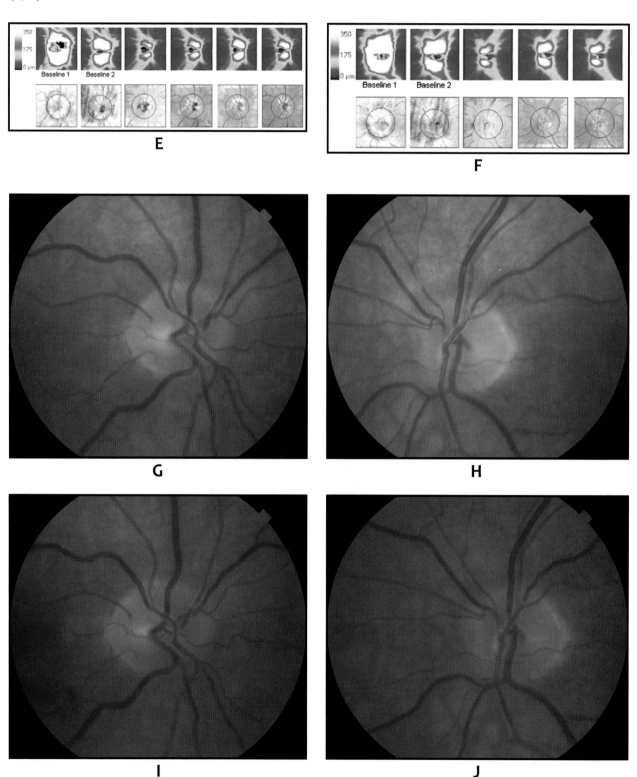

Case 13-13. Papilledema With Subretinal Fluid

Clinical Summary

A 21-year-old overweight female with a history of minocycline use over the previous 2 weeks developed positional headaches, transient visual obscurations, pulsatile intracranial noises, double vision, and decreased vision. Visual acuities are 20/40 on the right and 20/25 on the left. There is left lateral rectus dysfunction. Spinal tap shows intracranial pressure over 500 mm of water. Automated visual field testing (Humphrey program 30-2) pattern deviation shows enlargement of the blind spot and ring-like peripheral visual field loss on the left. The right visual field pattern deviation shows a similarly enlarged blind spot and an inferior arcuate scotoma (A).

On fundus examination, the right ONH is diffusely swollen with blurred margins 360 degrees, obscured peripapillary blood vessels, and flame-shaped hemorrhages (B). The left ONH shows similar abnormalities (C).

Optical Coherence Tomography

SD-OCT line scans show subretinal fluid apparently tracking from the edge of the optic discs on both sides (D, E).

SD-OCT RNFL thickness profile plot and quadratic analysis demonstrate 360-degree ONH swelling in both eyes (F).

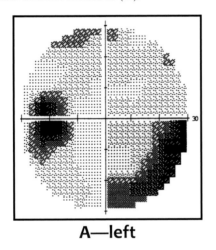

A—left

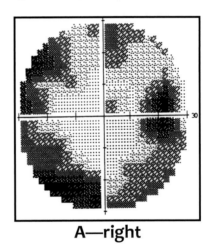

A—right

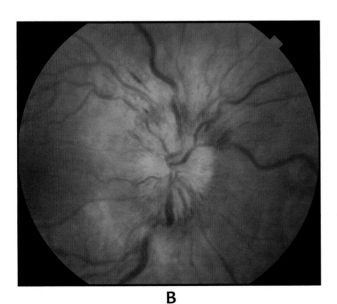

B

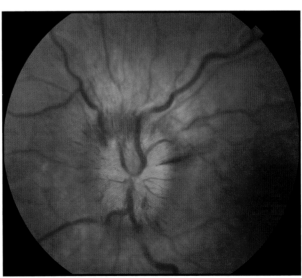

C

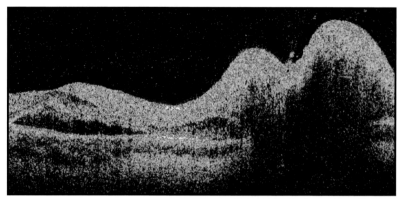

D

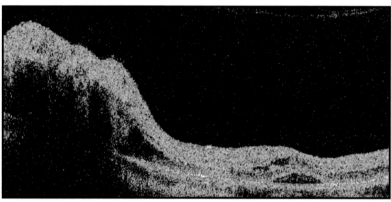

E

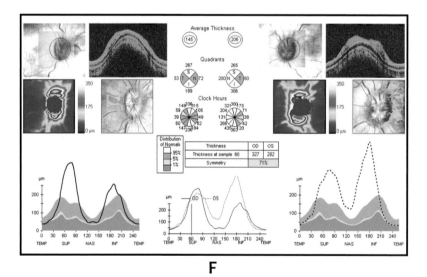

F

Follow-Up

At 2 years of follow-up, visual acuities are 20/20 on the right and 20/20 on the left. Her weight is stable, and she continues to take acetazolamide 500 mg twice a day. Automated visual field testing shows a significant improvement bilaterally with mild visual field loss inferiorly and nasally (G).

The optic nerves both appear pale without evidence of swelling on both sides (H, I).

At this time, SD-OCT RNFL thickness analysis shows mild RNFL thinning on the right side, especially on the thickness map, localized primarily to the superior nasal quadrant corresponding to the inferior nasal visual field defect (J).

Comment

This case illustrates how OCT demonstrates subfoveal and peripapillary fluid in some cases of papilledema, which can account for reduced visual acuity and can spontaneously return to normal as the papilledema resolves. Also, this shows the typical pattern of RNFL loss that occurs superonasally in papilledema.

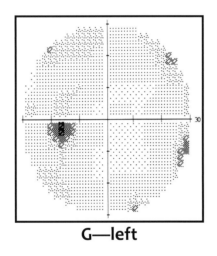

G—left

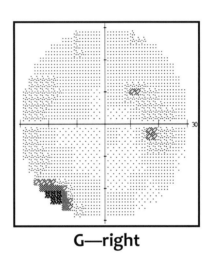

G—right

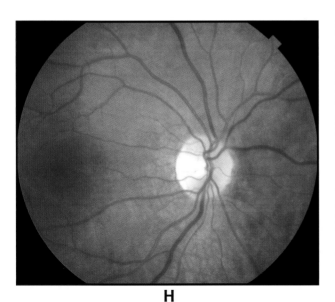

H

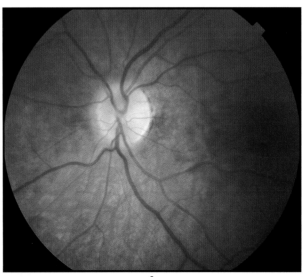

I

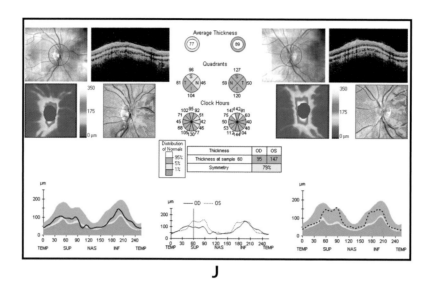

J

Case 13-14. Hypotony With Papilledema

Clinical Summary

A 50-year-old female with advanced glaucoma notes progressively worsening vision in her right eye 3 days after needle revision of a trabeculectomy bleb. On examination, her IOP measures less than 5 mm Hg. Her vision is hand motions on the right affected eye and 20/40 on the left. Funduscopic examination shows retinal folds and florid optic disc edema with flame hemorrhage and dilated tortuous blood vessels on the right side (A). The left optic nerve shows some glaucomatous cupping.

Optical Coherence Tomography

SD-OCT line scans show extensive retinal folds concentric to a large swollen ONH on the right and moderate cupping with no other abnormalities on the left (B).

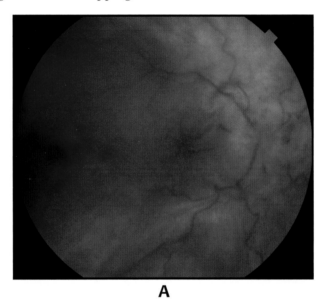

A

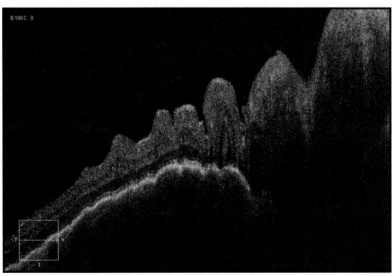

B

Case 13-15. Nonarteritic Anterior Ischemic Optic Neuropathy

Clinical Summary

A 46-year-old male notes blurred vision in the lower portion of his right visual field upon awakening. Visual acuities are 20/20 on the right and 20/20 on the left. Visual field testing shows inferior altitudinal loss on the right side and no abnormalities on the left (A).

There is a relative afferent pupillary defect. Fundus examination shows swelling of the right optic nerve with peripapillary hemorrhages (B) and crowding of the left optic disc (C).

Optical Coherence Tomography

SD-OCT line scans show elevation of the ONH on the right side (D) and crowding of the optic nerve on the left (E).

SD-OCT NFL analysis shows RNFL thickening on the right and mild apparent thickening consistent with crowding on the left (F).

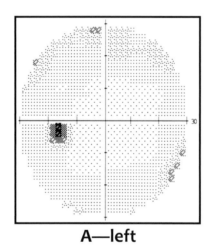

A—left

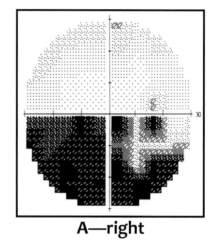

A—right

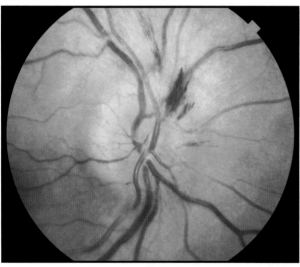

B

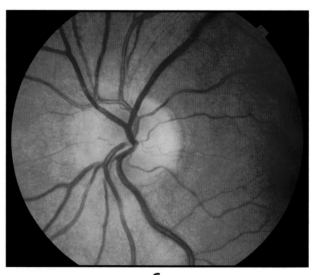

C

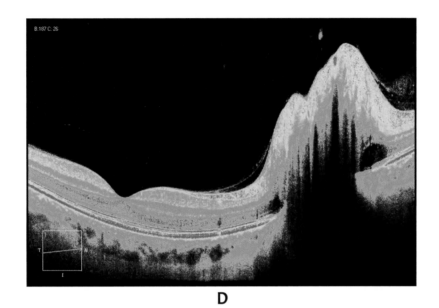

D

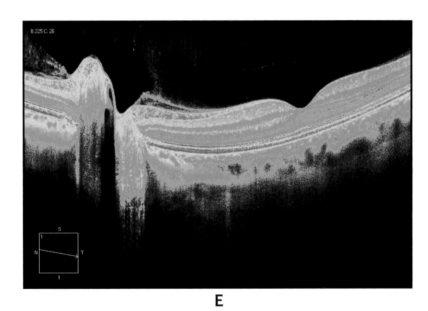

E

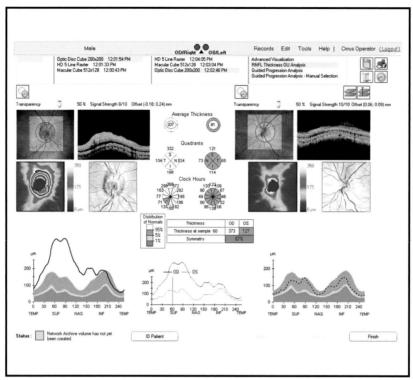

F

Case 13-16. Nonarteritic Anterior Ischemic Optic Neuropathy With Subretinal Fluid

Clinical Summary

A 36-year-old male notes acute loss of central vision in his right eye. Visual acuities are 20/400, there is decreased color perception, there is a relative afferent pupillary defect, and there are superior arcuate and inferior paracentral visual field defects on the right side (A).

Fundus examination shows optic disc swelling with peripapillary hemorrhages (B).

Optical Coherence Tomography

A TD-OCT line scan shows optic disc swelling with peripapillary as well as subfoveal fluid (C).

Follow-Up

Over the following several months, visual acuity improves to 20/80.

Comment

OCT demonstrates subfoveal fluid in some cases of anterior ischemic optic neuropathy accounting for decreased visual acuity, which can spontaneously resolve over time.

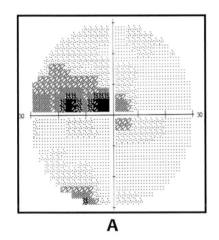

A

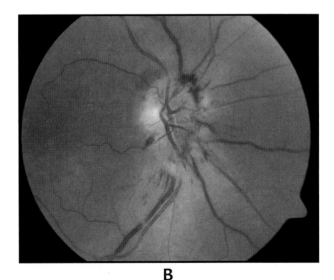

B

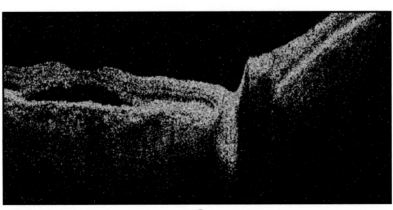

C

Case 13-17. Anterior Ischemic Optic Neuropathy/ Pseudo-Foster Kennedy Syndrome

Clinical Summary

A 42-year-old male awoke with loss of vision in the left eye 5 months before losing vision in the lower portion of the visual field in the right eye. He has hypertension but is otherwise healthy. Visual acuities are 20/30 on the right and 20/20 on the left. Visual field testing with Humphrey program 30-2 shows inferior altitudinal defects in both eyes (A).

Fundus examination shows swelling of the right ONH with peripapillary hemorrhages (B) and optic atrophy, especially superiorly on the left side (C).

Optical Coherence Tomography

SD-OCT line scans show disc elevation with a peripapillary area of hyporeflectance suggesting fluid on the right side (D). The left optic nerve shows evidence of crowding, and the RNFL appears thin (E).

SD-OCT NFL analysis shows generalized swelling on the right RNFL and loss of nerve fibers, especially superiorly, on the left (F).

Comment

OCT of anterior ischemic optic neuropathy allows for the study of the effects of pathologic optic nerve swelling on the RNFL and also the retina. It has the potential to show pre-ischemic optic nerve damage. Furthermore, OCT of ischemic optic neuropathy demonstrates the patterns and progression of RNFL loss over time and how these changes correspond to visual function, particularly the visual fields.

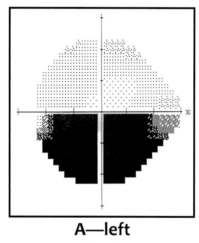

A—left

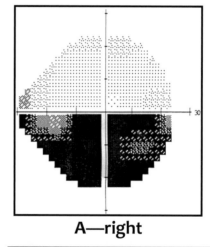

A—right

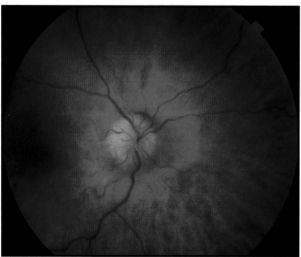

B

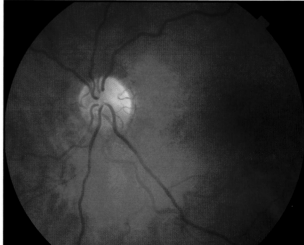

C

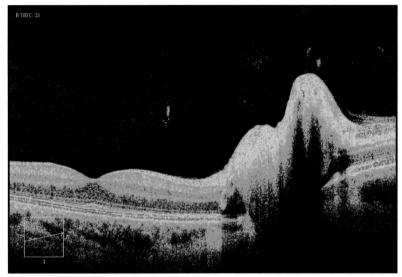

D

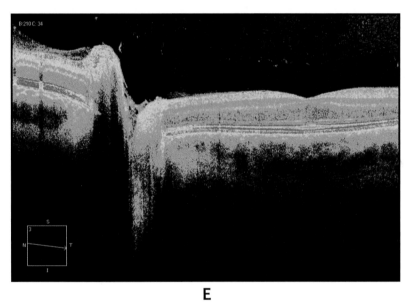

E

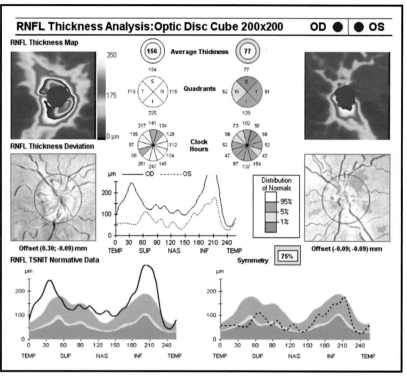

F

Case 13-18. Juvenile Diabetic Papillopathy

Clinical Summary

A 24-year-old female who had been insulin dependent for 15 years developed blurred vision in her left eye. This had been present for 3 months when she is evaluated. Visual acuities are 20/20 on the right and 20/30 on the left. Visual field testing shows enlargement of the blind spot in the left eye (A).

The right fundus shows minimal background diabetic microvascular changes. The left optic disc is very swollen (B).

Optical Coherence Tomography

OCT shows elevation of the ONH and macular thickening with apparent intraretinal and subretinal fluid best seen on the macular thickness map (C).

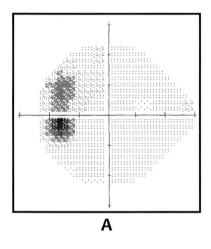

A

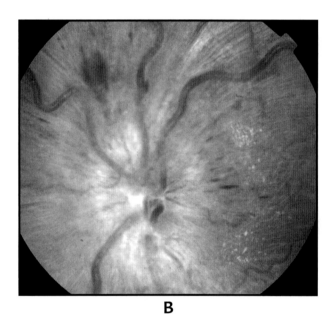

B

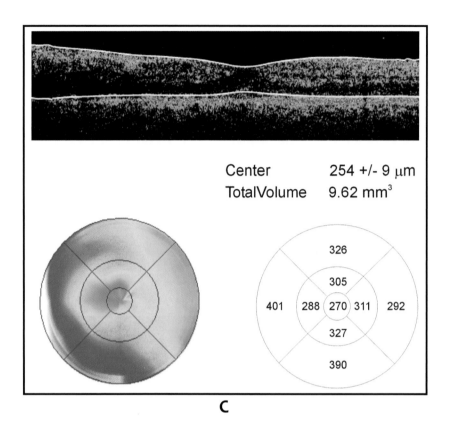

C

Case 13-19. *Neuroretinitis*

Clinical Summary

A 17-year-old female notes blurred vision in her right eye. She has some other nonspecific rheumatologic symptoms, but infectious disease and rheumatologic evaluations are unremarkable including Lyme and *Bartonella* titers. Visual acuities are 20/200 on the right and 20/20 on the left. There is a relative afferent pupillary defect on the right. The right visual fields show paracentral and superotemporal loss (A).

Fundus examination shows vitreous exudation obscuring part of the optic disc. Paton lines and radial macular folds with temporal partial starburst exudates radiating from the fovea are present (B).

Optical Coherence Tomography

SD-OCT line scan shows dense peripapillary vitreous condensations surrounded by points of hyperreflectivity corresponding to cells, ONH swelling, areas of hyporeflectivity under the peripapillary and foveal retina in which there are specks of hyperreflectivity, as well as lines of hyperreflectivity extending along Henle's fiber layer (C).

SD-OCT RNFL analysis shows a corresponding increase of RNFL thickness secondary to the optic nerve swelling. The algorithm for the detection of the boundaries of the RNFL may fail with greater disease pathology (D).

Follow-Up

She improves considerably on steroids and azithromycin.

Comment

OCT shows increased reflectance within subretinal fluid and in the vitreous indicating inflammatory cells as well as NFL and optic nerve swelling in neuroretinitis.

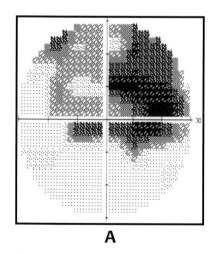

A

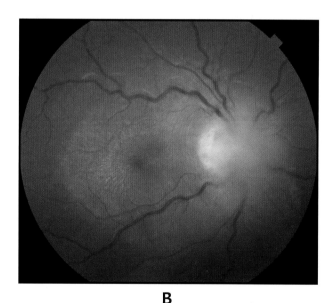

B

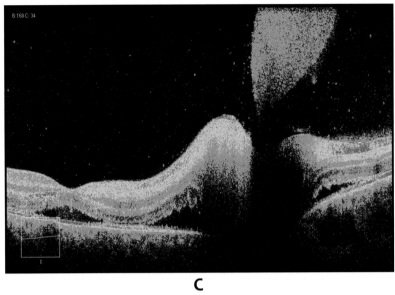

C

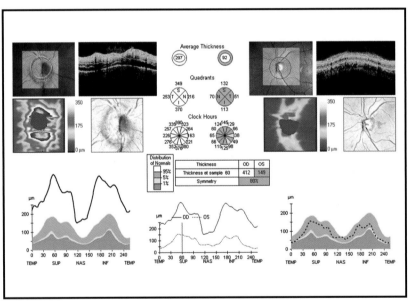

D

Case 13-20. Vitreopapillary Traction

Clinical Summary

A 62-year-old female is referred for possible papilledema involving the left eye. She is relatively asymptomatic. Visual acuity is 20/25 on the left side, and she has normal visual fields. Fundus examination shows blurring of the disc margins but no distinctive signs of edema or hemorrhage (A).

Optical Coherence Tomography

TD-OCT line scans show strands of persistent vitreopapillary attachment pulling the disc margins anteriorly with surrounding posterior vitreous separation (B).

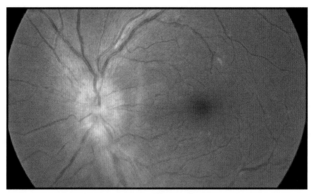

A

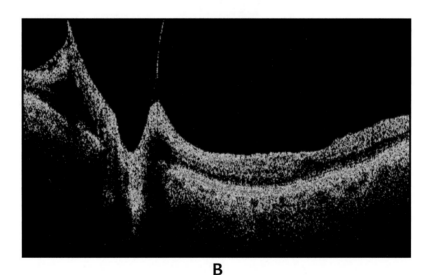

B

Case 13-21. Myelinated Nerve Fibers

Clinical Summary

A 27-year-old female is evaluated because of a possible ONH tumor noted by her optometrist. She is asymptomatic. Visual acuities are 20/20 on the right and 20/15 on the left. Visual fields show enlargement of the blind spot in the left eye only (A).

The right fundus shows a small cup and some blurring of the margins. The left disc shows fulminant myelin and possibly additional glial proliferation extending superiorly and inferiorly (B).

Optical Coherence Tomography

OCT shows marked thickening of the nerve fibers in the region of the apparent myelinated regions without evidence of more solid areas that might represent tumor (C).

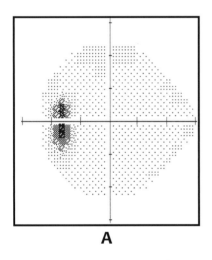

A

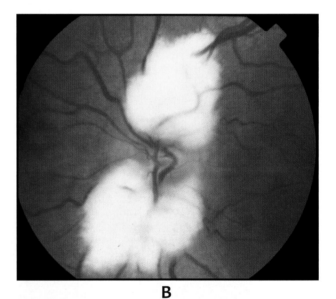

B

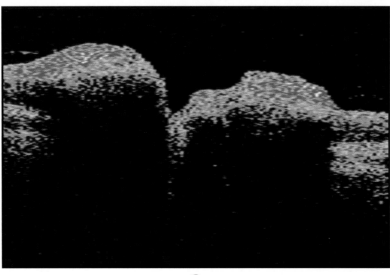

C

Case 13-22. Tilted Optic Discs

Clinical Summary

A 42-year-old female is found to have inferior temporal visual field defects on a routine eye exam. She is otherwise healthy and asymptomatic. Visual acuities are 20/20 on the right and 20/20 on the left. Visual fields show inferior temporal depression on the right and no abnormalities on the left (A).

Fundus examination on the right side shows an obliquely tilted optic nerve with a superior nasal elevation forming a ridge (B) as well as a colobomatous region temporally. Similar but less impressive findings are also apparent on the right side (C).

Optical Coherence Tomography

SD-OCT line scans show nasal ridge-like elevation and colobomatous depression of the temporal papillary sclera in both eyes (D, E).

RNFL thickness analysis shows thinning of the superior NFL on the right side corresponding to the visual field defect and somewhat similar but less impressive findings on the left side (F).

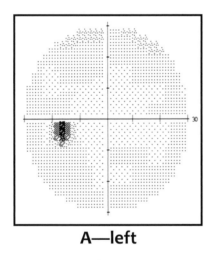

A—left

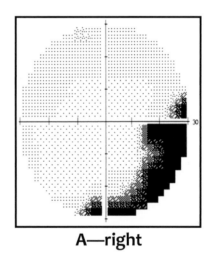

A—right

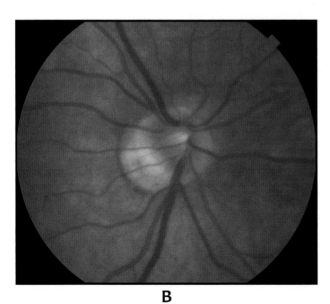

B

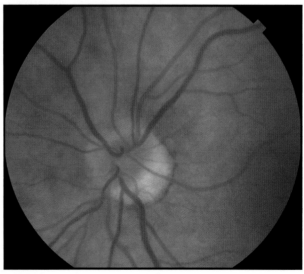

C

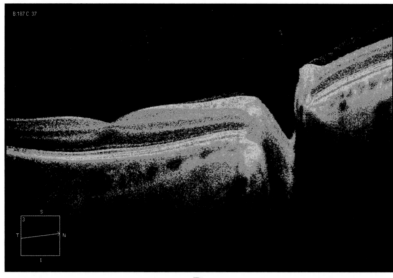

D

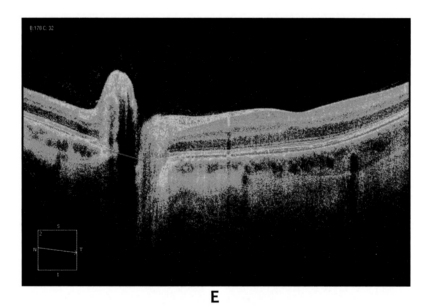

E

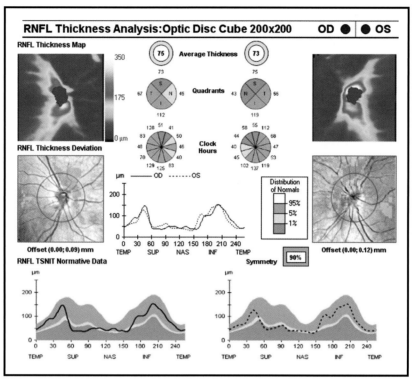

F

Case 13-23. Optic Nerve Hypoplasia

Clinical Summary

A 36-year-old female is evaluated because of a pituitary microadenoma. However, the tumor does not appear to be affecting the chiasm. Visual acuities are 20/20 on the right and 20/20 on the left. Automated visual field testing (Humphrey program 30-2) shows temporal depression bilaterally (A).

Fundus examination shows small optic nerves with a double-ring sign of exposed sclera (B, C).

Optical Coherence Tomography

SD-OCT line scans show small scleral canal measurements less than 850 μm on both eyes (D, E).

SD-OCT NFL analysis scans show sector RNFL thinning superiorly on the right and superonasally on the left (F). These findings are unrelated to the pituitary adenoma.

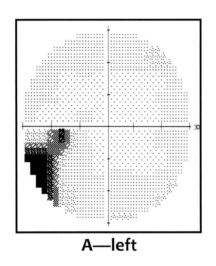

A—left

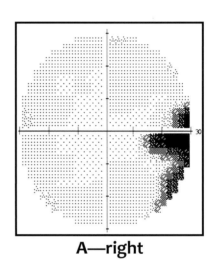

A—right

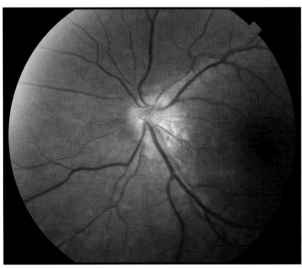

B

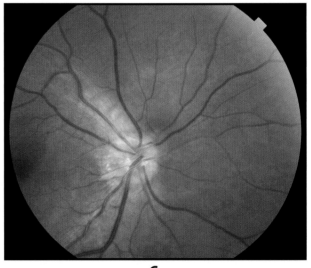

C

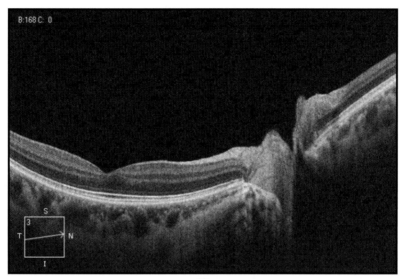

D

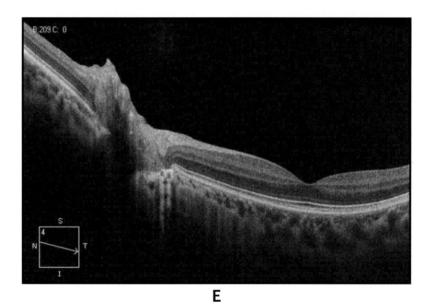

E

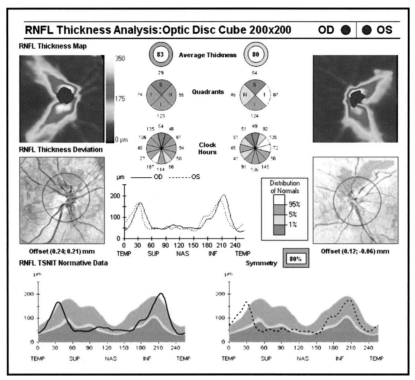

F

Case 13-24. Optic Pit

Clinical Summary

A 22-year-old female is found to have an optic pit on the right side on routine eye exam. There is associated macular retinoschisis. No subretinal fluid is found. Fundus examination shows a pit-like defect involving the optic disc as well as temporal peripapillary pigment epithelial atrophy secondary to previous retinal photocoagulation. There is also evidence of macular edema (A).

Optical Coherence Tomography

SD-OCT shows typical foveomacular schisis below the outer plexiform layer as well as retinal pigment epitheliopathy secondary to disruption of the peripapillary intermediary tissue at the temporal edge of the disc (B, C).

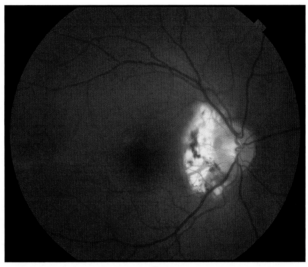

A

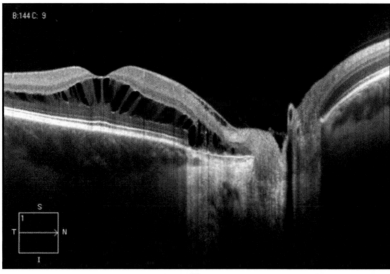

B

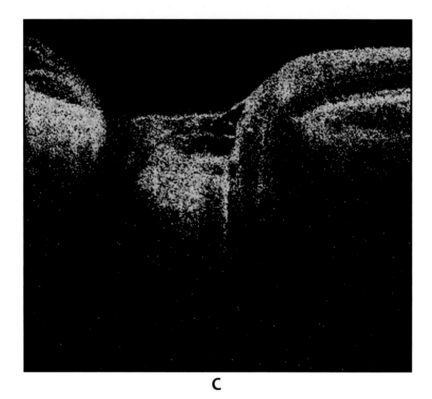

C

Case 13-25. Bilateral Optic Disc Coloboma

Clinical Summary

A 22-year-old male is found to have anomalous retinal and ONH findings on routine examination. Visual acuities are 20/40 on the right and 20/200 on the left. Fundus examination shows a large defect in the optic nerve with a dark patch of retinal pigment epithelial proliferation in the peripapillary region. Some of the pigmentary changes extend toward the macula, which appear elevated with cystic changes (A).

Optical Coherence Tomography

High-speed ultrahigh-resolution OCT shows a large central defect in the optic nerve (B) and a large intraretinal cystic area of schisis (C).

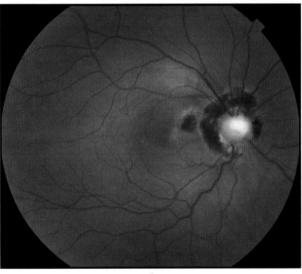

A

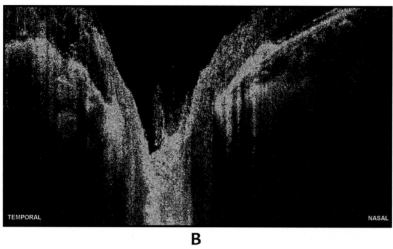

B

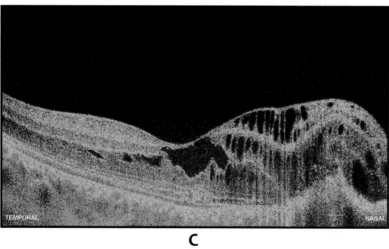

C

Case 13-26. Bergmeister's Papilla

Clinical Summary

A 22-year-old female is noted to have anomalous ONHs by an optometrist on routine examination. Visual acuities are 20/20 on the right and 20/20 on the left. Fundus examination shows prepapillary glial tissue in both eyes (A, B).

Optical Coherence Tomography

SD-OCT line scan shows elevation of the nasal portion of the optic disc with additional tissue anterior to normally patent central retinal vessels (C, D).

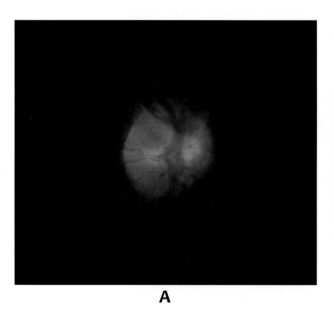

A

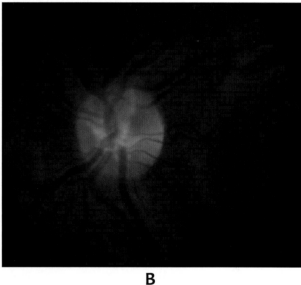

B

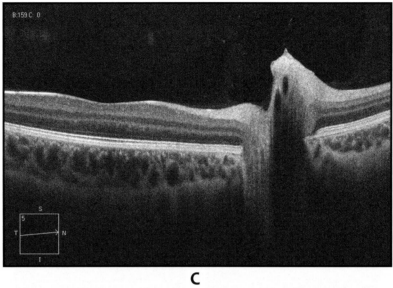

C

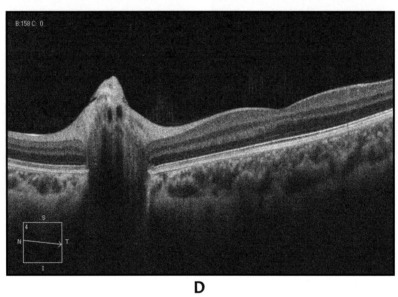

D

Case 13-27. Central Retinal Artery Occlusion

Clinical Summary

A 54-year-old male notes acute loss of central vision in his right eye. Visual acuities are counting fingers on the right and 20/25 on the left. Automated visual fields (Humphrey program 30-2) show a central scotoma in the right eye (A).

Fundus examination shows a cherry-red spot with surrounding ischemic retinal whitening (B).

Optical Coherence Tomography

SD-OCT of the macula shows intraretinal thickening in the macular region (C).

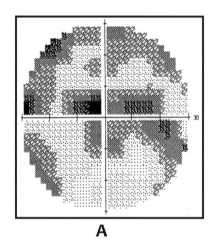

A

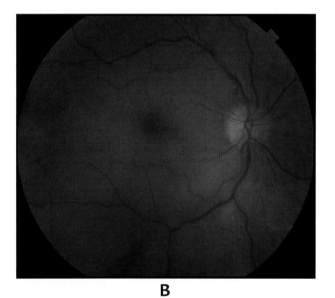

B

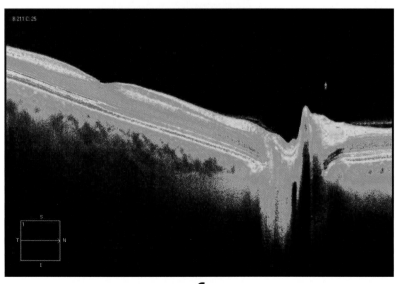

C

Follow-Up

Thirty-two months later, the vision is slightly improved. The fundus now appears more normal with a small peripapillary hemorrhage (D).

SD-OCT shows intraretinal thinning at this point (E).

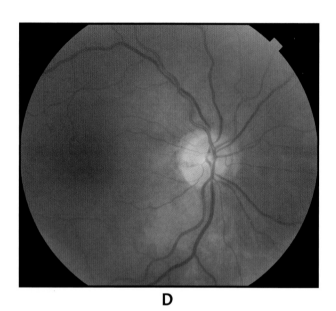

D

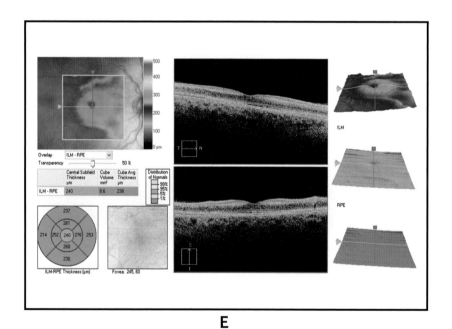

E

Case 13-28. Combined Hamartoma of the Optic Disc

Clinical Summary

A 14-year-old male notes blurred vision in the right eye and is referred by his pediatrician. Visual acuities are 20/80 on the right and 20/15 on the left. There is a relative afferent pupillary defect on the right side. Automated visual field testing (Humphrey program 30-2) shows an inferior and temporal defect approaching fixation (A).

Fundus examination shows grayish peripapillary tissue, which is elevated and not associated with hemorrhage (B). Fundus fluorescein angiography shows leakage and vascular autofluorescence with subsequent leakage and progressive staining in various portions of the peripapillary region (C).

Optical Coherence Tomography

SD-OCT line scans of the optic discs show elevation and enlargement of peripapillary tissue consistent with a mass growing within the retina, suggesting a combined hamartoma of the retina and retinal pigment epithelium (D).

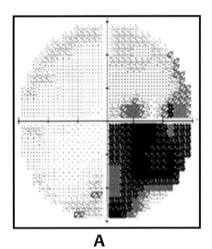

A

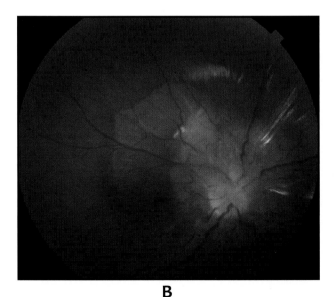

B

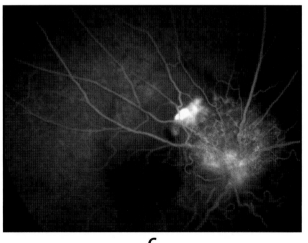

C

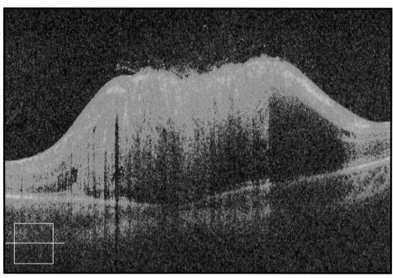

D

Anterior Segment Optical Coherence Tomography

Bing Qin, MD, PhD; Yan Li, PhD; and David Huang, MD, PhD

- Introduction
- Optical Coherence Tomography Devices
- Interpretation of Corneal Images
- Angle Assessment
- Refractive Surgery
- Corneal Pathologies and Surgeries

Introduction

Optical coherence tomography (OCT)[1] is capable of a higher speed and resolution than other noncontact corneal imaging modalities. As OCT technology improves, we are finding more and more applications for it in the management of corneal diseases and the planning of anterior eye surgeries.

Optical Coherence Tomography Devices

The most important advance in OCT technology was the transition from time-domain (TD) to Fourier-domain (FD) (also called *spectral-* [SD] or *frequency-domain*) detection. FD-OCT detects signal from the full depth range simultaneously. It is much more efficient than the serial scanning performed in TD-OCT. Therefore, FD-OCT is capable of a higher speed and signal than TD-OCT. The high speed reduces motion error and yields higher definition (more axial scans [A-scans] per image) images.

The fastest TD-OCT system, the Visante (Carl Zeiss Meditec, Inc, Dublin, CA), acquires 2000 A-scans per second, while the FD-OCT systems are roughly 10 to 20 times faster, with speeds between 17,000 to 52,000 A-scans per second (Table 14-1).

Another factor to consider is the wavelength. All current anterior segment OCT systems operate in the near infrared, at either 1310 or 830 to 850 nm. The longer wavelength of 1310 nm penetrates more deeply through the sclera, limbus, angle, and iris. The shorter wavelength range of 830 to 850 nm cannot penetrate the sclera or iris but offers much higher resolution (see Table 14-1). The 1310-nm systems cannot perform retinal imaging due to water absorption in the vitreous medium. The 830- to 850-nm OCT systems are generally also capable of retinal imaging. However, the hybrid retina/cornea platforms generally have limited anterior segment imaging width. To image the entire width and depth of the anterior chamber, it is necessary to have dedicated anterior segment scanning optics (Visante, SL-OCT [Heidelberg Engineering, GmbH, Heidelberg, Germany], Casia [Tomey Corp, Nagoya, Japan], see Table 14-1).

Finally, software is as important as hardware. The corneal OCT images shown in this chapter are obtained with the RTVue system (Optovue, Inc, Fremont, CA), which has software to map the corneal thickness and measure anterior and posterior corneal power.[2] The anterior chamber angle OCT images shown in this chapter are acquired with either

Schuman JS, Puliafito CA, Fujimoto JG, Duker JS, eds.
Optical Coherence Tomography of Ocular Diseases,
Third Edition (pp 549-562).

Table 14-1
Commercial Optical Coherence Tomography Systems Capable of Anterior Segment Imaging

Manufacturer	Device	Axial Resolution (μm)	Wavelength (nm)	Speed (A-scan/sec)	Type
Bioptigen, Inc (Research Triangle Park, NC)	3D SD-OCT	5	830	17,000	Fourier-domain
Canon/ Optopol Technology (Zawiercie, Poland)	Copernicus HR	3	850	52,000	Fourier-domain
Carl Zeiss Meditec, Inc (Dublin, CA)	Visante	18	1310	2,000	Time-domain
Carl Zeiss Meditec, Inc	Cirrus	5	830	27,000	Fourier-domain
Heidelberg Engineering, GmbH (Heidelberg, Germany)	SL-OCT	18	1310	200	Time-domain
OPKO, Inc (Miami, FL)	Spectral OCT SLO	5-6	830	27,000	Fourier-domain
Optovue, Inc (Fremont, CA)	RTVue	5	830	26,000	Fourier-domain
Tomey Corp (Nagoya, Japan)	Casia	10	1310	30,000	Fourier-domain

the RTVue system or Visante system to demonstrate OCT angle imaging at both 830- and 1310-nm wavelengths. We have extensive experience with the use of the RTVue and Visante in a wide range of corneal and anterior segment applications.

Interpretation of Corneal Images

Dewarping of Corneal Images

Anterior segment OCT images are distorted by refraction at several boundaries where the refractive index undergoes major changes. The distortion could be corrected by a "dewarping" algorithm performed in a computer.[3] Because of the cornea's dome-shaped structure, 2-dimensional images could be accurately dewarped if they are taken along meridional planes. The meridional lines pass through the corneal vertex. Therefore, corneal line scans should preferably

include the vertex, which appears as bright vertical flare on OCT images (Figure 14-1). Alternatively, one can also align the OCT scan on a meridian by making sure that the scan line is perpendicular to the limbus or the pupil. Accurate dewarping also requires that the OCT image contains the anterior corneal boundary.

Frame Averaging

Multiple frames, typically 8 to 16, can be accurately registered and automatically averaged to reduce the speckle and background noise (snow-like texture) and improve the signal-to-noise ratio of the image. Comparison of a single-frame image and frame-averaged image shows improved delineation of corneal layers in the averaged image (see Figure 14-1). Frame averaging is useful in the identification of thin structures with low contrast, such as the LASIK flap interface, Bowman's layer, corneal endothelium, and trabecular meshwork.

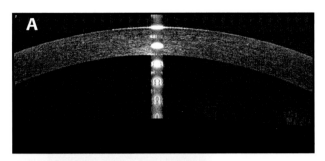

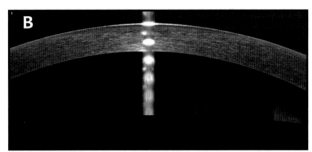

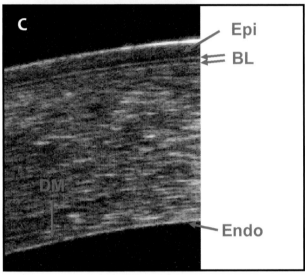

Figure 14-1. High-definition OCT image of a normal human cornea. (A) Single frame. (B) Average of 16 frames after registration. (C) Enlarged section of the frame-averaged image showing the epithelium (Epi), Bowman's layer (BL), Descemet's membrane (DM), and the endothelium (Endo). (Reprinted with permission from Huang D, ed. *RTVue Fourier-Domain Optical Coherence Tomography Primer Series: Cornea & Anterior Segment.* Fremont, CA: Optovue, Inc; 2008.)

Corneal Anatomy

In high-resolution, high-definition OCT images, one can clearly distinguish the epithelium, Bowman's layer, Descemet's membrane, and the endothelium (see Figure 14-1).

Mapping Corneal Thickness

The cornea can be mapped by raster or radial scans. Due to its dome shape, radial scans along meridional lines are best in providing shape and thickness measurements (Figure 14-2). The corneal thickness profile is measured by an automated algorithm that detects the anterior and posterior corneal boundaries on the cross-sectional images. A 6-mm diameter pachymetry map is formed by interpolation of the thickness profiles. We recommend using the pupil as the primary centration reference because the vertex can be shifted by surgery or disease. If the pupil is eccentric due to surgery or disease, then the vertex could be used as the centration landmark.

Corneal Power Measurement

High-speed OCT is able to directly measure the power of both anterior and posterior corneal surfaces. It is a logical improvement to conventional keratometry, which only measures the anterior surface. The corneal power measured by OCT is lower by 1.2 diopters compared to conventional keratometry using the conventional keratometric index of 1.3375.[4] The OCT measurement is probably more accurate, since the keratometric index was adapted by convenience and never adequately validated.[4,5] However, since most intraocular lens (IOL) power formulae are calibrated to conventional keratometry, OCT measurements need to be converted to the conventional keratometric equivalent before use in conventional IOL power formulae.

Angle Assessment

OCT systems working at 1310- and 830-nm wavelengths have been used to image the anterior chamber angle. The longer wavelength of 1310 nm penetrates more deeply through the sclera, limbus, angle, and iris (Figure 14-3).[6] Structures in the anterior chamber angle are clearly delineated including the scleral spur, ciliary body band, angle recess, and iris root.

The scleral spur marks the posterior boundary of the trabecular meshwork. It is highly reflective in 1310-nm OCT images. The quantitative angle parameters using the sclera spur as the landmark are as follows:

Figure 14-2. The RTVue pachymetry scan pattern (upper left) consists of 6-mm lines on 8 meridians. Each line consists of 1024 axial scans. The scan provides pachymetry maps shown both on a color scale (lower right) and in sector average (lower left). (Reprinted with permission from Huang D, ed. *RTVue Fourier-Domain Optical Coherence Tomography Primer Series: Cornea & Anterior Segment.* Fremont, CA: Optovue, Inc; 2008.)

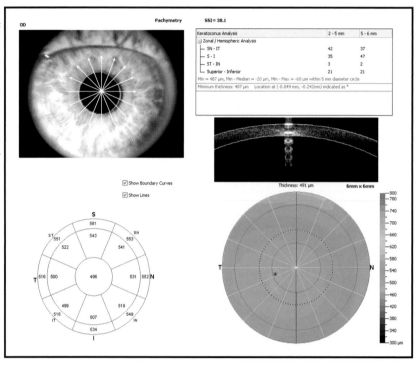

- **Angle opening distance by sclera spur at 500 or 750 μm (AOD-SS 500 or AOD-SS 750).** This parameter is defined as the linear distance between the trabecular meshwork and the iris at 500 or 750 μm anterior to the scleral spur. AOD-SS 500 is shown in Figure 14-4.
- **Angle recess area at 500 or 750 μm (ARA 500 or ARA 750).** The angle recess area is defined as the triangular area formed by the AOD-SS (the base), the angle recess (the apex), and the iris surface and the inner corneoscleral wall (sides of triangle). ARA 500 is shown in Figure 14-4.
- **Trabeculo-iris space area at 500 or 750 μm (TISA 500 or TISA 750).** This parameter is defined as the trapezoidal area with the following boundaries: anteriorly, the AOD-SS; posteriorly, a line drawn from the scleral spur perpendicular to the plane of the inner scleral wall to the opposing iris; superiorly, the inner corneoscleral wall; and inferiorly, the iris surface. TISA 500 is shown in Figure 14-4.

High-resolution OCT working at 830 nm cannot penetrate the sclera or iris, but it offers much higher resolution, which allows for visualization of very small anatomic details such as Schwalbe's line, Schlemm's canal, and the trabecular meshwork (Figures 14-5 and 14-6), which were not possible with previous generations of anterior segment OCT systems.[7,8]

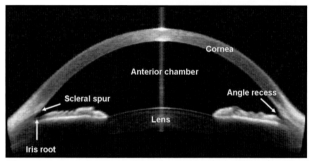

Figure 14-3. 1310-nm anterior segment OCT image illustrating structures in the anterior chamber angle. Eight frames have been averaged to obtain this image. (This article was published in *Ophthalmol Clin North Am*, 18, Radhakrishnan S, Huang D, Smith S, Optical coherence tomography imaging of the anterior chamber angle, 375-381, Copyright Elsevier 2005.)

The scleral spur cannot be clearly visualized on 830-nm wavelength images due to the greater scattering of light at the limbus. Schwalbe's line, which represents the termination of Descemet's membrane, however, is an anatomic feature that is consistently visible on all high-quality images (see Figures 14-5 and 14-6). Therefore, angle opening distance is best measured between Schwalbe's line and the anterior surface of the iris.

We have also used OCT to image the trabecular cleft after Trabectome (NeoMedix Corp, San Juan Capistrano, CA) surgery (Figure 14-7).

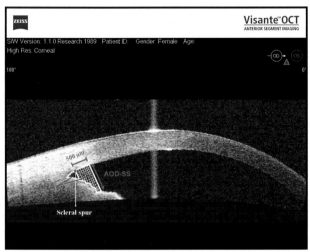

Figure 14-4. Visante OCT image of the anterior chamber angle illustrating the angle opening distance by scleral spur (AOD-SS), angle recess area (ARA), and trabeculo-iris space area (TISA). Note that the TISA does not include the area posterior to the scleral spur. (Reprinted with permission from Steinert R, Huang D, eds. *Anterior Segment Optical Coherence Tomography.* Thorofare, NJ: SLACK Incorporated; 2008.)

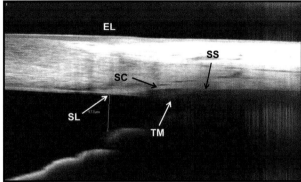

Figure 14-5. Cross-sectional OCT image of the nasal angle in a normal patient. The high resolution helps to visualize the termination of the endothelium and Descemet's membrane (Schwalbe's line [SL]). Also visible are the external limbus (EL), trabecular meshwork (TM), and the scleral spur (SS). The angle recess, iris root, and ciliary body are not visible due to blocking by the sclera. The angle opening distance between SL and the anterior surface of the iris (AOD-SL, yellow caliper line) was large, measuring 473 μm, indicating that the angle was open. (Reprinted with permission from Huang D, ed. *RTVue Fourier-Domain Optical Coherence Tomography Primer Series: Cornea & Anterior Segment.* Fremont, CA: Optovue, Inc; 2008.)

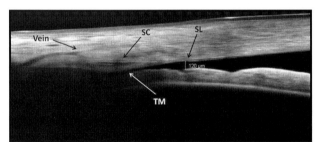

Figure 14-6. Cross-sectional OCT image of the nasal angle in an eye with narrow angle. Note the small distance between the trabecular meshwork (TM) and the iris, indicating a narrow, potentially occluded angle. The AOD-SL (dotted line) was narrow, measuring 120 μm. Also visible are Schlemm's canal (SC) and an aqueous collector vein. (Reprinted with permission from Huang D, ed. *RTVue Fourier-Domain Optical Coherence Tomography Primer Series: Cornea & Anterior Segment.* Fremont, CA: Optovue, Inc; 2008.)

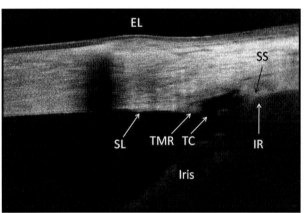

Figure 14-7. Cross-sectional OCT image of the nasal angle after Trabectome surgery. The shadowing in the peripheral cornea is caused by the limbal girdle of Vogt. The Trabectome removed the posterior trabecular meshwork, leaving a trabecular cleft (TC) of 374 μm in width and an anterior trabecular meshwork remnant (TMR). The iris root (IR) is very faint due to scleral shadowing but can be traced by contiguity with the iris. (Reprinted with permission from Huang D, ed. *RTVue Fourier-Domain Optical Coherence Tomography Primer Series: Cornea & Anterior Segment.* Fremont, CA: Optovue, Inc; 2008. Courtesy of Brian A. Francis, MD.)

Table 14-2
Cutoff Values for Optical Coherence Tomography Pachymetric Parameters

Pachymetric Parameters	Minimum	Minimum-Maximum	I-S	IT-SN
Cutoff (μm)	472	-62	-52	-51

I-S=inferior-superior octant difference, IT-SN=inferotemporal-superonasal octant difference.
The diagnostic cutoff threshold is 2.3 standard deviations below normal average (first percentile of normal distribution).
All measurements are made within the central 5-mm diameter of the map.

Refractive Surgery

LASIK Planning and Keratoconus Screening

Many refractive surgeons use ultrasound pachymetry or slit-based topography systems to measure central corneal thickness before LASIK. Although these are time-tested standards, the ultrasound probe only measures one point on the cornea at any one time. Any decentration in the manual probe placement could produce an overestimation of the central pachymetry because the peripheral cornea is thicker, or alternatively, it could miss peripheral thinning in cases of keratoconus. The OCT pachymetry map offers coverage over the central 6-mm diameter and automatically calculates the minimum thickness and the central thickness averaged over a central 2-mm diameter circle. Importantly, the measurement is centered over the pupil, which is also the landmark used for the excimer laser ablation. Pachymetric mapping by OCT is important in the planning of LASIK. It helps screen out patients with forme fruste keratoconus by detecting focal corneal thinning. It is also helpful in calculating the expected residual stromal bed thickness, which in standard practice is at least 250 μm in hopes of preventing post-LASIK ectasia. The reliability of TD-OCT pachymetric mapping has already been well established.[9] Although slit-scanning technology such as the Orbscan (Bausch & Lomb, Rochester, NY) and the Pentacam (Oculus, Wetzlar, Germany) can also produce a pachymetry map, these technologies have a tendency to underestimate corneal thickness in eyes that have undergone photorefractive keratectomy (PRK)[10-12] and LASIK[11-15] and in eyes with a corneal opacity.[16] This problem is especially relevant in retreatment procedures, when underestimation of corneal thickness could lead to an erroneous conclusion that further laser ablation would not be possible.

Keratoconus is the most important contraindication for laser refractive surgeries. Undetected corneal ectatic disorders can result in accelerated, progressive keratoectasia and unpredictable visual outcome after LASIK and PRK. Current detection of early-stage keratoconus (referred to as *forme fruste keratoconus* in the medical literature) relies primarily on Placido-ring-based corneal topography.[17-19] However, topography does not screen out all eyes at risk.[20] Corneal thinning is a characteristic feature of keratoconus. Studies show that the OCT pachymetric parameters listed in Table 14-2 are helpful in detecting keratoconic eccentric focal thinning patterns.[21] If one parameter is abnormal (lower than the cutoff value), the cornea is likely to have keratoconus. If 2 or more parameters are abnormal, then the eye is very likely to have keratoconus or other ectatic condition, such as pellucid marginal degeneration.[22]

LASIK Flap Measurement

To predict the residual stromal bed thickness, the surgeon needs to know the corneal thickness as well as the mean and standard deviation of the LASIK flap thickness for the microkeratome that will be used. We advise routine OCT scanning 1 week after LASIK to monitor the created flap thickness. At 1 week, surgically induced corneal hydration changes have mostly resolved, and the flap interface is still easily visible.[9] It is best to measure the flap thickness at this time before the interface reflectivity peak fades (Figure 14-8).

If the flap thickness is not measured at the 1-week post-LASIK visit, it is still possible to measure it at a later time. This is extremely useful to determine residual bed thickness calculations for any LASIK retreatment. Frame averaging of the OCT suppresses the speckle noise and enhances visualization of the flap interface (Figure 14-9). With this technique, it is sometimes possible to visualize the LASIK flap even 10 years later (Figure 14-10). In this

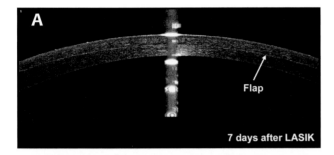

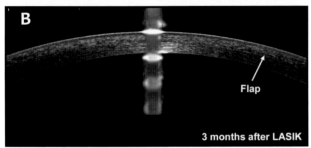

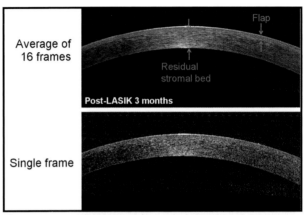

Figure 14-9. Three-month postoperative OCT image of a LASIK flap created by a mechanical microkeratome. The interface is more easily visible in the frame-averaged image (top, arrows) compared to the single-frame image (bottom). (Reprinted with permission from Huang D, ed. *RTVue Fourier-Domain Optical Coherence Tomography Primer Series: Cornea & Anterior Segment.* Fremont, CA: Optovue, Inc; 2008.)

Figure 14-8. OCT image of flap interface created with a mechanical microkeratome. (A) The interface has strong reflectivity 7 days after LASIK. (B) The interface is much fainter 3 months after LASIK, but it can still be seen and the flap thickness measured. (Reprinted with permission from Huang D, ed. *RTVue Fourier-Domain Optical Coherence Tomography Primer Series: Cornea & Anterior Segment.* Fremont, CA: Optovue, Inc; 2008.)

It is important to routinely monitor LASIK flap thickness because the actual result is often different from the microkeratome setting. For example, the Hansatome (Bausch & Lomb) typically produces flaps thinner than the nominal setting.[9] Even the femtosecond laser can occasionally create flaps that deviate significantly from the intended thickness, though on the whole the laser is more repeatable. In a consecutive series of 17 eyes, we found that the central flap thickness was 122.5 ± 8.5 µm (mean ± standard deviation), with a range of 113 to 144 µm using the 60 kHz Intralase femtosecond laser (Abbott Medical Optics Inc, Santa Ana, CA) set at 110-µm depth.

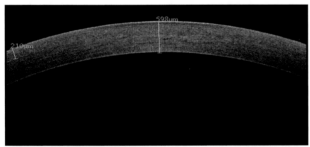

Figure 14-10. OCT image 10 years after LASIK. The flap interface is still visible in the periphery allowing measurement. (Reprinted with permission from Huang D, ed. *RTVue Fourier-Domain Optical Coherence Tomography Primer Series: Cornea & Anterior Segment.* Fremont, CA: Optovue, Inc; 2008. Courtesy of Perry Binder, MD.)

Post-LASIK Ectasia (Keratectasia)

Keratectasia after LASIK is most often caused by pre-existing forme fruste keratoconus or a thin residual posterior stromal bed.[20] It is similar to keratoconus in that the focal bulging and thinning tend to occur inferiorly or inferotemporally. However, the degree of thinning tends to be more severe in post-LASIK ectasia, as it is likely the result of both ectasia and laser ablation. In one example (Figure 14-11), the mechanically created flap was thick (204 to 225 µm) and the minimal corneal thickness was 194 µm based on OCT, far below the safe lower limit of 250 µm. This suggests that an excessively thick flap and insufficient residual stromal bed may

case, the flap thickness could be measured only in the periphery. Because the flap is relatively uniform, the surgeon could still estimate the central and minimum bed thickness by subtracting flap thickness from the central and minimum corneal thicknesses on the pachymetry map.

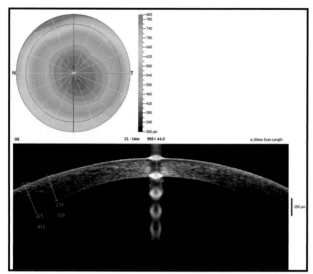

Figure 14-11. A case of keratectasia imaged 2 years after LASIK. (A) OCT pachymetry map showed a minimum thickness of 398 μm. (B) Frame-averaged horizontal section showed the central flap thickness and stromal bed thickness were both 204 μm. (Reprinted with permission from Huang D, ed. *RTVue Fourier-Domain Optical Coherence Tomography Primer Series: Cornea & Anterior Segment.* Fremont, CA: Optovue, Inc; 2008.)

have caused the keratectasia. It is important to note that the minimum corneal thickness on the Orbscan was only 320 μm, which usually indicates the ectasia was too advanced to be treated by intracorneal ring (ICR) segment implantation. However, the pachymetry map showed the minimum thickness to be 398 μm, which indicates a less severe degree of ectasia that might be amenable to ICR treatment rather than corneal transplantation. Of course, a rigid gas-permeable contact lens should be tried before any surgical intervention is considered. This case demonstrates the value of OCT in the evaluation and management of keratectasia.

Diffuse Lamellar Keratitis

In a case of bilateral diffuse lamellar keratoplasty after femtosecond laser-assisted LASIK, high-resolution OCT (Figure 14-12) revealed inflammation that involved the center of the cornea and the stroma on both sides of the flap interface.

Epithelial Ingrowth

Epithelial ingrowth appears as a moderately reflective area in the interface that contains highly reflective foci (equivalent to opaque "pearls" seen on

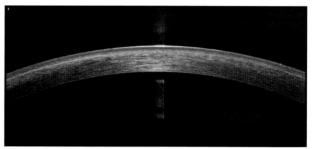

Figure 14-12. Diffuse lamellar keratitis, grade 3, 2 days after LASIK with femtosecond laser flap creation. The OCT image shows a hyperreflective flap interface. Stromal reflectivity was also increased in both the flap and bed, including the center. (Reprinted with permission from Huang D, ed. *RTVue Fourier-Domain Optical Coherence Tomography Primer Series: Cornea & Anterior Segment.* Fremont, CA: Optovue, Inc; 2008.)

slit-lamp examination [Figure 14-13]).[23] The thickness and width of epithelial ingrowth can be measured with OCT, which could be helpful in deciding whether surgical removal is necessary.

Interface Fluid Syndrome

In a case of post-LASIK interface fluid syndrome[21] associated with diffuse lamellar keratitis and steroid-induced ocular hypertension, OCT showed the interface fluid, epithelial ingrowth, and noncellular reflective deposits (Figure 14-14).

Photorefractive Keratectomy

High-resolution OCT provides the means for measuring epithelial hyperplasia and deposition of extracellular material that can be associated with clinical haze (Figure 14-15). The measurement of epithelial thickness and the opacity's depth could be helpful in the planning of a transepithelial PRK or phototherapeutic keratectomy (PTK) to correct irregular astigmatism or a residual refractive error.

Phakic Intraocular Lenses

Besides imaging the cornea and angle, OCT can also image the posterior chamber and lens. For example, OCT documented the presence of a good vault between an implantable collamer lens (Visian, STAAR Surgical Co, Monrovia, CA) and the natural crystalline lens (Figure 14-16). An adequate distance between the implanted lens and the crystalline lens is needed to avoid cataract formation.

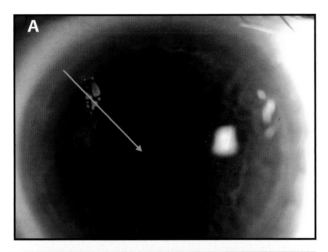

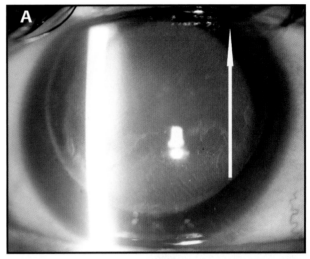

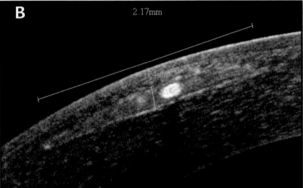

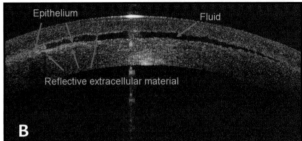

Figure 14-13. Epithelial ingrowth under a LASIK flap. (A) Slit-lamp photograph. (B) OCT sections along radial lines. The computer caliper measured the ingrowth to be 2.1 mm transversely and 124-μm thick. The characteristic opaque pearls within the ingrowth are visible in both images. (Reprinted with permission from Huang D, ed. *RTVue Fourier-Domain Optical Coherence Tomography Primer Series: Cornea & Anterior Segment.* Fremont, CA: Optovue, Inc; 2008.)

Figure 14-14. Interface fluid syndrome. (A) Slit-lamp photography on post-LASIK day 49 shows flap edema, interface fluid, and several zones of opacity. Inferiorly, there was a dense opacity. (B) OCT shows areas of epithelial ingrowth and fluid under the LASIK flap interspersed with streaks and pearls of clear material. The central and superior areas of fluid accumulation are associated with scattered granular haze. The arrow in A shows the OCT scan length and direction. (Reprinted with permission from Ramos JL, Zhou S, Yo C, Tang M, Huang D. High-resolution imaging of complicated LASIK flap interface fluid syndrome. *Ophthalmic Surg Lasers Imaging.* 2008;39[4 suppl]:S80-S82.)

Intracorneal Implants

Although slit-lamp examination can provide a rough sense of implant depth, OCT provides high-resolution images in which the depth of intracorneal implants can be precisely measured. Our experience shows that OCT provides more accurate measurement of depth than slit-lamp estimation.[24] This knowledge will help cornea surgeons improve their techniques while addressing depth-related problems earlier.

Intacs (Addition Technology, Des Plaines, IL) segments appear as dark spaces within the corneal stroma on OCT. In a case of Intacs implantation with femtosecond laser channel dissection, the depth of the implant was 62% according to OCT (Figure 14-17), close to the 70% target depth.

Corneal Pathologies and Surgeries

Corneal Opacities

OCT provides accurate measurements of the depth of corneal opacities. This can be helpful in the preoperative planning by allowing the surgeon to choose between an ablative therapy such as PTK if the residual stromal bed thickness will be greater than 250 μm or an excisional therapy such as anterior lamellar keratoplasty or penetrating keratoplasty if the residual stromal bed thickness will be less than

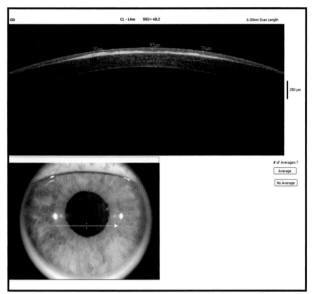

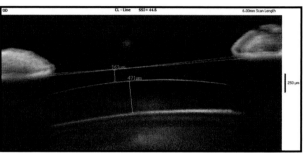

Figure 14-16. Horizontal OCT section showing good clearance of the sulcus-based phakic IOL over the natural crystalline lens. The central IOL thickness was 161 μm, and the distance between the IOL and the crystalline lens was 471 μm as measured by computer calipers (gold lines). (Reprinted with permission from Huang D, ed. *RTVue Fourier-Domain Optical Coherence Tomography Primer Series: Cornea & Anterior Segment.* Fremont, CA: Optovue, Inc; 2008. Courtesy of Juan Gabriel Ortiz [Imex].)

Figure 14-15. Horizontal OCT section (upper) after PRK showing severe subepithelial fibrosis under a thickened epithelium. The epithelial thickness varied from 30 to 95 μm. The direction of the scan is shown by the arrow on the video image (lower). (Reprinted with permission from Huang D, ed. *RTVue Fourier-Domain Optical Coherence Tomography Primer Series: Cornea & Anterior Segment.* Fremont, CA: Optovue, Inc; 2008. Courtesy of Stephen Trokel, MD, Harkness Eye Institute, Columbia University.)

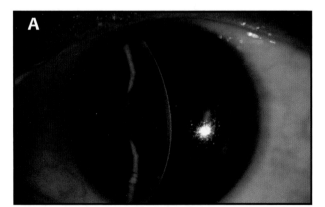

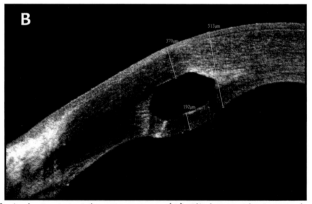

Figure 14-17. A single Intacs segment was implanted inferiorly to treat keratoconus. (A) Slit-lamp photograph shows the depth to be approximately 70%. (B) Radial OCT section of the implant. Implant depth is best measured at the inner edge to avoid distortion caused by refraction at the cornea-implant boundary. The depth from the anterior corneal surface to the inner edge of the segment was 513 μm, and the distance from the edge to the endothelium was 313 μm. The fractional depth was 62% (513 / [513 + 313]). (Reprinted with permission from Huang D, ed. *RTVue Fourier-Domain Optical Coherence Tomography Primer Series: Cornea & Anterior Segment.* Fremont, CA: Optovue, Inc; 2008.)

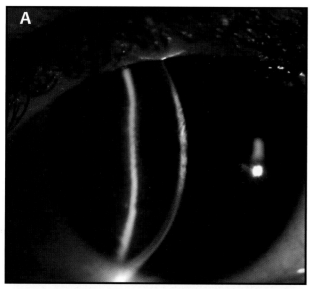

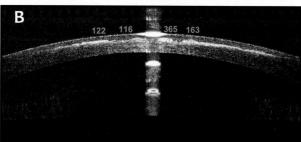

Figure 14-18. Corneal opacity. (A) Slit-lamp photograph of post-PRK haze. The photograph shows the presence of haze in the anterior stroma. (B) OCT of vertical sections of the cornea. Computer calipers were used to measure the opacity depth, epithelial thickness, and corneal thickness. The measured opacity depth ranged from 122 to 163 μm. (Reprinted with permission from Huang D, ed. *RTVue Fourier-Domain Optical Coherence Tomography Primer Series: Cornea & Anterior Segment.* Fremont, CA: Optovue, Inc; 2008.)

250 μm. The use of OCT in treatment planning is illustrated in the following examples.

Example 1

A 41-year-old male was referred for subepithelial haze 11 months after PRK enhancement for myopic regression in the left eye (Figure 14-18). The best spectacle-corrected visual acuity was reduced to 20/100. OCT images showed that the opacity was relatively deep (122 to 163 μm), and the central cornea was thin (365 to 368 μm). It was not possible to perform an ablative procedure to remove most of the opacity without maintaining at least 250 μm of residual stromal thickness. The eye was treated

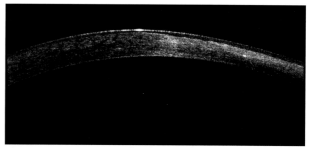

Figure 14-19. Horizontal OCT section of a corneal opacity secondary to contact lens-related bacterial keratitis. The scan showed that the opacity was full thickness. (Reprinted with permission from Huang D, ed. *RTVue Fourier-Domain Optical Coherence Tomography Primer Series: Cornea & Anterior Segment.* Fremont, CA: Optovue, Inc; 2008.)

with topical corticosteroid, and the resulting best-corrected visual acuity (BCVA) was 20/25.

Example 2

A 70-year-old female presented with a long-standing corneal scar secondary to contact lens-related bacterial keratitis. BCVA was 20/70 in the affected eye. OCT showed a full-thickness corneal opacity (Figure 14-19). The patient underwent penetrating keratoplasty.

Example 3

A 50-year-old female presented with granular corneal dystrophy and recurrent corneal erosion in both eyes. The left eye was worse, with a BCVA of 20/80. The OCT image showed multiple hyperreflective deposits in the anterior stroma under a layer of a subepithelial opacity (Figure 14-20). The OCT pachymetry map showed that PTK was a safe option with regard to residual thickness. Transepithelial PTK with adjunctive mitomycin-C was performed to remove the subepithelial opacity and smooth the anterior stromal surface. The postoperative BCVA in the left eye was 20/30.

Endothelial Keratoplasty

Since the inception of modern posterior lamellar keratoplasty in the late 1990s by Melles, the technique has undergone several cycles of refinement to Descemet's stripping automated endothelial keratoplasty (DSAEK).[25] The primary advantages of DSAEK over penetrating keratoplasty are a smaller and more secure wound, lower postoperative astigmatism, and faster visual rehabilitation.[26]

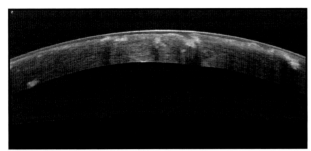

Figure 14-20. Horizontal OCT section from a granular dystrophy patient. The scan shows the presence of deposits in the anterior stroma. (Reprinted with permission from Huang D, ed. *RTVue Fourier-Domain Optical Coherence Tomography Primer Series: Cornea & Anterior Segment.* Fremont, CA: Optovue, Inc; 2008.)

Postoperative OCT scans can be used to monitor the detachment of the donor lenticule in patients with persistent postoperative corneal edema (Figure 14-21). It is also useful in tracking the postoperative corneal deturgescence, assessing the uniformity of the endothelial graft thickness, and measuring the postoperative posterior corneal curvature.

Femtosecond Laser-Assisted Keratoplasty

Penetrating keratoplasty is undergoing a phase of evolution thanks to the ability to make shaped incisions using a femtosecond laser such as the Intralase. A concern of traditional penetrating keratoplasty performed using trephine blades is the slow wound healing and the weak host-donor junction. Shaped incisions such as the zigzag, top hat, and mushroom configurations created using the femtosecond laser result in greater resistance to wound leakage when compared to traditional penetrating keratoplasty. The wound may also be stronger and heal faster due to the interlocking host-donor junction and greater wound contact area. Proper apposition of the interlocking wound can be visualized with OCT (Figure 14-22).

This chapter was based on studies supported by NIH grants R01 EY018184 and P30 EY03040; a grant from Optovue, Inc; a grant from Carl Zeiss Meditec, Inc; and the Charles C. Manger III, MD, Chair in Corneal Laser Surgery endowment (held by Dr. David Huang).

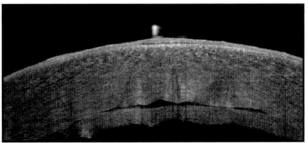

Figure 14-21. Horizontal OCT section showing detachment of donor lenticule 2 weeks following DSAEK. The 72-year-old female continued to have persistent postoperative edema 2 weeks after DSAEK OD. The scan shows a subtle detachment of the donor lenticule with overlying epithelial and stromal edema. The lenticule attached spontaneously resulting in an improvement in the edema at 1-month postoperative. (Reprinted with permission from Huang D, ed. *RTVue Fourier-Domain Optical Coherence Tomography Primer Series: Cornea & Anterior Segment.* Fremont, CA: Optovue, Inc; 2008.)

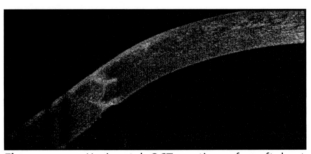

Figure 14-22. Horizontal OCT section of graft host junction 1 month after suture removal following femtosecond laser-assisted keratoplasty. The zigzag wound architecture is visible on OCT imaging. (Reprinted with permission from Huang D, ed. *RTVue Fourier-Domain Optical Coherence Tomography Primer Series: Cornea & Anterior Segment.* Fremont, CA: Optovue, Inc; 2008.)

References

1. Huang D, Swanson EA, Lin CP, et al. Optical coherence tomography. *Science.* 1991;254(5035):1178-1181.
2. Tang M, Li Y, Avila M, Huang D. Measuring total corneal power before and after laser in situ keratomileusis with high-speed optical coherence tomography. *J Cataract Refract Surg.* 2006;32(11):1843-1850.
3. Westphal V, Rollins AM, Radhakrishnan S, Izatt JA. Correction of geometric and refractive image distortions in optical coherence tomography applying Fermat's principle. *Opt Express.* 2002;10(9):397-404.
4. Bennett AG, Rabbetts RB. *Clinical Visual Optics.* 3rd ed. Oxford, England: Butterworth-Heinemann; 1998:387-388.

5. Gobbi PG, Carones F, Brancato R. Keratometric index, video-keratography, and refractive surgery. *J Cataract Refract Surg.* 1998;24(2):202-211.

6. Radhakrishnan S, Huang D, Smith S. Optical coherence tomography imaging of the anterior chamber angle. *Ophthalmol Clin North Am.* 2005;18(3):375-381.

7. Huang D, Li Y, Radhakrishnan S. Optical coherence tomography of the anterior segment of the eye. *Ophthalmol Clin North Am.* 2004;17(1):1-6.

8. Radhakrishnan S, Goldsmith J, Huang D, et al. Comparison of optical coherence tomography and ultrasound biomicroscopy for detection of narrow anterior chamber angles. *Arch Ophthalmol.* 2005;123(8):1053-1059.

9. Li Y, Netto MV, Shekhar R, et al. A longitudinal study of LASIK flap and stromal thickness with high-speed optical coherence tomography. *Ophthalmology.* 2007;114(6):1124-1132.

10. Boscia F, La Tegola MG, Alessio G, Sborgia C. Accuracy of Orbscan optical pachymetry in corneas with haze. *J Cataract Refract Surg.* 2002;28(2):253-258.

11. Fakhry MA, Artola A, Belda JI, et al. Comparison of corneal pachymetry using ultrasound and Orbscan II. *J Cataract Refract Surg.* 2002;28(2):248-252.

12. Prisant O, Calderon N, Chastang P, et al. Reliability of pachymetric measurements using Orbscan after excimer refractive surgery. *Ophthalmology.* 2003;110(3):511-515.

13. Chakrabarti HS, Craig JP, Brahma A, et al. Comparison of corneal thickness measurements using ultrasound and Orbscan slit-scanning topography in normal and post-LASIK eyes. *J Cataract Refract Surg.* 2001;27(11):1823-1828.

14. Iskander NG, Anderson Penno E, Peters NT, et al. Accuracy of Orbscan pachymetry measurements and DHG ultrasound pachymetry in primary laser in situ keratomileusis and LASIK enhancement procedures. *J Cataract Refract Surg.* 2001;27(5):681-685.

15. Kawana K, Tokunaga T, Miyata K, et al. Comparison of corneal thickness measurements using Orbscan II, non-contact specular microscopy, and ultrasonic pachymetry in eyes after laser in situ keratomileusis. *Br J Ophthalmol.* 2004;88(4):466-468.

16. Khurana RN, Li Y, Tang M, Lai MM, Huang D. High-speed optical coherence tomography of corneal opacities. *Ophthalmology.* 2007;114(7):1278-1285.

17. Li X, Rabinowitz YS, Rasheed K, Yang H. Longitudinal study of the normal eyes in unilateral keratoconus patients. *Ophthalmology.* 2004;111(3):440-446.

18. Erie JC, Patel SV, McLaren JW, et al. Effect of myopic laser in situ keratomileusis on epithelial and stromal thickness: a confocal microscopy study. *Ophthalmology.* 2002;109(8):1447-1452.

19. Maeda N, Klyce SD, Smolek MK, Thompson HW. Automated keratoconus screening with corneal topography analysis. *Invest Ophthalmol Vis Sci.* 1994;35(6):2749-2757.

20. Randleman JB, Russell B, Ward MA, et al. Risk factors and prognosis for corneal ectasia after LASIK. *Ophthalmology.* 2003;110(2):267-275.

21. Li Y, Tang M, Zhang X, et al. Pachymetric mapping with Fourier-domain optical coherence tomography. *J Cataract Refract Surg.* 2010;36:834-839.

22. Li Y, Meisler DM, Tang M, et al. Keratoconus diagnosis with optical coherence tomography pachymetry mapping. *Ophthalmology.* 2008;115(12):2159-2166.

23. Ustundag C, Bahcecioglu H, Ozdamar A, et al. Optical coherence tomography for evaluation of anatomical changes in the cornea after laser in situ keratomileusis. *J Cataract Refract Surg.* 2000;26(10):1458-1462.

24. Lai MM, Tang M, Andrade EM, et al. Optical coherence tomography to assess intrastromal corneal ring segment depth in keratoconic eyes. *J Cataract Refract Surg.* 2006;32(11):1860-1865.

25. Melles GR, Wijdh RH, Nieuwendaal CP. A technique to excise the descemet membrane from a recipient cornea (descemetorhexis). *Cornea.* 2004;23(3):286-288.

26. Thompson RW Jr, Choi DM, Price MO, et al. Noncontact optical coherence tomography for measurement of corneal flap and residual stromal bed thickness after laser in situ keratomileusis. *J Refract Surg.* 2003;19(5):507-515.

Section IV

Appendices

Physical Principles of Optical Coherence Tomography

Bernhard Baumann, PhD; James G. Fujimoto, PhD;
David Huang, MD, PhD; Jay S. Duker, MD; Eric Swanson, MS;
Carmen A. Puliafito, MD, MBA; and Joel S. Schuman, MD

- Introduction
- Optical Interferometry
- Low-Coherence Interferometry—Measurement of Light Echoes and Axial Resolution
- Principles of Fourier-Domain Optical Coherence Tomography—Measuring Echoes in the Spectral Domain
- Transverse Spatial Resolution
- Image Acquisition Time and Axial Scan Densities
- Three-Dimensional Optical Coherence Tomography Imaging
- Image Analysis and Display
- Image Averaging
- Advances in Optical Coherence Tomography Technology
- Conclusion

Introduction

Optical coherence tomography (OCT) is analogous to ultrasound imaging except that it measures the echo time delay and magnitude of light rather than sound.[1-3] OCT can achieve axial image resolutions of 1 to 10 µm, which is 1 to 2 orders of magnitude finer than standard clinical ultrasound. In tissues other than the eye, the maximum imaging depth is limited to approximately 2 to 3 mm by attenuation from light scattering. Although this depth is shallow when compared to other clinical imaging techniques, OCT can achieve resolutions 10x to 100x finer than conventional ultrasound, magnetic resonance imaging (MRI), or computed tomography (CT). OCT imaging has been termed *optical biopsy* because it provides images of tissue pathology in situ and in real time, without the need to remove and process specimens, which is required in excisional biopsy and histopathology.[4,5]

OCT imaging has several features that are attractive for medical imaging, including the following:
- OCT can perform imaging with resolutions approaching conventional histopathology.
- Imaging can be performed in situ and in real time.
- Imaging may be performed using a wide range of instruments such as ophthalmoscopes, microscopes, hand-held probes, endoscopes, catheters, laparoscopes, and needles.
- OCT can perform functional imaging such as spectroscopic imaging, Doppler blood flow imaging, and the measurement of blood oxygenation or tissue birefringence.
- Computer image-processing algorithms can be used to quantitatively assess OCT images and to generate objective diagnostic information.

Figure A-1 shows a collage of OCT images illustrating different applications.[1,5-9] OCT promises to have clinical applications in 3 general scenarios:

Schuman JS, Puliafito CA, Fujimoto JG, Duker JS, eds.
Optical Coherence Tomography of Ocular Diseases,
Third Edition (pp 565-590).
© 2013 SLACK Incorporated.

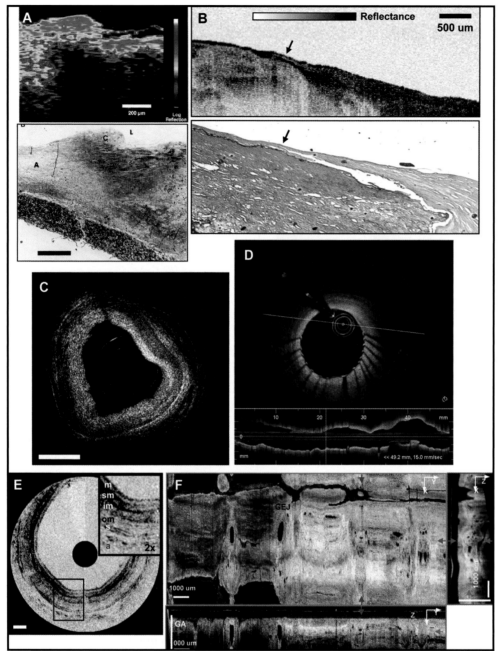

Figure A-1. (A) First demonstration of OCT imaging showing calcified arterial plaque. (Reprinted with permission from Huang D, Swanson EA, Lin CP, et al. Optical coherence tomography. *Science*. 1991;254:1178-1181.) (B) Early OCT image and histology illustrating vulnerable plaque with a thin intimal cap layer. (Reprinted with permission from Brezinski ME, Tearney GJ, Bouma BE, et al. Optical coherence tomography for optical biopsy: properties and demonstration of vascular pathology. *Circulation*. 1996;93:1206-1213.) (C) First demonstration of catheter-based intravascular imaging ex vivo. (Reprinted with permission from Tearney GJ, Brezinski ME, Boppart SA, et al. Catheter-based optical imaging of a human coronary artery. *Circulation*. 1996;94:3013.) (D) Example of state-of-the-art intravascular imaging in human patients. (Reprinted with permission from LightLab Imaging/St. Jude Medical.) (E) First demonstration of endoscopic OCT imaging in an animal. (Reprinted with permission from Tearney GJ, Brezinski ME, Bouma BE, et al. In vivo endoscopic optical biopsy with optical coherence tomography. *Science*. 1997;276:2037-2039.) (F) Example of state-of-the-art high speed endoscopic OCT imaging in human patients showing 3D-OCT and en face projection. (Reprinted with permission from Adler DC, Zhou C, Tsai TH, et al. Three-dimensional optical coherence tomography of Barrett's esophagus and buried glands beneath neosquamous epithelium following radiofrequency ablation. *Endoscopy*. 2009;41:773-776.)

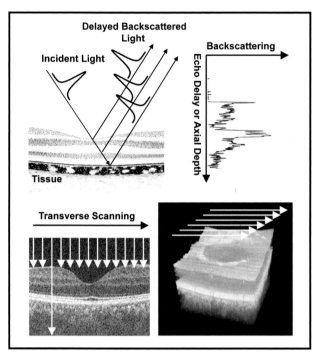

Figure A-2. OCT performs high-resolution, cross-sectional, and 3D imaging of the internal tissue structure by measuring the echo time delay and intensity of backscattered or backreflected light. (Top) Axial scans, measurements of backscattering versus depth, are the basic unit of OCT images. (Bottom left) 2D cross-sectional images are generated by transverse scanning the optical beam and sequentially acquiring axial scans. The data are displayed with a logarithmic grayscale or false-color scale representing intensity. (Bottom right) 3D or volumetric data sets can be acquired by recording a stack of images using a raster scan.

1. To image tissue pathology when excisional biopsy is hazardous or impossible, such as in ophthalmology or intravascular imaging
2. To guide interventional procedures
3. To reduce sampling errors and associated false negatives that can occur with excisional biopsy

Figure A-2 shows a schematic summarizing the principles of OCT imaging. A beam of light is directed onto the tissue or specimen to be imaged. The internal structure is measured noninvasively by measuring the echo delay time and magnitude of light, which is backreflected or backscattered from microstructural features at different depths. Two-dimensional (2D) imaging is accomplished by performing successive axial (longitudinal) measurements at different transverse positions and by displaying the resulting data as a 2D cross-sectional

image.[1,10-12] Three-dimensional (3D) imaging of tissues can be performed by recording a stack of such 2D images. This appendix provides detailed information on the physical principles of OCT, including how OCT detects echoes of light, as well as what determines the resolution, sensitivity, and speed of OCT imaging systems.

Optical Interferometry

In order to perform OCT imaging, it is first necessary to perform high-resolution measurements of the echo delay time of backreflected or backscattered light from inside tissue. Because light travels much faster than sound, direct electronic measurement of optical echoes is not possible. In OCT, measurements of optical echoes are performed using a correlation technique known as *low-coherence interferometry*. Low-coherence interferometry is a simple method that can measure distances to objects with high precision by measuring light reflected from them and correlating it with light that travels a known reference path delay.[13-15]

Light is a wave. A beam of light is composed of electric and magnetic fields that oscillate, periodically varying in time and in space.[13] Light can be characterized by its frequency, v, or its wavelength, λ. Light propagates with a characteristic velocity that is determined by the medium in which it is propagating. In a vacuum, the velocity of light is $c = 3 \times 10^8$ m/sec. In media such as water, vitreous, or glass, the velocity of light is slower than if it propagates in vacuum. The velocity of light in a medium is c/n, where n is the index of refraction of the medium. Because OCT measures echo time delays, the axial delay in an OCT image must be scaled by $1/n$ in order to obtain the physical dimension. This is analogous to ultrasound in which measurements of dimensions require knowledge of the sound-wave velocity.

Equation A-1 shows the mathematical form of the oscillating electric field in a light wave:

$$E(t) = E \cos [(2\pi v)t - (2\pi/\lambda)z] \qquad \text{(A-1.)}$$

Because light is a wave composed of oscillating electric and magnetic fields, a phenomenon known as *interference* can occur when 2 light beams originating from the same light source are combined. The electric and magnetic fields that compose the 2 light beams can add either constructively or destructively according to the relative phase of their oscillations. When 2 light beams are added so that their fields are in phase and tend to add, constructive interference occurs and the resulting light is more intense. Conversely, when beams of light are added so that their fields are out of phase and tend to cancel, destructive interference occurs and the resulting light is less intense.

An optical interferometer functions by adding or interfering the light waves from 2 light beams.[13] Figure A-3 shows a schematic diagram of a simple Michelson-type interferometer. A light wave is incident onto a partially reflecting mirror or beamsplitter that splits the light into 2 beams: one acts as a reference beam, while the other acts a measurement or signal beam. The light beams travel given distances in the 2 paths or arms of the interferometer. The measurement light beam is backreflected or backscattered from the tissue being imaged creating the signal light beam $E_{sample}(t)$, while the reference light beam $E_{reference}(t)$ is reflected from the reference mirror.

The signal and reference light beams are then interfered or added at the partially reflecting mirror (beamsplitter), and the intensity of the resulting interferometer output beam is measured by a photodetector. The output of the interferometer is light with an electric field $E_{out}(t)$ that is the sum of the fields from the signal and reference light beams. Equation A-2 gives the mathematical form of the electric field of the output light from the interferometer $E_{out}(t)$:

$$E_{out}(t) \sim E_{reference}(t) + E_{sample}(t) \qquad \text{(A-2.)}$$

The detector measures the intensity of the output light from the interferometer. The intensity of light is proportional to the square of the electric field. For the purposes of this analysis, let us assume that the reflected signal light beam consists of a single reflection at a given distance, rather than multiple echoes, as would be the case in an actual imaging measurement. If the length of the signal path is z_{sample} and the length of the reference path is $z_{reference}$, then the path difference is $\Delta z = z_{sample} - z_{reference}$. The output intensity from the interferometer will oscillate as a function of the path difference Δz because of interference effects. Equation A-3 gives the output intensity of the interferometer as a function of E_{sample}, $E_{reference}$, and Δz as:

$$I_{out}(t) \sim \tfrac{1}{4} \left| E_{reference} \right|^2 + \tfrac{1}{4} \left| E_{sample} \right|^2$$
$$+ \tfrac{1}{2} E_{reference} \, E_{sample} \cos \left[(2\pi/\lambda)(2\Delta z) \right] \qquad \text{(A-3.)}$$

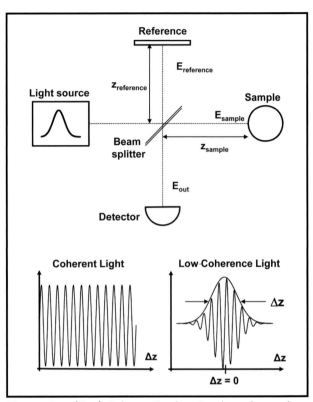

Figure A-3. (Top) Schematic showing how low-coherence interferometry measures echo delays. A beam from a light source is split into a reference and measurement beam by a partially reflecting mirror (beamsplitter). The measurement beam is backscattered or backreflected from tissue at a distance z_{sample} to produce an optical echo signal, while the reference beam is reflected from a mirror at a variable distance $z_{reference}$. The reference and sample light waves are combined and interfere. The interferometer output intensity is measured by a photodetector. (Bottom) If coherent light is used, then interference occurs between the reference and sample beams. The output intensity oscillates as the path length difference $\Delta z = z_{sample} - z_{reference}$ between the reference and sample paths is varied. In contrast, if low-coherence light is used, interference effects are only observed when the path length difference is less than the coherence length of the light. Coherence is a statistical property of the light and is related to statistical phase changes in the light waves. Low-coherence interferometry enables precise measurement of the echo delay of light.

If the position of the reference mirror is varied or scanned, the path length that the light travels in the reference arm will change, and the reference light will have a variable time delay. The reference light can add either destructively or constructively to the measurement light from the specimen. Interference will be observed in the output intensity as the length of the reference path is changed by translating the reference mirror. This is shown schematically in Figure A-3. The output signal oscillates between maximum and minimum as the total path difference traveled changes by one optical wavelength or the position of the reference mirror changes by one-half of an optical wavelength.

Low-Coherence Interferometry— Measurement of Light Echoes and Axial Resolution

If the light source used for the interferometer is coherent and has a long coherence length, then interference oscillations will be observed for a wide range of relative path length differences, Δz, of the reference and signal paths. However, for applications in optical ranging or OCT, it is necessary to precisely measure the absolute position of a structure within the tissue. In this case, light with a short-coherence length, or low-coherence light, is used. Strictly speaking, coherence is a statistical property of light; however, it is convenient to think of it as the ability of light to interfere. Low-coherence light is composed of an oscillating electric field that has rapid statistical changes in phase as a function of time and space. Low-coherence light is not a single frequency or wavelength but is composed of a distribution or bandwidth of multiple different frequencies or wavelengths. The coherence of light can be characterized by a distance, the coherence length, over which the light is coherent and does not have statistical phase discontinuities. The coherence length is inversely proportional to its frequency or wavelength content (bandwidth). The wider the wavelength range in the spectrum of the light source, the shorter its coherence length. Conceptually, it is also possible to think of low-coherence light as being composed of a continuous series of short optical pulses or fluctuations that have durations equal to the coherence length. This coherence length determines the axial resolution of OCT imaging.

When low-coherence light is used in the interferometer, interference only occurs when the path lengths of the reference and signal paths are closely matched to within the coherence length of the light (Δz is less than the coherence length). If the path lengths differ by a larger amount, then the fields from the 2 beams are not coherent or correlated, and there is no interference. This is shown schematically in Figure A-3 (bottom). When the interferometer paths are nearly matched in length, Δz small, complete destructive or constructive interference between the reference and signal beams is observed when the reference path length is scanned. However, when the path length difference, and hence the time delay difference, between the reference beam and the measurement beam is larger than the coherence length, no interference occurs. When the delay line in the reference arm is axially scanned, every backscattering or backreflecting site in the sample will produce an interference signal when the z_{sample} and $z_{reference}$ match. Scanning the reference path length measures the echoes of light sequentially.

The length Δz over which interference occurs is determined by the coherence length of the light and defines the axial resolution in OCT. Because low-coherence length light contains a spread of frequencies or wavelengths, it can also be characterized by its frequency or wavelength bandwidth. Theoretical calculations show that the axial resolution Δz is related to the wavelength bandwidth $\Delta\lambda$ by Equation A-4:

$$\Delta z = (2 \ln 2/\pi)(\lambda^2/\Delta\lambda) \qquad \text{(A-4.)}$$

Equation A-4 shows that the axial resolution Δz is inversely proportional to the full width at half maximum of the wavelength bandwidth $\Delta\lambda$ of the light source. A typical superluminescent diode light source for commercial ophthalmic OCT instruments operates in near-infrared wavelengths at ~840 nm and has a wavelength bandwidth of ~50 nm. This yields an axial resolution of ~6 μm in air. Because the speed of light is slower in tissue, the axial dimension is divided by the index of refraction of the tissue to give an axial resolution of ~4.5 μm. It is possible to significantly improve the axial resolution of OCT by using new light sources that have broader bandwidths and shorter coherence lengths. Axial image resolutions as fine as 1 to 3 μm have been achieved in research OCT systems using short-pulse laser light sources with bandwidths of 100 to 200 nm.[16-18]

The echo time delay of light can be determined by measuring the interference at the output of the interferometer as the reference arm path length is scanned. The interferometer effectively measures the echo time delay and magnitude of light by correlating the backreflected or backscattered light with reference light that has a known delay. Since each axial or depth profile is recorded as a function of time (ie, in the time domain [TD]), this type of OCT echo detection technique is referred to as *TD detection.*

In order to obtain high-quality OCT images, it is necessary to achieve extremely high detection sensitivities. For ophthalmic imaging, high sensitivity is required because the retina is nominally transparent and the intensity of weak backreflections and backscattering is extremely low. For imaging other tissues that are optically scattering, the sensitivity determines the maximum imaging depth in the tissue, because the incident light is attenuated by absorption and scattering in tissue. OCT uses a technique known as *optical heterodyne detection,* the same detection technique developed for optical communications systems. OCT can achieve high detection sensitivity to weak backreflected or backscattered light approaching detection limits set by fundamental quantum mechanical principles. The process of performing interferometry provides an amplification of weak optical signals. This can be seen by examining the expression (see Equation A-3) for the interferometer output intensity. The interference term of the output signal is proportional to $E_{reference}E_{sample}$. This is the result of interference of the electric field E_{sample} from the backreflected or backscattered beam from the tissue, multiplied by the electric field $E_{reference}$ of the reference beam. The signal from the tissue E_{sample} can be weak, but it is multiplied by the strong electric field $E_{reference}$ from the reference beam, thereby increasing the magnitude of the oscillating interference term measured by the photodetector. In addition, the interferometer measures the field of the backscattered or backreflected light rather than the intensity. Since the intensity of light is given by the square of its electric field, a high sensitivity and dynamic range can be achieved. For example, a detection sensitivity of 10^{-5} for the electric field corresponds to a sensitivity of 10^{-10} for the intensity.

Figure A-4 shows a schematic of how the echo time delay and magnitude are measured from the interferometer output signal as the path length difference is scanned.[19] The reference mirror is usually scanned at a constant velocity, v, which causes interference to be generated at a frequency $2v/\lambda$. The scanning reference mirror can also be thought of as Doppler shifting the reflected reference light beam. When this reference light interferes with the signal light, the interference oscillates at the Doppler frequency $2v/\lambda$. The axial profile of the echo time delay, the axial scan (A-scan), can be measured by electronically filtering and demodulating the photodetector signal. The process of demodulation cor-

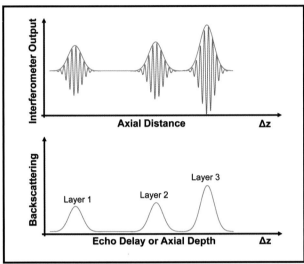

Figure A-4. Measurement of an axial scan, echo magnitude versus time delay or depth, from the interferometer output signal. The echo signal can be measured by demodulating or extracting the envelope (red line) of the interference signal. The interferometer output is proportional to the product of the sample and reference fields, so the interferometer measures the field of the echo light wave. The measurement is closely related to a technique known as optical heterodyne detection, which is used in optical communications and enables very high detection sensitivities.

responds to detecting the envelope of the interference signal. The interferometer measures the field of the backscattered or backreflected signal versus delay or depth so that the intensity of the light is the square of the interference envelope.

Since the principles of operation of OCT are similar to optical communications systems, the performance of OCT systems can be calculated using well-established methods in optical communications theory.[19] The signal-to-noise ratio (SNR) for the detected signal is given by Equation A-5:

$$SNR = 10\log\,(\eta P/2h\nu NEB) \qquad \text{(A-5.)}$$

In Equation A-5, η is the photodetector quantum efficiency, P is the power in the detected signal, $2h\nu$ is the photon energy, and NEB is the noise equivalent bandwidth of detection system. The sensitivity of the OCT imaging is proportional to the amount of available power in the signal and is inversely proportional to the bandwidth of the detection. Faster image acquisition or higher resolution imaging requires a broader detection bandwidth since there are more data. Therefore, there is a tradeoff in signal-to-noise performance or sensitivity. For typical measurement parameters, OCT systems have a signal-to-noise performance of up to ~100 dB, which means that backscattered or backreflected intensities as small as 10^{-10} of the probe beam's incident intensity can be detected. In ophthalmic imaging, high sensitivity is required in order to visualize weak backscattering or backreflecting structures in the retina and vitreous. A decrease in signal-to-noise performance means that structures such as the outer nuclear layer of the retina or reflections from epiretinal membranes or vitreal anomalies appear dark and are difficult to visualize.

Principles of Fourier-Domain Optical Coherence Tomography— Measuring Echoes in the Spectral Domain

While the first OCT systems were based on interferometric detection by scanning a reference delay as a function of time, recently a new generation of OCT systems have been developed that rely on a different type of interferometric detection. Instead of scanning the reference delay and detecting the depth of the backscattered light, the axial scan depth profiles can also be measured by analyzing the spectrum of the output from the interferometer. This approach is known as *spectral* (SD) or *Fourier* (FD) *-domain detection* and was first proposed in 1995.[20] In 2002, SD/FD-OCT was demonstrated for retinal imaging.[21] In 2003, multiple groups working independently demonstrated that SD/FD detection has a significant sensitivity advantage over the earlier generations of OCT using TD detection.[22-24] This increase in sensitivity enables imaging at ~50x to 100x higher imaging speeds. Today, almost all commercial OCT systems are based on SD/FD detection and the increased imaging speeds enable significant improvements in image quality as well as the acquisition of 3D volumetric data sets.

Figure A-5 shows a schematic of how SD/FD detection works. SD/FD detection is somewhat similar to MRI in that it encodes different spatial positions as different frequencies. The system differs from first-generation OCT interferometers using TD detection (see Figure A-3) in 2 ways. First, the reference mirror is in a fixed position and it is not necessary for the reference delay to be scanned in order to acquire an axial depth profile. In SD/FD-OCT, light backscattered from different axial depths is essentially detected simultaneously. Second, a spectrometer is used to record the interference signal at the interferometer output. The spectrometer separates the light into its different wavelength or frequency components using a prism or diffraction grating. The spectrum is then detected by a high-speed line scan camera that records the output interference spectra.

It can be seen from the last term of Equation A-3 that the interferometer output signal E_{out} depends on the wavelength λ of the light in the interferometer. In other words, for a given path length difference Δz, different wavelengths will interfere constructively or destructively. Therefore, when a low-coherence light source having a broad band of wavelengths or frequencies is used as the input to the interferometer, the output spectrum will be modulated dependent on the path length difference Δz.[13] For a given wavelength λ, the spectral interference signal at the interferometer output is shown in Equation A-6:

$$S_{out}(\lambda, \Delta z) \sim 2\sqrt{S_{reference}(\lambda)}\sqrt{S_{sample}(\lambda)}\cos[(2\pi/\lambda)(2\Delta z)] \quad \textbf{(A-6.)}$$

where $S_{reference}$ and S_{sample} denote the spectral components of the light returning from the reference and sample arm, respectively. Modulation in the spectrum caused by the cosine interference term occurs with a frequency that is proportional to the delay Δz. Therefore, different echo delays are encoded as different frequencies. Figure A-5 (bottom left) shows this modulation in the interference spectrum for 2 different delays Δz. Each modulation frequency of the spectrum corresponds to a given Δz, and the modulation frequency increases for longer path length differences. The magnitude of the modulation at a given frequency is proportional to the light intensity backscattered from the corresponding depth.

In order to extract depth or axial scan profiles from the spectral interference signal, a frequency analysis is performed. Mathematically, the link between the SD and TD is the Fourier transform, which given an oscillating signal, computes the frequency components.[13]

As shown in Equation A-7, using the Fourier transform, FT, of the spectrum at the interferometer output, the A-scan signal can be calculated as:

$$\text{Fourier Transform} \left[S_{out}(\lambda, \Delta z) \right] \xrightarrow{FT} I_{out}(\Delta z) \quad \textbf{(A-7.)}$$

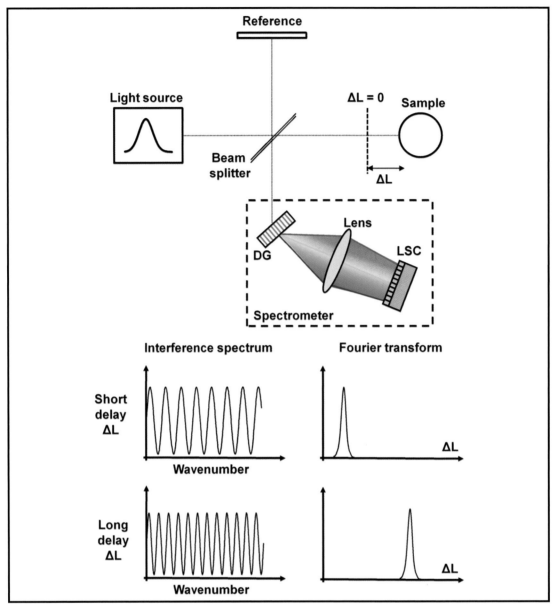

Figure A-5. (Top) Schematic showing how SD/FD detection works. Light from a broadband, low-coherence light source is used with a Michelson-type interferometer. Backscattered light from different depths in the sample is recombined with light from a known reference path. A spectrometer measures the spectrum of the interferometer output signal. The spectrometer separates the light into its spectral components by a diffraction grating (DG) and images the spectrum onto a line scan camera (LSC). (Bottom left) Path length differences Δz between the sample arm and the fixed reference arm length produce a periodic modulation of the interference spectrum. This modulation occurs because constructive and destructive interference occur at different wavelengths or frequencies for the same Δz. Equivalently, the Michelson interferometer acts as a wavelength or frequency filter. The modulation frequency of the spectrum is proportional to Δz. For a short delay Δz, the spectral modulation will be at a lower frequency, whereas for a long delay, the modulation frequency will be higher frequency. (Bottom right) Using the Fourier transform, the modulation frequency of the interference spectrum can be extracted to generate an axial scan, a measurement of echo magnitude versus delay or depth. SD/FD detection measures the entire axial depth scan signal from a single interference spectrum and therefore achieves much higher sensitivity than TD detection.

Since the spectral interference signal can cover a large range of modulation frequencies encoding backscattered signals from a variety of different depths, a single readout of the spectrometer line scan camera yields the spectral data necessary to calculate an axial scan.

Since SD/FD detection essentially detects all of the echoes of light simultaneously rather than sequentially as in TD detection, it has a dramatic improvement in sensitivity. The line scan camera can be read very rapidly, enabling a very rapid axial scan repetition rate, typically 20,000 to 50,000 Hz.

Increasing the path difference Δz between the interferometer sample and reference arms results in higher frequency modulation on the output spectrum. The maximum axial distance, Δz_{max}, that can be measured is limited by the resolution of the spectrometer and the number of pixels, N, on the line scan camera. As shown in Equation A-8, Δz_{max} corresponds to the modulation frequency with a period of 2 pixels:

$$\Delta z_{max} = N\lambda^2/(4\Delta\lambda) \qquad \text{(A-8.)}$$

where $\Delta\lambda$ is the spectral range covered by the camera pixels. For a fixed number of pixels N (usually 1024 or 2048), the maximum achievable depth range is limited by the spectral range covered since Δz_{max} is inversely proportional to $\Delta\lambda$.

The axial resolution in SD/FD-OCT is determined by the coherence length of the light source (see Equation A-4) similar to TD-OCT. In order to achieve a short coherence length and fine axial resolution, a very broadband light source is required. A high axial resolution requires a broad spectrometer bandwidth; however, a large depth measurement range requires a high spectrometer resolution. The choice of the light source and spectrometer design therefore involves a tradeoff between axial resolution and axial measurement range. For example, using a broadband light source with a bandwidth of ~100 to 150 nm at 800-nm wavelengths yields an axial resolution of 2 to 3 µm; however, the axial measurement range will be only Δz_{max} 1 to 2 mm. This limited axial measurement range makes the instrument alignment more difficult in the presence of axial eye motion and is one of the reasons why ultrahigh-resolution OCT instruments have not been developed for general clinical use. In standard commercial clinical OCT ophthalmic systems employing light sources with a bandwidth of ~50 nm, the axial resolution is ~5 to 6 µm, but the axial measurement range is longer Δz_{max} ~2 to 3 mm.[16-18]

Mirror Image Artifacts

Although SD/FD detection enables dramatic improvement in imaging speed, it is subject to artifacts that are not present in TD detection. The modulation frequency in the interference spectrum, S_{out} (see Equation A-6), is proportional to the path length difference Δz between the sample and reference beams in the interferometer. However, the modulation frequency and interference spectrum are the same for positive and negative path length differences. Therefore, optical echo signals originating from backscattering at $+\Delta z$ and $-\Delta z$ depths are indistinguishable because they yield the same modulation frequency in S_{out}. Therefore, these signals will overlap in the axial depth scan, resulting in a "mirror image" artifact where structures that are symmetric about the zero delay depth, $\Delta z = 0$, appear reflected. In order to avoid these mirror image artifacts, the OCT instrument is usually aligned such that all retinal or anterior eye structures are within a depth range that is either only positive or only negative Δz. However, in cases when the retina is tilted at an angle or where there are axially elevated structures such as epiretinal membranes or vitreous detachments, features can cross the zero delay, $\Delta z = 0$, generating mirror image artifacts (Figure A-6). When interpreting OCT images, it is important to recognize that these mirror image artifacts result from the Fourier/spectral detection and are not real structures.

Sensitivity Variation With Axial Position

In addition to mirror image artifacts, SD/FD detection also has the property that the detection sensitivity varies with the axial position of the backscattering or backreflection signal in the image.[24-26] Lower spectral modulation frequencies can be resolved better than higher ones, which results in decreased sensitivity for larger positive or negative delays Δz. Structures will appear brightest near the zero delay, $\Delta z = 0$, and become dimmer when they are moved toward larger delays, $\Delta z = \Delta z_{max}$. The increased sensitivity close to $\Delta z = 0$ can be used to enhance the sensitivity to features posterior to the retinal pigment epithelium (RPE) or anterior to the retina by placing the zero delay below the choroid or in the vitreous, respectively.[27]

SD/FD-OCT can detect all backscattering signals from different depths simultaneously rather than sequentially as it is done in TD detection. In

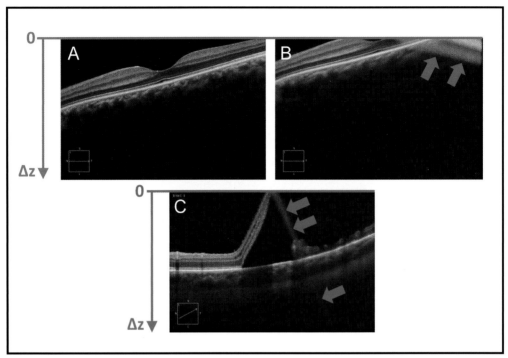

Figure A-6. Mirror image artifacts in SD/FD-OCT. SD/FD detection has the disadvantage that light echoes from positive and negative delays cannot be distinguished. When tissue structures cross the zero delay depth, $\Delta z = 0$, they appear reflected about the zero, generating a mirror image. (A) Artifact-free OCT image where all retinal structures are located on one side of the zero delay. (B) Portions of the tilted retina cross the zero delay and appear as overlapping mirrored structures marked by red arrows. (C) Mirror artifact of an elevated retina in a patient with retinoschisis. Special care must be exercised in interpreting these images.

addition, SD/FD-OCT operates without scanning the reference delay as it is required in time-domain OCT. The parallel detection of all of the echoes results in a dramatic increase in detection sensitivity. The detection sensitivity of SD/FD-OCT is improved by ~20 dB compared to TD detection, yielding significantly higher SNR.[22-24] This enables OCT imaging ~50 to 100 times faster compared with previous-generation TD-OCT systems. While TD systems were able to acquire several hundreds of axial scans per second, current commercially available SD/FD ophthalmic OCT systems operate at ~20,000 to 50,000 axial scans per second. Higher acquisition speed reduces motion artifacts in OCT images and allows an increased number of axial scans or transverse pixels per image, yielding high-definition images that can be acquired in a fraction of a second. Alternatively, sequences of cross-sectional images or raster scans can be acquired within a few seconds. This enables acquisition of 3D-OCT volumetric data sets in a time comparable to that of previous OCT scan protocols that only acquired several individual images.

Transverse Spatial Resolution

Image resolution is an important parameter that governs OCT system performance. In OCT, the axial (longitudinal) and transverse resolutions are determined by completely different physical mechanisms. It was shown in Equation A-4 that the axial image resolution depends upon the coherence length of the light source, which varies inversely as the bandwidth of the light source.

In contrast, the transverse resolution in OCT imaging is determined by the same principles as the transverse resolution in conventional optical microscopy. The transverse resolution is given by the spot size of the focused OCT imaging beam. The minimum focal spot size, Δx, of an optical beam is determined by the diffraction properties of light and the focusing parameters used. Equation A-9 gives

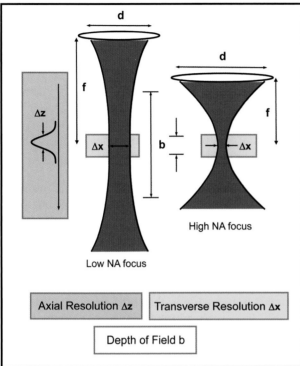

Figure A-7. Image resolution in OCT. The transverse resolution in OCT images is determined by the transverse spot size of the optical beam. This spot size is governed by the focusing optics, the diameter, d, of the incident beam, and the focal length, f, of the focusing lens. A small focusing angle or numerical aperture, NA, results in a small transverse spot size, Δx, and a long depth of focus, b. Conversely, a large focusing angle or a large numerical aperture, NA, results in a small transverse spot size but a short depth of focus, b. The axial or longitudinal resolution is given by the coherence length of the light source and is independent of the focusing optics. In ophthalmology, this enables OCT imaging to achieve extremely high axial resolutions despite the limited pupil size of the eye.

an expression for the focused spot size, Δx, for an optical beam with a diameter, d, incident upon a lens with focal length, f:

$$\Delta x = (4\lambda/\pi)(f/d) \qquad \text{(A-9.)}$$

This result follows from optical diffraction theory and is well known in microscopy. The focused spot size is proportional to the focal length of the focusing lens and inversely proportional to the diameter of the incident beam. Stated another way, the focused spot size is inversely proportional to the numerical aperture of the beam. This means that in

order to achieve a small spot size, it is necessary to have a large beam diameter and a short focal length lens, or equivalently a high numerical aperture. Figure A-7 shows 2 different focusing conditions with large and small transverse spot sizes, which correspond to low and high numerical aperture focusing conditions, respectively.

There is a tradeoff between the transverse resolution and the depth of field in OCT imaging. This is similar to microscopy, where higher magnification microscope objectives have very short depths of field. As shown in Equation A-10, the depth of field or depth range where the beam is in focus is characterized by a parameter known as the confocal parameter, b:

$$b = \pi(\Delta x)^2/2\lambda \qquad \text{(A-10.)}$$

Smaller spot sizes, which improve the transverse resolution, have a shallower depth of field. The depth of field decreases with the square of the focused spot size.

Figure A-7 shows schematically the relationship between focused spot size and depth of field for low and high numerical aperture focusing. These focusing conditions define 2 limiting cases for OCT imaging. Typically, OCT is performed with low numerical aperture focusing because it is desirable to have a large depth of field and to use low-coherence interferometry to achieve axial (longitudinal) resolution. In this limit, the depth of field is longer than the coherence length. In contrast to conventional microscopy, OCT can achieve high axial resolution independently of the focusing conditions and depth of field. This feature is particularly powerful in ophthalmic applications where the available numerical aperture is limited by the pupil of the eye.

The smallest spot size that can be achieved on the retina is also limited by optical aberrations in the eye. The maximum beam diameter that can be incident in the eye without significant aberrations is typically limited to ~3 to 4 mm and the smallest focal spot is approximately 5 to 7 μm. For clinical applications, it is desirable to be able to perform OCT imaging without dilating the pupil. In addition, a larger depth of field is desired so that the instrument focus is not overly sensitive. Typical ophthalmic OCT systems have a ~1-mm diameter beam incident on the eye, which results in a ~20-μm spot size on the retina. Much smaller transverse spot sizes of approximately 2 to 3 μm can be achieved using adaptive optics techniques.[28,29] Adaptive optics technology was originally developed for astronomy and uses a deformable mirror and a wavefront sensor in order to correct for aberrations in the eye and obtain enhanced transverse resolutions.

In applications other than ophthalmology, it is possible to focus with high numerical aperture and to achieve fine transverse resolutions at the expense of a reduced depth of focus. This operating regime is typical for conventional microscopy or confocal microscopy. Depending upon the coherence length of the light, the depth of field can be shorter than the coherence length. In this case, the depth of field can be used to differentiate backscattered or backreflected signals from different depths. The interferometric detection enhances image contrast and penetration depth by rejecting unwanted out-of-focal plane scattered light. This regime of operation is called *optical coherence microscopy.*[30]

Image Acquisition Time and Axial Scan Densities

Current commercial OCT devices using SD/FD detection can record several tens of thousands of axial scans per second, which allows the acquisition of densely sampled data sets within a few seconds. Rapid acquisition in ophthalmic imaging is important in order to minimize image distortion artifacts from residual eye motion, as well as to improve patient comfort during the examination. The image acquisition time is directly related to the sensitivity—increasing the imaging speed decreases the OCT instrument's signal-to-noise performance. In principle, the signal-to-noise performance could be improved by using higher incident optical power, as shown in Equation A-5. However, there is a maximum permissible light exposure determined by safety standards, such as the American National Standards Institute (ANSI) standards for laser exposure. The maximum permissible exposure depends upon the wavelength, the spot size, the duration of exposure, as well as repeated exposures. Because OCT instruments have extremely high detection sensitivities, low power levels of ~750 µW can be used for retinal imaging with infrared light at 800-nm wavelengths, which are well within safe exposure limits. Thus, the image acquisition time is determined by a combination of the safe incident power and the signal-to-noise requirements that are necessary to achieve sufficient quality images for clinical applications. Axial scan density in an image and the number of images per data set are therefore limited and may be chosen differently dependent on the clinical application.

It is important to note that the fundamental optical resolution of an OCT instrument is different from the pixel size or pixel density in an OCT image. The pixel density in an OCT image is analogous to pixel density in digital photography. The image must have sufficient pixel density in order to visualize small features with a given resolution. Figure A-8 shows a schematic describing pixel density and size in the axial and transverse directions.

OCT images are generated by acquiring successive axial measurements (axial scans) of backreflection or backscattering versus depth at different transverse positions. Therefore, the number of pixels in the transverse direction is equal to the number of axial scans. If the OCT image has N_x transverse pixels (axial scans) and is L_x wide in the transverse direction, then the pixel size in the transverse direction is L_x/N_x. For example, a typical OCT retinal image is 6-mm wide in the transverse direction and has 512 transverse pixels (axial scans), so the pixels are 6 mm/512 = 11.7-µm wide. If larger numbers of axial scans are acquired, corresponding to additional transverse pixels, the pixel size becomes smaller and the density of pixels increases. For example, a typical "high-definition" OCT retinal image is 6-mm wide and has 4096 transverse pixels (axial scans), so the pixels are 6-mm/4096 = 1.5-µm wide. However, in this limit where the number of axial scans is high, the image resolution is governed by the optical resolution of the instrument. In contrast to the pixel size, the transverse resolution for a typical retinal image is determined by the focused spot size on the retina and is typically ~20 µm. In order to utilize the full instrumental resolution, the size of the pixels must be smaller than the instrument resolution. However, the image resolution is ultimately governed by the optical resolution rather than the pixel size.

The pixel density in the axial (longitudinal) direction is governed by a different mechanism than in the transverse direction. In TD-OCT systems, the number of pixels, N_z, is determined by the speed at which the computer can record the electronic signal from the axial scan of backscattering or backreflection versus depth. However, in SD/FD-OCT, the number of axial pixels is given by the spectrometer design. In particular, the spectral resolution of the spectrometer and the line scan camera determines both the axial imaging range (see Equation A-8) and pixel density in the axial direction. For a line scan camera with N pixels, the axial scan will consist of $N_z = N/2$ pixels after the Fourier transform is used to generate the axial scan from the interference spectrum. This is because the Fourier transform process

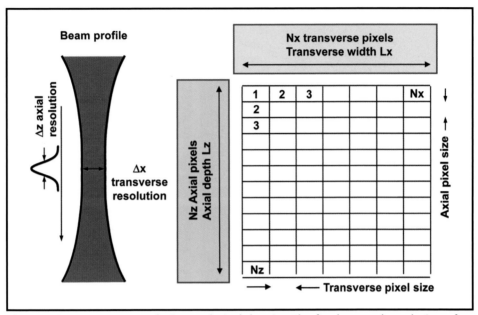

Figure A-8. OCT image resolution and pixel density. The fundamental resolution of an OCT instrument can be different from the pixel resolution in an image. The number and size of the pixels in transverse direction is determined by the number of axial scans in the OCT image. Since the axial scan rate of an OCT device is limited, there is a tradeoff between the transverse pixel density and image acquisition time. The number of pixels in axial direction is determined by other factors, such as the computer data acquisition speed in TD-OCT systems or the spectrometer configuration in SD/FD-OCT setups. In order to resolve a small feature in an image, the pixel size must be sufficiently small or there must be a large enough number of pixels in an image.

extracts both positive and negative frequencies from the interference spectrum, resulting in a loss of one-half of the available pixels in the axial scan. If the OCT image has Nz axial pixels and is Lz deep in the axial direction, then the pixel size is Lz/Nz in the axial direction. For example, a typical clinical OCT instrument has a spectrometer and line scan camera designed to enable a 2-mm axial image range and has a 2048-pixel camera. Therefore, the number of pixels in the axial direction is 1024, and given the 2-mm axial range, the pixel size is 2 mm/1024 = 1.9 µm in axial depth. In contrast, the optical axial (longitudinal) resolution of the typical retinal image is given by the coherence length of the light source and is typically ~6 µm.

Image acquisition time increases in proportion to the number of transverse pixels or axial scans in an image. If the instrument operates at an axial scan repetition rate of R, then the image acquisition time, T, is given by T = Nx/R. The acquisition time is the number of axial scans or transverse pixels, Nx, in the image, divided by the axial scan repetition rate, R, of the instrument. If higher numbers of transverse pix-

els are desired, more axial scans are necessary and the image acquisition time increases proportionally. Transverse oversampling (ie, acquiring more axial scans per spot size given by Equation A-9) increases the SNR in an image and reduces speckle noise by averaging axial scans. If only low-transverse resolution imaging is necessary (eg, if only topographic information is required), then the number of transverse pixels may be reduced and the image acquisition time will be proportionally faster.

OCT instruments have a maximum axial scan rate (number of axial scans per second), so that the tradeoff between the pixel density and acquisition speed is an important factor in determining the imaging protocols. Figure A-9 shows OCT images with low transverse pixel density versus high transverse pixel density images with 200, 512, and 4096 transverse pixels, respectively. The images were recorded using the Cirrus HD-OCT (Carl Zeiss Meditec, Inc, Dublin, CA) with an axial scan repetition rate, R, of 27,000 axial scans per second. The low transverse pixel density, fast-acquisition image of Figure A-9A is 6-mm wide and has 200 transverse pixels, thus the

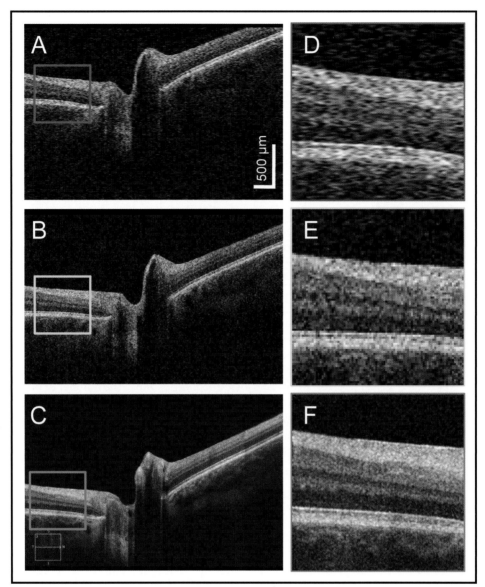

Figure A-9. Tradeoff between transverse pixel density and image acquisition speed. (A) OCT image of the optic nerve head with 200 transverse pixels acquired in 7.4 ms. (B) Image with a higher number of transverse pixels, 512 axial scans, acquired in 19.0 ms. (C) A high transverse pixel density, high-definition image consisting of 4096 axial scans, acquired in 151.7 ms. (D, E) The enlargements of the retinal image cross sections on the right show the reduced graininess and smoother appearance for higher transverse pixel densities. Note that it takes 8 and 20 times longer to acquire the high-density image (C) than the images with lower transverse pixel densities, (A) and (B), respectively.

transverse pixel spacing is 6 mm/200 = 30 µm and the image is acquired in T = 200/27,000 = 7.4 ms. Figure A-9B contains 512 axial scans, which corresponds to a transverse pixel spacing of 6 mm/512 = 11.7 µm and an image acquisition time of T = 512/27,000 = 19.0 ms. The high transverse pixel density, slow

acquisition image of Figure A-9C has 4096 transverse pixels, so the transverse pixel spacing is 6 mm/4096 = 1.5 µm and the image is acquired in T = 4096/27,000 = 0.152 sec. Note the grainier appearance of the low transverse pixel density image. Images with higher or lower numbers of transverse pixels can also be acquired, and acquisition times will vary accordingly. In nonophthalmic imaging applications, higher incident optical powers can be used so that image acquisition speeds can be dramatically increased.

These examples illustrate an important fundamental tradeoff between the transverse pixel density of the image and the acquisition speed. In ophthalmic imaging, a larger number of transverse pixels is desirable in order to improve the visualization of retinal features; however, high-definition images require a longer acquisition time, thus artifacts from eye motion can increase when recording a sequence of images. A more precise registration of OCT images to positions on the fundus is possible by acquiring images rapidly because eye motion artifacts are reduced. However, because of a corresponding reduction in the transverse pixel density, the image appears grainier.

Three-Dimensional Optical Coherence Tomography Imaging

The high image acquisition speeds of modern OCT systems enable the acquisition of cross-sectional images as well as 3D data sets of the human retina in vivo. As shown in Figure A-2, 3D data sets consist of a series of cross-sectional (B-scan) images covering a certain sample volume. This scan pattern, consisting of sequential cross-sectional images, separated in the perpendicular direction, covers an area of the retina and is known as a *raster scan*. Most OCT instruments perform the raster scan by acquiring cross-sectional images in the horizontal (temporal-nasal) direction, which are sequentially offset in the vertical (superior-inferior) direction. The acquisition speed of the OCT instrument limits the maximum number of axial scans that can be acquired during an allowed image acquisition time. The total number of axial scans in a 3D data set is the number of axial scans per image, Nx, times the number of B-scan images, Ny, in the raster scan pattern. A volumetric data set can consist of a small number of highly oversampled B-scan images (Nx > Ny) or of a larger number of B-scans, where each is made up of fewer axial scans in order to provide isotropic sampling in the 2 directions (Nx = Ny).

Different diagnostic or monitoring applications may require differently sampled volumes. When it is necessary to resolve small focal features such as drusen, a higher sampling density is required

per cross-sectional image (B-scan). In addition, a larger number of cross-sectional images should also be acquired to have a higher sampling density in the perpendicular direction. Therefore, in high-definition 3D-OCT imaging the number of axial scans required increases as the square of axial scan density, since the axial scans must be performed in 2D (Nx x Ny). Although SD/FD-OCT instruments have dramatically higher imaging speeds than previous TD technology, these speeds are still not fast enough to obtain high sampling density in 3D data sets within a reasonable acquisition time.

Therefore, in order to visualize retinal features, anisotropic raster scan protocols are used, which acquire cross-sectional images (B-scans) with large numbers of axial pixels (Nx) and with a small number of cross-sectional images (Ny). For example, a typical raster scan acquisition acquires cross-sectional images with 512 axial scans per image, but only 128 cross-sectional images. Assuming a 6-mm x 6-mm area of the retina is imaged with a horizontal raster pattern, this corresponds to a 6 mm/512 = 12 µm pixel size in the horizontal direction and a 6 mm/128 = 47 µm pixel size in the vertical direction. The low sampling density in the vertical direction means that cross-sectional images extracted from the 3D data set in this direction will have large pixel sizes and poorer resolution than horizontal cross-sectional images.

For other applications, such as mapping the retinal nerve fiber layer (RNFL) thickness during glaucoma assessment, an isotropic raster scan pattern with axial scans equally spaced in x- and y- direction is used. The isotropic sampling provides a smoother map of the RNFL thickness. For example, a typical isotropic raster scan acquires B-scans in the horizontal direction consisting of 200 axial scans per image with 200 B-scans in the vertical direction. Assuming a 6-mm x 6-mm area of the papillary region is imaged, this corresponds to a 6 mm/200 = 30 µm pixel size in both the horizontal and vertical directions. Although each B-scan of this isotropically sampled data set has a low number of pixels and therefore does not allow good quality cross-sectional visualization of small retinal features, the gross morphology of the RNFL can still be assessed. However, since the isotropic scan pattern gives a pixel size that is the same in the horizontal and vertical directions, this scan pattern is well suited to map structures that have comparable feature sizes in both horizontal (temporal-nasal) and vertical (superior-inferior) directions. Thus, the RNFL thickness can be mapped with higher fidelity than it would be possible using an anisotropic raster scan pattern.

Current commercially available SD/FD-OCT devices offer a variety of different scan patterns for 3D imaging of the retina.[31,32] For volumetric imaging covering an area of 6 mm x 6 mm around the fovea, the Cirrus HD-OCT employs a Macular Cube scan composed of 128 B-scans of 512 axial scans each. The 3D Macular scan pattern available with Optovue's (Fremont, CA) RTVue-100 images a similar region (6 mm x 6 mm) using 101 frames of 513 axial scans. The total acquisition times for these volumetric scans are 2.5 sec and 2.2 sec for the Cirrus HD-OCT and the RTVue-100, respectively. The axial scan density, L_x/N_x, in each cross-sectional image is ~12 µm, and the spacing between consecutive image frames, L_y/N_y, is 47 µm and 59 µm, respectively, for the 2 devices. The RTVue-100 provides a similar pattern for imaging the optic disc (3D Disc scan: 101 frames of each 513 axial scans over an area of 6 mm x 6 mm). A more isotropic pattern consisting of 200 frames with 200 axial scans is available for imaging the optic nerve with the Cirrus HD-OCT (Optic Disc Cube 200 x 200, 6 mm x 6 mm). Here, the axial scan density in each frame and the spacing between frames are both 6 mm/ 200 = 30 µm ($N_x = N_y$).

Macular 3D scan patterns:
- Zeiss Cirrus: Macular Cube 512 x 128, 128 x 512, 6 mm x 6 mm, 2.5 s
- Optovue RTVue: 3D Macular, 101 x 513, 6 mm x 6 mm, 2.2 s
- Heidelberg (Heidelberg, Germany) Spectralis: Macula, 25 x 1024 (each averaged from 49 frames), 20 x 20 degrees

Optic disc 3D scan patterns:
- Zeiss Cirrus: Optic Disc Cube 200 x 200, 200 x 200, 6 mm x 6 mm, 1.5 s
- Optovue RTVue: 3D Disc, 101 x 513, 6 mm x 6 mm, 2.2 s
- Heidelberg Spectralis: Optic Nerve Head (ONH), 73 x 384 (each an average of 9 frames), 15 x 15 degrees, 6.3 s (estimated)

Image Analysis and Display

Viewing and interpreting 3D-OCT data can be challenging, since a 3D data set may contain several hundreds of B-scans. Browsing through each individual image is time consuming and although each image is registered to the en face fundus view, it can be difficult to conceptualize the 3D structure of the retinal pathology.

Commercial OCT devices offer automated software tools for quantitative assessment of retinal morphology. The software in most clinical OCT systems is able to detect the major retinal layers and their boundaries. In order to analyze macular morphology, determining the inner limiting membrane (ILM), the boundary between vitreous and neural retina, is important. At the posterior boundary of the neural retina, different OCT devices have different standards for the segmentation of different retinal layers. For example, the Zeiss Stratus OCT segments the junction of the inner and outer photoreceptor segments. The Optovue RTVue and Zeiss Cirrus provide automated delineation of the RPE (Figure A-10A). The Heidelberg Spectralis OCT provides segmentation of Bruch's membrane.

Elevation maps of layer boundaries or single retinal layers can be generated by plotting the axial position detected by the segmentation algorithm. Elevation maps of single retinal layers such as the RPE map shown in Figure A-10B enable visualization of disorders that affect the morphology of a particular retinal layer. For example, in the early stages of age-related macular degeneration (ARMD), the RPE may be focally elevated due to underlying deposits and drusen. RPE elevation maps such as Figure A-10B reveal the positions of larger drusen from the entire 3D data set and enable quantitative mapping.

By computing the axial distance between 2 segmented layer surfaces or positions, thickness maps can be generated. For example, the retinal thickness maps offered by the analysis software tools of commercial OCT devices are calculated as the difference between the axial ILM position and the position of the posterior boundary of the neural retina (Figure A-10C). Note that different devices use different layers—photoreceptor inner/outer segments junction, RPE, or Bruch's membrane—as a posterior boundary. As a result, different retinal thicknesses will be computed and care should be taken when comparing retinal thickness measurements taken with different OCT devices.[31,32]

Changes in the RNFL thickness are an important indicator for glaucoma diagnosis and progression.[33] An important feature of modern OCT devices is their ability to measure RNFL thickness by segmenting the anterior and posterior RNFL boundary. By computing the axial distance between the 2 boundaries, thickness maps and profiles can be generated and compared to normative data. For example, subsets of the RNFL thickness analysis

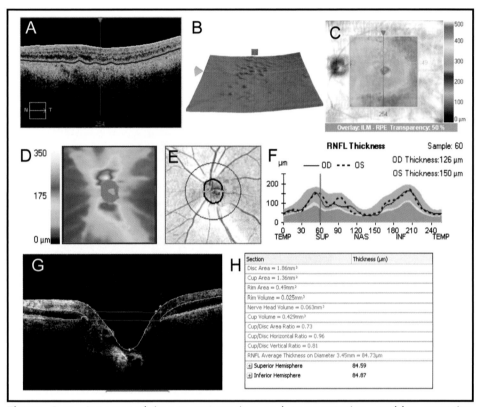

Figure A-10. Automated image processing and segmentation enables quantitative assessment of retinal features—examples from commercial OCT devices. (A) Automatic delineation of retinal layers such as the ILM and RPE using the Zeiss Cirrus HD-OCT in a patient with ARMD. (B) The layer positions can be used to generate RPE elevation maps for visualization of drusen. (C) En face fundus maps of retinal thickness can be computed from the segmented layer positions. (D) En face fundus map showing RNFL thickness in a healthy patient. RNFL thickness can be compared to a normative database using deviation maps (E) or cirumpapillary RNFL thickness profiles (F). (G, H) Examples of automated assessment of optic disc dimensions using the Optovue RTVue optic disc analysis software.

provided by the Cirrus OCT are shown in Figures A-10D through F.

The 3D imaging capabilities of state-of-the-art OCT systems enable ophthalmologists to extract clinically relevant parameters such as RNFL thickness or macular volume. Commercial OCT devices also offer software tools that can measure the dimensions of anatomical features as well as assess pathological changes quantitatively. Figures A-10G and H show an example of the optic disc analysis of the Optovue RTVue, which provides an automatic measurement of the geometric dimensions of the disc, such as cup volume, cup-to-disc ratios, and disc area.

Acquiring dense 3D data sets enables the extraction of cross-sectional images with arbitrary position and orientation. For example, en face images perpendicular to the OCT beam direction can be displayed. More sophisticated software also enables extraction and display of images along curved surfaces. For example, the analysis software of the Zeiss Cirrus allows the segmented layer positions of the ILM or RPE to be used as a backbone to extract en face images from the 3D data. In addition, fundus projection images can be generated by summing the intensity of the OCT signals in a user-defined depth range between layer boundaries or arbitrarily chosen surfaces (Figure A-11). Such fundus projection images can increase the contrast of backscattering retinal structures such as vessels or the NFL as well as improve visualization of pathological features such as drusen or edema.

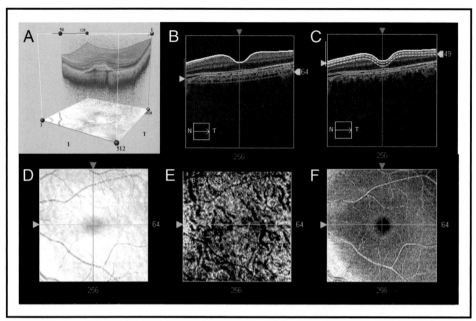

Figure A-11. Display of 3D-OCT volumetric data. (A) 3D rendering of volumetric OCT data of the macular region of a patient with central serous retinopathy. En face fundus projection maps can be generated by summing the intensity of the OCT axial signal in a user-defined depth range between layer boundaries or arbitrarily chosen surfaces (indicated by dashed lines in B and C). Examples of a healthy eye, showing summation over the entire depth range (D) as well as for summing over ranges indicated in (B) and (C) to enhance contrast in the choroidal (E) and retinal vessel structures (F). All images were generated using the Zeiss Cirrus HD-OCT.

Many commercial devices offer software with 3D volume rendering features that enable the operator to visualize the 3D retinal structure as well as to rotate the view and crop the displayed volume (see Figure A-11). Most instruments have software that enables arbitrary cross-sectional planes to be selected and displayed. While it is hard to identify small features and lesions in 3D renderings, rendering provides an overview of the general retinal morphology. However, 3D rendering requires viewing the data on the OCT instrument or a networked computer and therefore is more time intensive than using a single- or multiple-page printout in a patient record. Therefore, the ultimate clinical utility of 3D rendering is still undetermined. However, rendering can be used as an educational tool and can help the clinician explain disease patterns and progression to patients.

Image Averaging

An important feature of modern OCT systems is the ability to enhance image contrast and sensi-tivity by averaging multiple images. Although the sensitivity of OCT instruments is very high, the image contrast is limited and signal levels can be low in patients with ocular opacities or when imaging deep structures such as the choroid. Contrast in OCT images is limited by speckle noise, which produces a grainy or textured appearance of scattering structures such as the different retinal layers. The phenomenon of speckle noise occurs because tissue structures have small irregularities on the submicron scale corresponding to optical wavelengths.[34] When light scatters from these tissues, there is partial constructive and destructive interference in the scattering. This speckle noise produces a discontinuous appearance of the retinal layers, making delineation of layer boundaries more difficult.

As previously mentioned, the high acquisition speeds of OCT systems can be used to acquire high sample densities in the transverse direction (high-definition images). The high density of axial scans produces an averaging effect, which reduces the speckle noise and increases sensitivity. However, image quality can be improved even further by acquiring and averaging multiple cross-sectional images at the

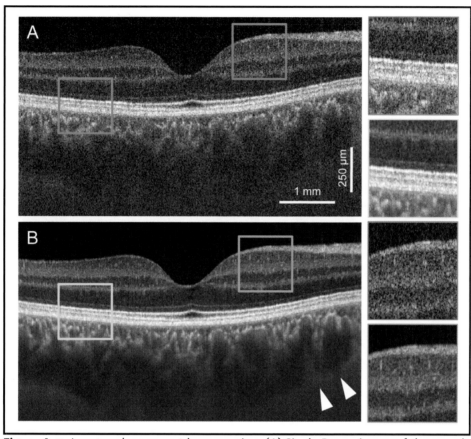

Figure A-12. Image enhancement by averaging. (A) Single B-scan image of the macula with 2048 transverse pixels. (B) Result from averaging 8 images. Note the significant signal-to-noise improvement and reduced speckle noise in the averaged image. Deep structures in the choroid can be observed (arrowheads). Enlarged images on the right show improved visibility of the retinal layer structure and better contrast of small features such as capillaries.

same location. After aligning these images to remove any shifts due to eye motion between successive B-scans, an averaged image can be computed that will exhibit higher SNR and a smoother appearance of tissue structures. It is important to point out that image averaging does not improve the axial resolution of the instrument, which is determined by the light source. However, since speckle noise produces discontinuities of fine retinal structures, reducing noise by image averaging improves the continuity of structures, yielding a significant improvement in image quality. This generates the perception that the images have improved resolution.

The effect of image averaging is demonstrated in Figure A-12. Figure A-12A shows a single B-scan image consisting of 2048 axial scans. Figure A-12B shows an averaged image generated from 32 repeated images. The averaged image has a uniformly

black background in the vitreous, showing that the noise floor is reduced. The signal level for deep structures in the choroid is enhanced, thus allowing visualization of vascular features as deep as the sclera. At the same time, the continuity and contrast of the layered structure of the retina is increased. Small features such as capillaries can be visualized and also the fine features of the external limiting membrane appear as a continuous line.

The newest versions of clinical OCT systems such as the Zeiss Cirrus HD-OCT ("enhanced HD" scan) or the Optovue RTVue-100 "line" scan pattern, averaging 16 images of 1024 A-lines in 0.039 sec) offer the ability to repeatedly record B-scan images at the same retinal location and generate averaged images.

Averaging decreases noise by approximately the square root of the number of images averaged. For example, a 4x increase in the number of images averaged produces a 2x decrease in noise. However, increasing the number of images to be averaged will increase the image acquisition time proportionally. Transverse eye motion will ultimately limit the number of B-scans that can be recorded at the same retinal location. Some instruments address this issue by using eye tracking.[35] The Spectralis OCT allows the user to set the number of B-scans to be averaged between 1 and 100 images. This device incorporates a retinal tracker, a device that measures and dynamically compensates for transverse eye motion. The retinal tracker stabilizes the OCT imaging beam on the retina such that the same position on the retina is scanned in multiple images. In instruments without eye tracking, the total acquisition time is limited to 2 to 3 sec due to eye motion. However, the stabilization against transverse eye motion achieved by retinal tracking enables the recording of OCT data over extended time periods of many seconds. In this manner, it is possible not only to acquire averaged cross-sectional images (B-scans) in a single location, but also a series of averaged B-scans covering 3D volumes of the retina. Examples of 3D patterns offered by the Spectralis OCT are the "dense" preset covering a field of 20 x 20 degrees with 49 frames, each of which consists of an average of 16 images of 512 axial scans, or the "ONH" preset, which acquires 73 images of 384 axial scans and averaged from 9 frames over a field of view of 15 x 15 degrees. The spacing between consecutive B-scans is ~120 and ~60 μm for the dense and ONH patterns, respectively.

The recent advances in OCT image acquisition speed have enabled the acquisition of several averaged cross-sectional images per second or a 3D data set within a few seconds. However, there is still a tradeoff between either recording a smaller number of densely sampled or averaged B-scan images or acquiring sparsely sampled, isotropic 3D data sets within a time frame suitable for imaging in clinical routine. With currently available OCT systems, densely sampled 3D data sets, which then would enable extracting high-definition cross-sectional images in any arbitrary direction, still cannot be acquired. New developments that enable even faster acquisition speeds, combined with advanced image-processing algorithms, may ultimately solve this problem and pave the way for the next generation of clinical OCT devices in ophthalmology.

Advances in Optical Coherence Tomography Technology

While OCT has become an indispensable tool for diagnostic imaging and monitoring disease progression in the clinic, development of new OCT techniques, pushing the limits of resolution, speed, and contrast, is still an active area of research in biomedical optics. The ability of OCT to perform high-speed, real-time, volumetric imaging with micrometer scale resolution has enabled clinical applications not only in ophthalmology, but also for cardiovascular and endoscopic imaging. Using broadband light sources, the axial image resolution has been improved dramatically down to 1 to 3 μm, thus enabling imaging approaching the cellular level.

In ophthalmic imaging, axial image resolutions as fine as 2 to 3 μm have been demonstrated using TD-OCT and SD/FD-OCT.[17,36-38] Figure A-13 shows an example of the first ultrahigh-resolution OCT images obtained in 2001.[17] Ultrahigh-resolution OCT improved the visualization of internal retinal architectural morphology, enabling visualization of all of the major internal retinal layers. Early ultrahigh-resolution OCT imaging studies provided important information to confirm the interpretation of standard-resolution OCT images. Using SD/FD detection enables high-speed image acquisition, and ultrahigh-resolution images can be recorded within a fraction of a second.[36-38] Although ultrahigh-resolution OCT has been used extensively in research instruments, several factors have limited its commercial development and availability. The first factor is cost. Ultrahigh-resolution OCT requires broadband light sources. The earliest ultrahigh-resolution OCT studies were performed using femtosecond lasers. This technology can generate very broad bandwidths of 200 to 300 nm around 800 nm, corresponding to axial resolutions of 1 to 2 μm, but it is much too expensive for clinical use. The development of advanced superluminescent diode light sources dramatically reduced the cost of ultrahigh-resolution OCT. By combining or multiplexing 2 or more superluminescent diodes emitting at different wavelengths, it is possible to generate bandwidths of more than 100 nm around 800 nm, yielding axial resolutions approaching 3 μm. These light sources are still more expensive than single superluminescent diodes that can generate bandwidths of ~50 nm. However, in addition to cost, a more critical limitation occurs because SD/FD-OCT has a limited

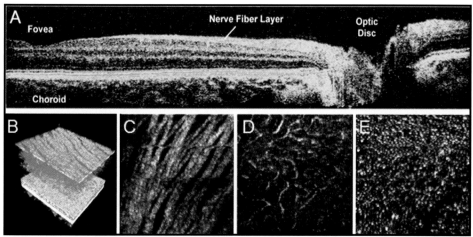

Figure A-13. Ultrahigh-resolution (UHR) OCT. (A) Using broadband light sources, the axial resolution can be significantly improved. In this UHR-OCT image, fine details of the retinal structure can be resolved with an unprecedented axial resolution of 3 μm. Transverse optical resolution in OCT images is limited by ocular aberrations. Using AO, wavefront distortion can be measured and ocular aberrations compensated, thus enabling high transverse resolution. Combining AO-OCT and UHR-OCT achieves isotropic resolutions of 2 to 3 μm. (Reprinted by permission from Macmillan Publishers Ltd: *Nature Medicine.* Drexler W, Morgner U, Ghanta RK, Kärtner FX, Schuman JS, Fujimoto JG. Ultrahigh-resolution ophthalmic optical coherence tomography, 7[4], Copyright 2001.) (B) 3D rendering of retinal volume recorded with UHR-AO-OCT. En face images extracted from this volume show nerve fiber bundles (C), capillary networks (D), and cone photoreceptors (E). (Figures B-E reprinted with permission of Dr. Boris Považay and Dr. Wolfgang Drexler.)

number of axial pixels and varying sensitivity with axial range. Therefore, increasing the axial image resolution reduces the available imaging range, making image acquisition difficult in patients with axial eye motion. For these reasons, most commercial OCT instruments have been designed to operate with 5- to 7-μm axial resolution.

As noted previously, the transverse image resolution in OCT is determined by the focused spot size of the OCT beam on the retina. Smaller spot sizes, with correspondingly reduced depth of field, can generally be achieved by increasing the diameter of the incident beam onto the cornea. However, the eye has optical aberrations that limit the smallest focal spot size. Transverse image resolution in retinal OCT can be greatly improved by combining OCT with adaptive optics (AO), a method that was originally developed for imaging in astronomy. In AO-OCT, the optical aberrations in the cornea and lens are characterized by measuring the wavefront (or phase) of a light beam that is directed into the eye and reflected from the retina. Aberrations in

the optical phase are then dynamically compensated using a deformable mirror in the incident light beam.[39-41] The deformable mirror operates by adjusting the phase of the incident light beam in order to cancel phase aberrations from the cornea and lens. In this manner, the spot size on the retina can be improved from 15 to 20 μm down to ~4 μm. Features such as individual cone photoreceptor cells, capillaries, and individual nerve fiber bundles have been imaged using AO-OCT (Figures A-13B through E). Combined with ultrahigh-resolution OCT, retinal features can be imaged in vivo with isotropic resolution on the few-micron scale in both axial and transverse directions.

Further advances have also been made in imaging speed. Using the newest generation of SD/FD-OCT based on new high-speed CMOS (complementary metal oxide semiconductor) line scan cameras, it is possible to perform retinal imaging at more than 300,000 axial scans per second, factors of 5x to 10x faster than standard commercial instruments.[42] Other FD detection methods enable even higher imaging speed. SD/FD detection uses an interferometer with a broadband light and the entire spectral interferogram is detected simultaneously. However, there is another FD detection method that uses a frequency-swept light source. This method is known as *swept-source/FD-OCT* (or *optical frequency-domain imaging*).[43-46] In swept-source/FD-OCT, a narrow bandwidth light source is used where the frequency or wavelength is rapidly swept across a broad spectral range as a function of time. The interference signal is recorded as a function of time using a detector at the output of the interferometer. Each sweep of the laser generates an axial scan, and the image acquisition rates are determined by the repetition rate of the laser sweep. Swept-source/FD detection does not require a spectrometer or line scan camera. Compared to SD/FD detection, which uses a spectrometer, swept-source OCT systems exhibit significantly better sensitivity roll-off characteristics and support larger axial depth measurement ranges because they are not limited by spectrometer resolution. The majority of commercial OCT systems and clinical studies have been performed using SD/FD-OCT rather than swept-source OCT. However, record imaging speeds have been achieved using special high-speed swept lasers based on FD mode locking.[47,48] Retinal imaging with swept-source OCT was demonstrated at ~250 kHz[49,50] using a FD mode locking swept laser and at 400 kHz using dual beam imaging with a commercial swept laser.[51]

OCT image penetration into deeper retinal layers such as the choroid is limited by the high scattering of melanin in the RPE for near infrared wavelengths close to the visible light range as well as by water absorption in the vitreous for wavelengths near 950 nm as well as for wavelengths longer than ~1200 nm. As an alternative to the 840-nm wavelength range usually used for retinal OCT imaging, imaging using the 1050-nm wavelength range has recently been proposed. The 1050-nm wavelength is in a water absorption window in the vitreous, and the maximum bandwidth that can be used is approximately 100 nm, limiting axial image resolutions to the ~5-μm level. However, studies have shown that this wavelength range enables the visualization of deep structures in the choroid and optic nerve and is less sensitive to scattering from ocular opacities compared with shorter wavelengths.[52-54] Imaging at 1050 nm can be performed using spectral as well as swept-source/FD-OCT and currently is an active topic in OCT research.

OCT provides comprehensive structural information about the retina and anterior eye. However,

there is also considerable interest developing OCT techniques that can perform functional imaging. Integrated structural and functional imaging would be a powerful tool since many diseases may have functional changes that precede structural changes. Doppler OCT enables the measurement of blood flow velocities in retinal arteries and veins. Scattering from flowing blood produces a phase shift of the scattered light beam, which can be detected as a function of time. High-speed SD/FD-OCT methods have been developed to generate angiography-like maps and 3D images of retinal and choroidal vasculature in vivo.[55-57] Quantitative Doppler techniques allow measurement of total retinal blood flow, which is a key parameter for understanding the pathophysiology of diseases such as diabetic retinopathy, glaucoma, or ARMD (Figure A-14).[58-61]

Polarization sensitive (PS) OCT is another functional imaging technique that provides additional, tissue-inherent contrast based on the optical polarizing properties of different biological structures.[62,63] In the eye, birefringent structures such as the NFL, depolarizing tissues such as the RPE, and polarization-preserving structures such as the photoreceptor layer, can be distinguished in PS-OCT images.[64] The depolarizing characteristic of the RPE can be used to segment this layer. The RPE is of interest in ARMD where it plays a key role in disease progression, but is often hard to identify solely based on its reflectivity (Figures A-14A and B).[65,66] NFL birefringence can be measured and mapped using PS-OCT and might be an important marker for glaucoma diagnostics in addition to the total NFL thickness (Figure A-14C).[67-69] In the anterior segment, structures such as sclera, conjunctive tissue, and trabecular meshwork can be distinguished by their polarization properties.[70,71] These functional imaging methods are very promising but still in the research phase. The outcomes of clinical studies will govern whether they are developed to a level suitable for widespread clinical use in commercial instruments.

Conclusion

OCT is a powerful imaging modality that can have applications in a wide range of areas in addition to ophthalmology. The ability to perform "optical biopsy" (ie, visualizing tissue morphology in situ and in real time) promises not only to improve the understanding of disease pathogenesis, but also to increase the sensitivity and specificity of diagnosis and enable guidance of

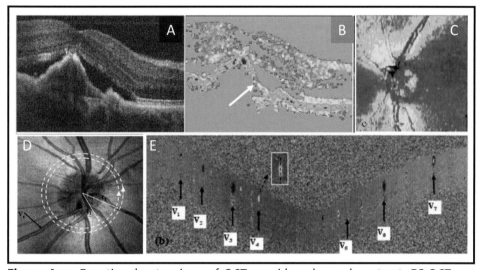

Figure A-14. Functional extensions of OCT provide enhanced contrast. PS-OCT can distinguish structures based on their intrinsic polarization properties. In particular, in the pathologic retina, it is difficult to identify highly scattering layers such as the photoreceptor layer and RPE solely based on backscattered intensity (A). However, the depolarizing character of pigmented tissues such as the RPE can be used to segment these structures in PS-OCT images (B). PS-OCT can also be used to investigate the birefringent RNFL, which may be an important marker for glaucoma. (Figures A and B reprinted with permission from Ahlers C, Götzinger E, Pircher M, et al. Imaging of the retinal pigment epithelium in age-related macular degeneration using polarization-sensitive optical coherence tomography. *Invest Ophthalmol Vis Sci.* 2010;51[4]:2149-2157.) (C) PS-OCT en face fundus map of phase retardation in the RNFL. (Reprinted with permission from Götzinger E, Pircher M, Baumann B, Hirn C, Vass C, Hitzenberger CK. Analysis of the origin of atypical scanning laser polarimetry patterns by polarization-sensitive optical coherence tomography. *Invest Ophthalmol Vis Sci.* 2008;49:5366-5372.) (D) Doppler OCT enables blood flow measurement in the retina. (E) Using circumpapillary Doppler OCT scans around the optic disc, total retinal blood flow can be calculated. (Figures D and E reprinted with permission from Wang Y, Bower BA, Izatt JA, Tan O, Huang D. Retinal blood flow measurement by circumpapillary Fourier domain Doppler optical coherence tomography. *J Biomed Opt.* 2008;13[6]:064003-1–064003-9.)

interventional procedures. This appendix has provided a more detailed description of the physical principles of how OCT instruments operate, how images are generated and displayed, and what fundamental factors limit OCT imaging performance. OCT technology remains an active area of investigation in itself, with continuing advances in performance as well as development of new methods and protocols for displaying and analyzing 3D-OCT datasets and assessing functional processes in vivo. The realization of the full clinical potential of this exciting technology relies on structured and systemic clinical studies that will determine its applications and efficacy.

References

1. Huang D, Swanson EA, Lin CP, et al. Optical coherence tomography. *Science.* 1991;254:1178-1181.
2. Fujimoto JG, Pitris C, Boppart SA, Brezinski ME. Optical coherence tomography: an emerging technology for biomedical imaging and optical biopsy. *Neoplasia.* 2000;2:9-25.
3. Fujimoto JG. Optical coherence tomography for ultrahigh resolution in vivo imaging. *Nat Biotechnol.* 2003;21:1361-1367.
4. Fujimoto JG, Brezinski ME, Tearney, et al. Optical biopsy and imaging using optical coherence tomography. *Nat Med.* 1995;1:970-972.
5. Brezinski ME, Tearney GJ, Bouma BE, et al. Optical coherence tomography for optical biopsy. Properties and demonstration of vascular pathology. *Circulation.* 1996;93:1206-1213.
6. Tearney GJ, Brezinski ME, Boppart SA, et al. Catheter-based optical imaging of a human coronary artery. *Circulation.* 1996;94:3013.

7. Tearney GJ, Brezinski ME, Bouma BE, et al. In vivo endoscopic optical biopsy with optical coherence tomography. *Science*. 1997;276:2037-2039.

8. Adler DC, Zhou C, Tsai TH, et al. Three-dimensional optical coherence tomography of Barrett's esophagus and buried glands beneath neosquamous epithelium following radiofrequency ablation. *Endoscopy*. 2009;41:773-776.

9. Aguirre AD, Chen Y, Bryan B, et al. Cellular resolution ex vivo imaging of gastrointestinal tissues with optical coherence microscopy. *J Biomed Opt*. 2010;15:016025.

10. Swanson EA, Izatt JA, Hee MR, et al. In vivo retinal imaging by optical coherence tomography. *Opt Lett*. 1993;18:1864-1866.

11. Izatt JA, Hee MR, Swanson EA, et al. Micrometer-scale resolution imaging of the anterior eye in vivo with optical coherence tomography. *Arch Ophthalmol*. 1994;112:1584-1589.

12. Hee MR, Izatt JA, Swanson EA, et al. Optical coherence tomography of the human retina. *Arch Ophthalmol*. 1995;113:325-332.

13. Born M, Wolf E, Bhatia AB. *Principles of Optics: Electromagnetic Theory of Propagation, Interference and Diffraction of Light*. 7th expanded ed. Cambridge, England: Cambridge University Press; 1999.

14. Youngquist R, Carr S, Davies D. Optical coherence-domain reflectometry: a new optical evaluation technique. *Opt Lett*. 1987;12:158-160.

15. Gilgen HH, Novak RP, Salathe RP, Hodel W, Beaud P. Submillimeter optical reflectometry. *IEEE J Lightwave Tech*. 1989;7:1225-1233.

16. Drexler W, Morgner U, Kartner FX, et al. In vivo ultrahigh-resolution optical coherence tomography. *Opt Lett*. 1999;24:1221-1223.

17. Drexler W, Morgner U, Ghanta RK, Kärtner FX, Schuman JS, Fujimoto JG. Ultra-high-resolution ophthalmic optical coherence tomography. *Nat Med*. 2001;7:502-507.

18. Povazay B, Bizheva K, Unterhuber A, et al. Submicrometer axial resolution optical coherence tomography. *Opt Lett*. 2002;27:1800-1802.

19. Swanson EA, Huang D, Hee MR, Fujimoto JG, Lin CP, Puliafito CA. High-speed optical coherence domain reflectometry. *Opt Lett*. 1992;17:151-153.

20. Fercher AF, Hitzenberger CK, Kamp G, Elzaiat SY. Measurement of intraocular distances by backscattering spectral interferometry. *Opt Commun*. 1995;117:43-48.

21. Wojtkowski M, Leitgeb R, Kowalczyk A, Bajraszewski T, Fercher AF. In vivo human retinal imaging by Fourier domain optical coherence tomography. *J Biomed Optics*. 2002;7:457-463.

22. Choma MA, Sarunic MV, Yang CH, Izatt JA. Sensitivity advantage of swept source and Fourier domain optical coherence tomography. *Opt Express*. 2003;11:2183-2189.

23. De Boer JF, Cense B, Park BH, Pierce MC, Tearney GJ, Bouma BE. Improved signal-to-noise ratio in spectral-domain compared with time-domain optical coherence tomography. *Opt Lett*. 2003;28:2067-2069.

24. Leitgeb R, Hitzenberger CK, Fercher AF. Performance of Fourier domain vs. time domain optical coherence tomography. *Opt Express*. 2003;11:889-894.

25. Yun SH, Tearney GJ, Bouma BE, Park BH, De Boer JF. High-speed spectral-domain optical coherence tomography at 1.3 microns wavelength. *Opt Express*. 2003;11:3598-3604.

26. Bajraszewski T, Wojtkowski M, Szkulmowski M, Szkulmowska A, Huber R, Kowalczyk A. Improved spectral optical coherence tomography using optical frequency comb. *Opt Express*. 2008;16:4163-4176.

27. Spaide RF, Koizumi H, Pozonni MC. Enhanced depth imaging spectral-domain optical coherence tomography. *Am J Ophthalmol*. 2008;146:496-500.

28. Zawadzki RJ, Cense B, Zhang Y, Choi SS, Miller DT, Werner JS. Ultrahigh-resolution optical coherence tomography with monochromatic and chromatic aberration correction. *Opt Express*. 2008;16:8126-8143.

29. Fernandez EJ, Hermann B, Povazay B, et al. Ultrahigh resolution optical coherence tomography and pancorrection for cellular imaging of the living human retina. *Opt Express*. 2008;16:11083-11094.

30. Izatt JA, Hee MR, Owen GM, Swanson EA, Fujimoto JG. Optical coherence microscopy in scattering media. *Opt Lett*. 1994;19:590-592.

31. Wolf-Schnurrbusch UEK, Ceklic L, Brinkmann CK, et al. Macular thickness measurements in healthy eyes using six different optical coherence tomography instruments. *Invest Ophthalmol Vis Sci*. 2009;50:3432-3437.

32. Pierro L, Giatsidis SM, Mantovani E, Gagliardi M. Macular thickness interoperator and intraoperator reproducibility in healthy eyes using 7 optical coherence tomography instruments. *Am J Ophthalmol*. 2010;150:199-204.

33. Schuman JS, Hee MR, Puliafito CA, et al. Quantification of nerve fiber layer thickness in normal and glaucomatous eyes using optical coherence tomography. *Arch Ophthalmol*. 1995;113:586-596.

34. Schmitt JM, Xiang SH, Yung KM. Speckle in optical coherence tomography. *J Biomed Opt*. 1999;4:95-105.

35. Ferguson RD, Hammer DX, Paunescu LA, Beaton S, Schuman JS. Tracking optical coherence tomography. *Opt Lett*. 2004;29:2139-2141.

36. Leitgeb RA, Drexler W, Unterhuber A, et al. Ultrahigh resolution Fourier domain optical coherence tomography. *Opt Express*. 2004;12:2156-2165.

37. Wojtkowski M, Srinivasan VJ, Ko TH, Fujimoto JG, Kowalczyk A, Duker JS. Ultrahigh-resolution, high-speed, Fourier domain optical coherence tomography and methods for dispersion compensation. *Opt Express*. 2004;12:2404-2422.

38. Cense B, Nassif N, Chen TC, et al. Ultrahigh-resolution high-speed retinal imaging using spectral-domain optical coherence tomography. *Opt Express*. 2004;12:2435-2447.

39. Hermann B, Fernandez EJ, Unterhuber A, et al. Adaptive-optics ultrahigh-resolution optical coherence tomography. *Opt Lett*. 2004;29:2142-2144.

40. Zhang Y, Cense B, Rha J, et al. High-speed volumetric imaging of cone photoreceptors with adaptive optics spectral-domain optical coherence tomography. *Opt Express*. 2006;14:4380-4394.

41. Zawadzki RJ, Choi SS, Jones SM, Oliver SS, Werner JS. Adaptive optics-optical coherence tomography: optimizing visualization of microscopic retinal structures in three dimensions. *J Opt Soc Am A Opt Image Sci Vis*. 2007;24:1373-1383.

42. Potsaid B, Gorczynska I, Srinivasan VJ, et al. Ultrahigh speed spectral/Fourier domain OCT ophthalmic imaging at 70,000 to 312,500 axial scans per second. *Opt Express*. 2008;16:15149-15169.

43. Chinn SR, Swanson EA, Fujimoto JG. Optical coherence tomography using a frequency-tunable optical source. *Opt Lett*. 1997;22:340-342.

44. Lexer F, Hitzenberger CK, Fercher AF, Kulhavy M. Wavelength-tuning interferometry of intraocular distances. *Appl Opt*. 1997;36:6548-6553.

45. Yun SH, Tearney GJ, De Boer JF, Iftimia N, Bouma BE. High-speed optical frequency-domain imaging. *Opt Express*. 2003;11:2953-2963.

46. Oh WY, Yun SH, Tearney GJ, Bouma BE. 115 kHz tuning repetition rate ultrahigh-speed wavelength-swept semiconductor laser. *Opt Lett*. 2005;30:3159-3161.

47. Huber R, Adler DC, Fujimoto JG. Buffered Fourier domain mode locking: unidirectional swept laser sources for optical coherence tomography imaging at 370,000 lines/s. *Opt Lett.* 2006;31:2975-2977.

48. Huber R, Wojtkowski M, Fujimoto JG. Fourier domain mode locking (FDML): a new laser operating regime and applications for optical coherence tomography. *Opt Express.* 2006;14:3225-3237.

49. Huber R, Adler DC, Srinivasan VJ, Fujimoto JG. Fourier domain mode locking at 1050 nm for ultra-high-speed optical coherence tomography of the human retina at 236,000 axial scans per second. *Opt Lett.* 2007;32:2049-2051.

50. Srinivasan VJ, Adler DC, Chen Y, et al. Ultrahigh-speed optical coherence tomography for three-dimensional and en face imaging of the retina and optic nerve head. *Invest Ophthalmol Vis Sci.* 2008;49:5103-5110.

51. Potsaid B, Baumann B, Huang D, et al. Ultrahigh speed 1050 nm swept source/Fourier domain OCT retinal and anterior segment imaging at 100,000 to 400,000 axial scans per second. *Opt Express.* 2010;18:20029-20048.

52. Unterhuber A, Povazay B, Hermann B, Sattmann H, Chavez-Pirson A, Drexler W. In vivo retinal optical coherence tomography at 1040 nm-enhanced penetration into the choroid. *Opt Express.* 2005;13:3252-3258.

53. Lee ECW, De Boer JF, Mujat M, Lim H, Yun SH. In vivo optical frequency domain imaging of human retina and choroid. *Opt Express.* 2006;14:4403-4411.

54. Yasuno Y, Hong YJ, Makita S, et al. In vivo high-contrast imaging of deep posterior eye by 1-micron swept source optical coherence tomography and scattering optical coherence angiography. *Opt Express.* 2007;15:6121-6139.

55. Makita S, Hong Y, Yamanari M, Yatagai T, Yasuno Y. Optical coherence angiography. *Opt Express.* 2006;14:7821-7840.

56. An L, Subhush HM, Wilson DJ, Wang RK. High-resolution wide-field imaging of retinal and choroidal blood perfusion with optical microangiography. *J Biomed Opt.* 2010;15:026011.

57. Szkulmowska A, Szkulmowski M, Szlag D, Kowalczyk A, Wojtkowski M. Three-dimensional quantitative imaging of retinal and choroidal blood flow velocity using joint spectral and time domain optical coherence tomography. *Opt Express.* 2009;17:10584-10598.

58. Makita S, Fabritius T, Yasuno Y. Quantitative retinal-blood flow measurement with three-dimensional vessel geometry determination using ultrahigh-resolution Doppler optical coherence angiography. *Opt Lett.* 2008;33:836-838.

59. Wang Y, Lu A, Gil-Flamer J, Tan O, Izatt JA, Huang D. Measurement of total blood flow in the normal human retina using Doppler Fourier-domain optical coherence tomography. *Br J Ophthalmol.* 2009;93:634-637.

60. Wehbe H, Ruggeri M, Jiao S, Gregori G, Puliafito CA, Zhao W. Automatic retinal blood flow calculation using spectral domain optical coherence tomography. *Opt Express.* 2007;15:15193-15206.

61. Singh ASG, Kolbitsch C, Schmoll T, Leitgeb RA. Stable absolute flow estimation with Doppler OCT based on virtual circumpapillary scans. *Biomed Opt Express.* 2010;1:1047-1059.

62. Hee MR, Huang D, Swanson EA, Fujimoto JG. Polarization-sensitive low-coherence reflectometer for birefringence characterization and ranging. *J Opt Soc Am B.* 1992;9:903-908.

63. De Boer JF, Milner TE, van Gemert MJC, Nelson JS. Two-dimensional birefringence imaging in biological tissue by polarization-sensitive optical coherence tomography. *Opt Lett.* 1997;22:934-936.

64. Pircher M, Götzinger E, Leitgeb R, Sattmann H, Findl O, Hitzenberger C. Imaging of polarization properties of human retina in vivo with phase resolved transversal PS-OCT. *Opt Express.* 2004;12:5940-5951.

65. Götzinger E, Pircher M, Geitzenauer W, et al. Retinal pigment epithelium segmentation by polarization sensitive optical coherence tomography. *Opt Express.* 2008;16:16410-16422.

66. Ahlers C, Götzinger E, Pircher M, et al. Imaging of the retinal pigment epithelium in age-related macular degeneration using polarization-sensitive optical coherence tomography. *Invest Ophthalmol Vis Sci.* 2010;51:2149-2157.

67. Cense B, Chen TC, Park BH, Pierce MC, De Boer JF. Thickness and birefringence of healthy retinal nerve fiber layer tissue measured with polarization-sensitive optical coherence tomography. *Invest Ophthalmol Vis Sci.* 2004;45:2606-2612.

68. Götzinger E, Pircher M, Baumann B, Hirn C, Vass C, Hitzenberger CK. Analysis of the origin of atypical scanning laser polarimetry patterns by polarization-sensitive optical coherence tomography. *Invest Ophthalmol Vis Sci.* 2008;49:5366-5372.

69. Yamanari M, Miura M, Makita S, Yatagai T, Yasuno Y. Phase retardation measurement of retinal nerve fiber layer by polarization-sensitive spectral-domain optical coherence tomography and scanning laser polarimetry. *J Biomed Opt.* 2008;13:014013.

70. Götzinger E, Pircher M, Sticker M, Fercher AF, Hitzenberger CK. Measurement and imaging of birefringent properties of the human cornea with phase-resolved, polarizationsensitive optical coherence tomography. *J Biomed Opt.* 2004;9:94-102.

71. Miyazawa A, Yamanari M, Makita S, et al. Tissue discrimination in anterior eye using three optical parameters obtained by polarization sensitive optical coherence tomography. *Opt Express.* 2009;17:17426-17440.

Optical Coherence Tomography Scanning and Image-Processing Protocols

Gadi Wollstein, MD; Lindsey S. Folio, MS, MBA;
Jessica E. Nevins, BS; Hiroshi Ishikawa, MD;
Carmen A. Puliafito, MD, MBA; James G. Fujimoto, PhD; and Joel S. Schuman, MD

- Line and Radial Scan Protocols
- Circle Scan Protocols
- Compound Radial and Concentric Circles Scan Protocols
- Three-Dimensional Cube Raster Scan Protocols
- Eye Motion Tracking
- Image-Processing Protocols
- Repeated Scan (Image) Averaging
- Segmentation
- C-Mode
- Circumpapillary Retinal Thickness and Retinal Thickness Map
- Optic Nerve Head
- Macula
- Progression Analysis
- Anterior Segment Optical Coherence Tomography Scan Protocols

The fast scanning rate provided by spectral-domain optical coherence tomography (SD-OCT) allows a wide variety of scan patterns or protocols to be employed. These patterns can vary from a single linear line, multiple parallel lines, densely packed parallel frames in a raster pattern, or a combination of scan patterns, such as linear and circular scans. In addition, the enhanced resolution of SD-OCT enables advanced image processing such as tissue sampling in any desirable location within the scanning region or detailed layer segmentation. In this appendix, we provide a succinct summary of the most common scan patterns and image-processing protocols available by different SD-OCT devices, in order to allow the reader to choose the most appropriate scan for his or her needs among the myriad options. The following descriptions of scan and image-processing protocols are intended to be general and unspecific to any particular OCT device and default parameter value.

Line and Radial Scan Protocols

The line scan is composed of sequential individual axial scans (A-scans) acquired while scanning the OCT beam in a transverse direction to form a B-scan or optical cross section of the structure of interest. The length and the density of A-scans along the line vary among the various commercial devices. The line scan protocol is mainly used for detailed visualization of structures sampled along the line, which is most relevant for retinal pathologies. Line scanning is usually performed in the horizontal direction producing an OCT image along the temporal-nasal axis, but line scanning can also be performed vertically or radially.

The raster line protocol consists of a series of parallel and equally spaced line scans. The spacing between the linear scans and the length of the linear scans vary among the commercial devices and can be adjusted in some of them. Raster scanning is usually

Schuman JS, Puliafito CA, Fujimoto JG, Duker JS, eds.
Optical Coherence Tomography of Ocular Diseases,
Third Edition (pp 591-596).
© 2013 SLACK Incorporated.

performed with horizontal priority, rapidly scanning the OCT beam in the horizontal direction to produce B-scans with vertical offsets between consecutive horizontal B-scans in order to cover a region of the fundus. The raster scan pattern typically generates a set of temporal-nasal cross-sectional B-scan images that are offset in the superior-inferior direction. This scanning protocol is mostly used for detailed visualization of pathology expanding beyond the single linear scan but still of limited size. The cube scan, described below, is a variant of the raster scan.

The cross-hair scan protocol consists of 2 perpendicular linear scans that intersect at their centers. This type of scan is also used to align the OCT instrument to the patient's eye because it is sensitive to the centering of the OCT beam through the pupil.

The radial lines protocol consists of a series of linear scans centered through a common point (fovea or center of optic nerve head [ONH]) oriented at equally spaced angles. The number and length of the radial scans vary among the devices. This scan allows the acquisition of data from a relatively wide region, but it should be noted that the sampling lines are densely spaced closer to the center point and widely spaced away from the center. More interpolation is necessary between lines at farther distances away from the center point. Therefore, a localized small abnormality occurring in the periphery of the scan might be undetected.

Circle Scan Protocols

A circular scan is conceptually similar to a linear scan except that the OCT beam is scanned in a circular transverse pattern. This scan protocol images a cylindrically shaped cross section of the retina and is typically displayed as a flat image, as if the cylindrically shaped cross-sectional image was cut and unfolded to make it flat.

This circular scan pattern was the most important scan pattern with time-domain (TD) OCT devices for glaucoma evaluation, because if it is centered around the ONH (circumpapillary scan) it intercepts all of the retinal nerve fibers emanating from the ONH and therefore enables comprehensive measurement. The circular scan is image processed using segmentation algorithms in order to identify the boundaries of the nerve fiber layer (NFL) and measure its thickness. The NFL thickness is reported as an average over the entire circumpapillary scans, as hemifield, quadrant, or by clock hour or sector. The same scan pattern is offered by several SD-OCTs, but it should be noted that even though the sampling of the retina is performed in similar locations, TD- and SD-OCT measurements are not interchangeable because different retinal features are used to identify the outer retinal boundary. Three consecutive scans are automatically acquired after positioning the scan at the desirable location, and the average of the 3 scans is reported. A proportional circle protocol, provided by some devices, allows the operator to account for optic disc size variability by altering the aiming circle radius and multiplication factor.

A few SD-OCT devices also provide multiple circle scans. The number of circles and diameter of each circle vary among the devices. The concentric rings protocol is composed of consecutive circle scans that proceed with increasing diameter. The spacing between circles and the diameter of the circles can be adjusted.

Compound Radial and Concentric Circles Scan Protocols

Compound scan protocols perform a combination of radial and concentric circle scans with concentric circular scans centered on the intersection point of the radial scans. These scan protocols were created with the intention of improving the registration of the circular scans to the ONH. The concentric circular scans can map the NFL at multiple radial distances from the ONH, while the radial scans provide a position reference to the center of the ONH in order to account for patient eye movement. However, during the time lag between the beginning of the acquisition of the radial scans and the end of the acquisition of the circular scans, some eye movement might occur that can impair accurate registration of the scans.

Three-Dimensional Cube Raster Scan Protocols

The 3-dimensional (3D) cube raster is created from a series of parallel B-scans that are offset by a small amount in the perpendicular direction and captured in rapid succession. Cube raster scans are typically performed by rapidly scanning the OCT beam in the horizontal temporal-nasal direction with sequential small offsets in the vertical superior-inferior direction. The intention of a 3D cube raster scan is to obtain volumetric data. However, because of instrument acquisition speed limitations, this means that the density of A-scans in any direction is significantly less than for the individual linear scans mentioned previously. Therefore, the quality of B-scan or cross-sectional images extracted from the 3D cube raster scan is usually significantly reduced. However, the 3D cube raster scan protocol is well suited for generating en face OCT images or maps of retinal layer thicknesses or elevations. The volumetric data allow post-processing of any desired area or view within the scanned region. The cube data also enables registration of the data set using alignment of blood vessels and other en face structural landmarks from images acquired in multiple visits.

Scans are typically performed on the macula or the ONH regions, and the scanning region size and density vary among the devices. Some devices acquire images as an isometric scan, where the distance between the A-scan sampling points is consistent and pixel size is identical in both x- and y-directions. Other devices provide asymmetric scans, where the distance between pixels is different in x- and y-directions. Asymmetric scan patterns are often used when it is desirable to display individual cross-sectional B-scan images from the volumetric raster scan data. However, this approach prioritizes one scan direction over the other. For example, scanning with a high A-scan density in the horizontal direction and a low A-scan density in the vertical direction will yield high-quality horizontal cross-sectional images at the expense of lower quality vertical images. Finally, the scanned region can also be square versus rectangular. A rectangular orientation is sometimes useful for capturing features in the macula and optic disc in a single scan protocol.

3D cube scans are the prime scanning type for glaucoma, retina, and neuro-ophthalmic evaluations because of their ability to cover large areas in a single scan and their wide range of post-processing options.

Eye Motion Tracking

Eye motion tracking is used for the correction of eye movements occurring during scanning. When eye motion is identified, the position of the previously completed B-scan is adjusted and repeated and scanning resumes from that frame. Eye tracking systems incorporated into commercially available devices typically measure eye motion using an independent view of the fundus obtained from an integrated scanning laser ophthalmoscope or video camera. They are capable of correcting most movement, although the measurement of eye motion has limited accuracy and there is a limited response time for the tracking adjustment so that small or rapid eye movements are often not well corrected. Because eye motion is tracked and scans are repeated, the duration can be substantially extended in patients with excessive eye movement.

Image-Processing Protocols

All acquired images are processed for optimized visualization by reducing background noise and utilizing an indexed color or grayscale. The scan image false-color or grayscale contains the log of the OCT signal values from 0 to 255. The background as well as the maximum signal level (equivalent to setting the image brightness and contrast) is typically set automatically in order to display the image for optimal viewing.

Median smoothing blends the OCT image colors and averages out noise by using the median values of the signal values in a given region. Gaussian smoothing, which is slightly more sophisticated than median smoothing, blends the OCT image colors and averages out noise by calculating a moving average of the signal values in a given region according to a Gaussian function. The peripheral points in the region are weighted less than those more central, and higher resolution details may be lost.

Most retinal images are presented so that the image size is stretched vertically to allow easier visualization of details within the cross section. This is done because retinal images typically span a several-millimeters transverse range, while the retina is only a few hundred microns in thickness. Displaying the images with the correct vertical and horizontal aspect ratio would result in the retina appearing very thin, making interpretation of pathology difficult. At the same time, it is important to remember that the stretched display can produce distortion of tomographic features. Tilting of the retina or the cup depth in the disc appears progressively exaggerated depending on the vertical stretching used in the image display. Since the vertical and horizontal scales are different in the OCT images, care must be taken when measuring dimensions of retinal features. Instruments having software calipers or rulers for measuring dimensions automatically account for asymmetric display effects.

OCT fundus images, also known as *en face images*, are created by summing OCT signal values along depth in each A-scan. This essentially displays the light that is backscattered or backreflected from different depths and forms 2-dimensional images from the region of interest, which resemble clinical biomicroscopic examination or standard fundus photos. There are also variations of OCT fundus imaging where only the OCT signal from specific depths is summed and displayed. This is known as *projection* or *C-mode* OCT fundus imaging and is described later in this appendix.

Repeated Scan (Image) Averaging

Repeated scan (image) averaging is used to increase the image quality by reducing the noise level and speckle (graininess or texture) as well as improving the signal. Averaging is most useful in the linear and radial scan protocols because the averaging does not substantially increase the total scan time duration of the original short scan pattern duration. Averaging is less applicable for longer duration scan patterns, such as the 3D cube scans, because it will substantially prolong scan acquisition leading to eye movement artifacts in the transverse and axial directions as well as patient blinking, which causes deterioration in image quality.

Segmentation

Segmentation enables differentiation and measurement of retinal layer structures in the region of interest. Two examples of commonly used segmentation for images acquired from the posterior eye are the retinal nerve fiber layer (RNFL) in the peripapillary region and retinal layers in the macula. The segmentation is automatically performed by identification of certain landmarks in the signal profile of each A-scan and transversely in the B-scan or volume. Segmentation enables detection of abnormal thickness in certain layers, quantification, and advanced post-processing. However, in the presence of severely deformed structures associated with advanced pathology, segmentation may fail because the typical landmarks required for the segmentation are not present. Therefore, it is recommended to routinely inspect the segmentation performance to ensure its validity.

C-Mode

C-mode or projection OCT fundus imaging sums and displays the OCT signal from a specific A-scan depth range. This contrasts with OCT fundus imag-

ing, which sums the signal from the entire depth range. For example, many SD-OCT devices identify the position of the retinal pigment epithelium (RPE) and can display en face or projection images of the OCT signal from specific depth ranges with respect to the RPE. This display feature can be used to selectively enhance the contrast or sensitivity to specific retinal features. For example, displaying signal only from the RPE level gives information about whether the RPE is intact or elevated from its normal position. Displaying signal from the choriocapillaris or choroid level gives information about light penetration through the RPE into the chorid and is sensitive to areas of geographic atrophy. Projection OCT fundus imaging is a relatively new feature, and guidelines for interpreting these images are still under development. However, the use of en face imaging has the powerful advantage that it enables 3D-OCT data to be viewed analogously with standard fundus photographs, fluorescein angiography, or fundus autofluoroescence.

Circumpapillary Retinal Thickness and Retinal Thickness Map

After applying the segmentation analysis on each of the B-scans, the RNFL thickness is reported along a circle surrounding the ONH. The thickness profile along the circle is provided with comparison to thickness measurements in a normative healthy population. This comparison improves the ability to detect locations with excessive thickening or marked thinning of the RNFL. The typical configuration of the circumpapillary RNFL thickness profile is often described as a double-hump pattern with thickened areas adjacent to the ONH poles and thinning in the temporal and nasal aspects. It should be noted that RNFL measurements are not interchangeable because there can be differing thickness measurements among the various SD-OCT devices. In addition to the visual presentation of the RNFL profile, thickness measurements are provided for the entire circle, hemifields, quadrants, and in smaller sectors. Many of the SD-OCT devices also provide RNFL thickness maps of the entire peripapillary region. This allows detection of abnormalities located outside the sampled circle of the circumpapillary scan. Thickness measurements are compared with thickness values from a healthy population and reported as a deviation map highlighting locations of thickness abnormalities.

Optic Nerve Head

Various scan patterns are offered among the different SD-OCT devices for imaging the ONH region. The common patterns include raster scans, radial scans, and the combination of radial and circular scans. The disc margin is conventionally defined as the termination of the RPE layer, and some devices automatically identify this location, while others require manual delineation. The cup is defined by a plane parallel to the plane connecting the disc margins with a fixed offset that varies among the different devices. All devices provide quantification of ONH structures including disc, rim, and cup areas as well as cup-to-disc ratios.

Enhanced Depth Imaging

SD-OCT instruments have a varying sensitivity as a function of depth. Sensitivity is highest for structures that are closer to the reference zero delay position and decreases for structures that are further from this position. In addition, SD detection cannot distinguish between positive or negative delays with respect to the reference zero delay position. If retinal features cross the zero delay position, they appear as if they are reflected about the zero, the "mirror image" artifact. For conventional imaging, the reference zero delay position is typically positioned in front of the retina in the vitreous because it is desirable to have the highest sensitivity for weak signals from vitreal abnormalities or detachments. However, it is also possible to position the zero delay in back of the retina in order to enhance sensitivity to deeper structures, enhanced depth imaging (EDI). EDI is useful for imaging structures deep within the eye, including choroidal and ONH features, such as the lamina cribrosa. EDI is available with all scan patterns, but at the time of writing this appendix, it is used for visualization purposes only and automated quantifiable analysis is not provided.

Macula

Scanning of the macular region can be performed using various scan patterns, including linear scans, cross-hair scans, multiple parallel line scans, radial scans, or raster scans. While linear scans are beneficial for detailed visualization along the scan line, other scan patterns provide structural information of the entire macular region. All devices are capable of reporting the macular retinal thickness encompassing the entire retina spanning from the inner limiting layer to the photoreceptors or RPE complex. However, the precise layer that is used as the outer retina boundary varies among the SD-OCT devices, making it difficult to compare total retinal thickness measurements between the devices. In addition to total retinal thickness, some of the devices provide the thickness measurements in predefined sectors.

Advanced segmentation analysis offered by some devices is capable of identifying several of the intraretinal layers separately. This segmentation is based on identifying typical patterns in the signal profile of each B-scan. The individual layers that are segmented by the various devices vary, and there is a balance between the desire to quantify as many possible layers and the robustness of the segmentation analysis. Identification and quantification of specific retinal layers improve the ability to detect structural changes in diseases affecting only specific layers. An example of such a disease is glaucoma, where the ganglion cell layer is prone to the glaucomatous effect, and quantification of this layer can improve disease detection. In addition to providing quantitative summary parameters of the layers, some devices provide thickness maps of individual layers and deviation maps from a population of healthy individuals.

Another macular feature offered by some devices is C-mode sections described previously. These en face views enable visualization of specific depth levels within the macula. One such example is a C-mode section at the RPE layer that highlights the presence of drusen as irregular "bumps" in the plane.

The EDI scanning method is used in cases where attention is focused on the outer retina or choroid. This scanning method provides a higher sensitivity to signals from the deeper layers and enables visualization of choroidal features and thickness.

Progression Analysis

The ability of SD-OCT to provide accurate quantification of ocular structures enables the detection of structural changes over time. Most SD-OCT devices provide progression analysis for the RNFL thickness in glaucoma assessment. However, at the time of writing this appendix, limited analysis is offered for macular structures. At present, this analysis includes a side-by-side summary of scans acquired over time, as well as a quantitative thickness subtraction map. However, concrete effort is underway by the manufacturers to provide in-depth longitudinal analysis tools that are expected to be available commercially shortly.

Anterior Segment Optical Coherence Tomography Scan Protocols

Anterior segment OCT scanning enables the visualization of the anterior chamber angle and anterior segment structures, such as the cornea, iris, and anterior lens. Devices with this scan capability use a longer wavelength and higher power than other OCT devices.

The various devices offer several common scan patterns, including the following:

- Line scans are typically repeated in the same location to generate an average image with an improved signal-to-noise ratio. This scan is optimized to provide highly detailed visualization along the scan line.
- Pachymetry scan is a set of radial linear scans that provides a comprehensive set of corneal thickness measurements over a selected area of the central cornea.
- Cross scan is a set of 2 perpendicular linear scans that intersect in the center of each scan.
- Raster scan is a set of parallel linear scans that images at equal distances to cover an adjustable size of the central cornea.
- 3D cornea scan consists of a set of parallel linear scans as well as a few coarse raster scans. The raster scans are used for z-axis alignment. The scan lengths are adjustable.

In addition to dedicated anterior segment SD-OCT devices, several conventional SD-OCT devices have the ability to provide anterior segment scanning by employing customized add-on apparatuses. These devices provide similar scan patterns as described previously.

The quantitative information provided by the various devices varies substantially. Corneal thickness and topographic mapping are often provided. Some devices provide quantification of the angle, but capabilities and features vary considerably between devices from different manufacturers.

Financial Disclosures

Dr. Bernhard Baumann has no financial or proprietary interest in the materials presented herein.

Dr. Vanessa Cruz-Villegas has not disclosed any relevant financial relationships.

Dr. Janet Davis is on the advisory board for Xoma, and she receives grant support from Santen.

Dr. Jay S. Duker is on the advisory board for scientific information for Paloma Pharmaceuticals, Inc. He is a consultant for clinical trial design for Alcon; EMD Serono, Inc; Genentech, Inc; Merck; Novartis; QLT Inc; Regeneron; and ThromboGenics, Inc. Dr. Duker receives grant support from Carl Zeiss Meditec, Inc; Optovue, Inc; and Topcon Medical Systems, Inc (in the form of devices supplied to Tufts Medical Center). He is a shareholder in EyeNetra, Hemera Biosciences, and Ophthotech.

Dr. Harry W. Flynn Jr is a consultant for Alimera, Pfizer, and Santen.

Lindsey S. Folio has no financial or proprietary interest in the materials presented herein.

Dr. James G. Fujimoto receives royalties from intellectual property owned by MIT and licensed to Carl Zeiss Meditec, Inc; Optovue, Inc; and LightLab Imaging/St. Jude Medical. He is also an advisor for Optovue and has stock options in Optovue.

Dr. Thomas R. Hedges III has no financial or proprietary interest in the materials presented herein.

Dr. David Huang has a significant financial interest in Optovue, Inc. He also has a significant interest in Carl Zeiss Meditec, Inc. Optovue and Carl Zeiss Meditec are companies that may have a commercial interest in the results of this research and technology. These potential conflicts of interest have been reviewed and managed by Oregon Health and Science University.

Dr. Hiroshi Ishikawa has no financial or proprietary interest in the materials presented herein.

Dr. Matthew D. Lazzara has no financial or proprietary interest in the materials presented herein.

Dr. Yan Li has a significant financial interest in Optovue, Inc, which is a company that may have a commercial interest in the results of this research and technology. This potential conflict of interest has been reviewed and managed by Oregon Health and Science University.

Dr. Elias C. Mavrofrides has no financial or proprietary interest in the materials presented herein.

Dr. Carlos Mendoza-Santiesteban has no financial or proprietary interest in the materials presented herein.

Jessica E. Nevins has no financial or proprietary interest in the materials presented herein.

Dr. Carmen A. Puliafito is a consultant for Carl Zeiss Meditec, Inc, and receives royalties for intellectual property owned by Massachusetts Institute of Technology and Massachusetts Eye and Ear Infirmary and licensed to Carl Zeiss Meditec.

Dr. Bing Qin has no financial or proprietary interest in the materials presented herein.

Dr. Adam H. Rogers has no financial or proprietary interest in the materials presented herein.

Dr. Philip J. Rosenfeld has received a research grant and honoraria for lectures from Carl Zeiss Meditec, Inc.

Dr. Joel S. Schuman receives royalties for intellectual property owned by Massachusetts Institute of Technology and Massachusetts Eye and Ear Infirmary and licensed to Carl Zeiss Meditec, Inc. He receives grant/research support from the NIH.

Dr. Heeral R. Shah has no financial or proprietary interest in the materials presented herein.

Eric Swanson is a cofounder of Advanced Ophthalmology Diagnostics, which was acquired by Carl Zeiss Meditec, Inc, and served as the initial basis of Zeiss's ophthalmic OCT product line. Mr. Swanson is a cofounder of LightLab Imaging, which was aquired by St. Jude Medical. He is a holder of numerous OCT patents that are licensed to various companies around the world. Mr. Swanson is the editor of www.octnews.org.

Dr. Steven N. Truong has no financial or proprietary interest in the materials presented herein.

Dr. Natalia Villate has no financial or proprietary interest in the materials presented herein.

Dr. Gadi Wollstein has no financial or proprietary interest in the materials presented herein.

Index